B. Höfling, A. v. Pölnitz (Eds.)

E. Erdmann, G. Steinbeck, B. E. Strauer (Co-Eds.)

Interventional Cardiology and Angiology

With contributions by

Th. v. Arnim · U. Babic · D. Backa · H. Bardenheuer
P. Dartsch · J. S. Douglas · R. Erbel · G. Fontaine
W. Grundfest · R. Haberl · M. P. Heintzen · V. Hombach
K. R. Karsch · S. B. King · E. Kreuzer · R. Moosdorf
B. Reichart · P. Schanzenbächer · H. E. Scherer
P. Serruys · C. Vallbracht

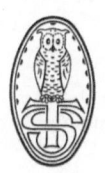 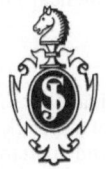

Springer-Verlag Berlin Heidelberg GmbH

The Editors:

Prof. Dr. B. Höfling
Dr. A. v. Pölnitz
Medizinische Klinik I
Klinikum Großhadern
Marchioninistraße 15
8000 München

CIP-Titelaufnahme der Deutschen Bibliothek

Interventional cardiology and angiology / B. Höfling ; A. v. Pölnitz (eds.). E. Erdmann ... (Co eds.).
With contr. by Th. v. Arnim ...
   ISBN 978-3-662-12116-0   ISBN 978-3-662-12114-6 (eBook)
   DOI 10.1007/978-3-662-12114-6
NE: Höfling, Berthold [Hrsg.]; Arnim, Thomas von [Mitverf.]

Copyright © 1989 by Springer-Verlag Berlin Heidelberg

Ursprünglich erschienen bei Dr. Dietrich Steinkopff Verlag GmbH & Co. KG, Darmstadt 1989
Softcover reprint of the hardcover 1st edition 1989
Medical Editorial: Sabine Müller – Copy Editing: James C. Willis – Production: Heinz J. Schäfer

Preface

The acquisition of knowledge often follows the application of new methodology. The history of clinical cardiology could be viewed as the result of new methods, confirming or negating previously developed hypotheses. New methods, in turn, have their roots in basic biological and technical science.

For example, the historical innovation by Einthoven in 1895 resulted from basic anatomical work (Purkinje, 1845; His, 1893), electrophysiological studies (Waller 1889; Matteuci and Du Bois-Reymond, 1843), and advances in registration technology (Marey, 1876). The past 100 years have seen an integration of additional diagnostic techniques (infarct recognition, identification of HIS-bundle structures and bypass tracts, ischemia monitoring by continuous ST-segment registration) which have led to improved medical and operative therapy. Today we are witness to the growth of interventional cardiology, which plays an increasingly important role in patient management.

The focus of this volume is on percutaneous techniques which are currently in use in interventional cardiology and, in addition, on future developments such as the application of laser energy and ablative techniques.

G. Riecker

Introduction

This book reports on a symposium held at the University Hospital of Munich – Klinikum Großhadern in July, 1988 which focussed on the current state of balloon angioplasty, as well as on the many new techniques and approaches which are quickly becoming an integral part of interventional cardiology and angiology.

In the field of *balloon angioplasty,* which is well established and has become a routine procedure within cardiology, work is centered on the optimization of the technique with minor, but very effective improvements in materials and catheter design. Important advances are also being made in the fields of computerized imaging and stenosis quantification. We have chosen to focus on the "ischemic state" of angioplasty, a somewhat untapped scientific model, and present work on the biochemical markers of ischemia and potential myocardial salvage afforded by the technique.

Balloon valvuloplasty has recently received much enthusiastic attention as a percutaneous therapeutic modality, perhaps because of the surprisingly effective use of balloon angioplasty for the treatment of coronary heart disease. We have therefore critically examined the indications for balloon valvuloplasty and attempted a synthesis with the field of cardiothoracic surgery.

A special focus has naturally been given to the vast array of *new interventional techniques* for vessel reconstruction, some of which have perhaps all too quickly urged their way into clinical application. Stenting, mechanical approaches such as atherectomy and rotational devices, as well as high-energy techniques such as laser and high frequency, were examined in detail. In addition, some of these techniques offer new approaches to the study of the atherosclerotic process and that of restenosis, by providing percutaneously removed plaque material. We have thus also presented results of initial evaluation of such material with histology and cell culture.

Supportive diagnostic methods, such as angioscopy and vascular Doppler imaging may come to play an increasingly important role in interventional cardiology and angiology, and these approaches have also been discussed.

Finally, the field of *arrhythmia control* has seen new advances with the interventional approach both to diagnostic as well as to therapeutic issues, with percutaneous mapping and catheter ablation gaining increasing application.

Special thanks must be given to the distinguished chairmen who integrated these highly specialized fields of interventional cardiology and angiology and helped us gain a perspective on their role in modern cardiology.

B. Höfling

Contents

X

4. Interventional techniques for arrhythmia control

The authors

PD Dr. Th. v. Arnim
Krankenanstalt Rotes Kreuz
Nymphenburger Str. 163
8000 München 19

Dr. Uros U. Babic
Cardiovascular Center
„Dr. Dragisa Misovic"
YU 11000 Belgrad
Yugoslavia

Dr. D. Backa
Department für Medizin I
Klinikum Großhadern
Marchioninistr. 15
8000 München 70

Dr. H. J. Bardenheuer
Institut für Anästhesiologie
Klinikum Großhadern
Universität München
Marchioninistr. 15
8000 München 70

Dr. Peter C. Dartsch
Physiologische Klinik I
Universität Tübingen
Gmelinstr. 5
7400 Tübingen

Dr. John S. Douglas, Jr.
Emory University Hospital
Room C430
1364 Clifton Road, N.E.
Atlanta, Georgia 30322
USA

Dr. E. Erdmann
Medizinische Klinik I
Klinikum Großhadern
Universität München
Marchioninistr. 15
8000 München 70

Dr. G. Fontaine
Hôpital Jean Rostand
39–41 rue Jean Le Galleu
F-94206 Ivry Cedex
France

Dr. Warren S. Grundfest
Department of Surgery
Cedars-Sinai Medical Center
Los Angeles, CA 90048
USA

Dr. R. Haberl
Medizinische Klinik I
Klinikum Großhadern
Marchioninistr. 15
8000 München 70

Dr. Matthias P. Heintzen
Medizinische Klinik und Poliklinik B
der Universität
Moorenstraße 5
4000 Düsseldorf

Dr. K. J. Henrichs
II. Medizinische Klinik
Universität Mainz
Langenbeckstr. 1
6500 Mainz 1

Prof. Dr. V. Hombach
Abt. für Kardiologie, Angiologie,
Pneumologie
der Universität
Robert-Koch-Str. 8
7900 Ulm

Prof. Dr. B. Höfling
Medizinische Klinik I
Klinikum Großhadern
Marchioninistr. 15
8000 München 70

Dr. K. R. Karsch
Medizinische Klinik
Abteilung für Kardiologie
Universität Tübingen
Otfried-Müller-Str. 10
7440 Tübingen

Dr. S. B. King
The Emory Clinic
Cardiovascular Laboratory
1365 Clifton Road, N.E.
Atlanta, Georgia 30322
USA

Prof. Dr. E. Kreuzer
Herzchirurgische Klinik der Univ.
Klinikum Großhadern
Marchioninistr. 15
8000 München 70

Dr. R. Moosdorf
Klinik für Herz- und Gefäßchirurgie
am Zentrum der Justus-Liebig-Universität
Klinikstr. 29
6300 Gießen

Prof. Dr. B. Reichart
Head of Cardiothoracic Surgery
University of Cape Town
Medical School, Observatory 7925
Cape Town
South Africa

Priv. Doz. Dr. P. Schanzenbächer
Med. Univ. Klinik
Josef Schneider Str. 2
8700 Würzburg

Dr. Timothy A. Sanborn
Division of Cardiology – Box 1030
One Gustave L. Levy Place
New York, NY 10029
USA

Dr. Hans-Eberhard Scherer
Medizinisch Klinik (Kardiologie)
Zentralkrankenhaus „Links der Weser"
Senator-Weßling-Str. 1
2800 Bremen

Dr. P. W. Serruys
Catheterization Laboratory,
Erasmus University
Thoraxcenter, Bd 144
P.O. Box 1738
NL-3000 DR Rotterdam
The Netherlands

Dr. P. W. Serruys
Catheterization Laboratory
Thoraxcenter
P.O. Box 1738
NL-3000 DR Rotterdam
The Netherlands

Dr. John B. Simpson
Sequoia Hospital
Dept. of Cardiology
Redwood City, CA
USA

Prof. Dr. G. Steinbeck
Medizinische Klinik I der Univ.
Klinikum Großhadern
Marchioninistr. 70
8000 München 70

Dr. C. Vallbracht
Zentrum für Innere Medizin
Abt. für Kardiologie
Theodor-Stern-Kai 7
6000 Frankfurt/M

Current and future techniques in interventional cardiology and angiology

B. Höfling, A. v. Pölnitz

Department of Medicine I, Klinikum Großhadern, University of Munich, Munich, FRG

Building on basic balloon angioplasty, the past 10 years have seen remarkable progress in the field of instrumental techniques. Most branches of medicine, and in particular that of cardiovascular disease, have been affected by these new techniques. These new therapeutic concepts can be grouped together under the heading "Interventional Cardiology and Angiology". The most important established and a variety of still experimental techniques are summarized in Table 1.

The reason for the development of so many new techniques lies in an effort to be less invasive than open-heart surgery and more effective than medical therapy. This can be achieved for example with the use of balloon dilatation instead of bypass operation, percutaneous valvuloplasty to postpone valve replacement in critically ill patients, or catheter ablation to avoid more invasive surgical therapy of medically intractable arrhythmias.

In addition, new methods are also needed to counteract problems with established procedures. For example, occlusion of bypassed segments is a common occurence shortly after bypass surgery. The loss of graft patency continues over time, occurring

Table 1. Interventional cardiology and angiology
– established and newly developed methods.

Revascularization
  Balloon angioplasty
  Atherectomy
  Mechanical ablation of plaque
  Microembolization
  Aspiration
  High energy
  – laser
  – radio-frequency
  – sonographic
  – spark erosion
  Assisting devices
  – perfusion catheters
  – stents
  – angioscopy
  – counterpulsation
  – cardiopulmonary support

Other Indications
  – valvuloplasty
  – catheter ablation
  – shunt occlusion

in 10–20% of grafts in the first year and 1–3% every subsequent year (1). Internal mammary grafting, with a significantly better patency rate (2) is one solution, but one could also view PTCA as another, since balloon dilatation can be more reconstructive than bypass surgery. However, balloon dilatation has its own well known limitations such as tight and long stenoses, total occlusions or tortuous vessels. New catheter systems can help to overcome these limitations, and several companies now produce highly flexible, low profile systems which have excellent trackability (e.g. micro-Hartzler) and allow easy passage of stenoses, which were not passable with the systems available just a few years ago. Other low-profile catheters have excellent pushability (Medtronic Omniflex) and new modes of exchangability have been created, as with the monorail catheters, or by use of a long or extension wire technique.

Naturally, difficulties such as acute occlusion and restenosis remain problematic for the field of balloon angioplasty and are most probably related to intimal trauma during dilation or residual plaque material within the vessel. Therefore, new catheter techniques which focus on this problem are being developed, which use mechanical or high energy to remove or ablate plaque material.

Mechanical angioplasty

The Kaltenbach-Vallbracht group has developed a low-speed rotational angioplasty device (3) which has been used successfully in the periphery and testing in the coronary system is now underway. There are also rotary ablaters which use burr tips with diamond blades to ablate the plaque tissue; evaluation of effluate has shown that more than 90% of ablated particles were smaller than 8 microns (4). An interesting and promising device was developed by Kensey et al. (5), in which the tip of the catheter has an integrated rotating cam with a fine lateral jet spray which keeps the rotating cam centered and cools the vessel as it is heated by the mechanical action. In addition, the circular jet spray may contribute to lumen dilation and smoothening of its inner surface. In a series of dog experiments, recanalization of diseased human arterial imponates in the carotid position could be so treated without embolization.

Rotational atherectomy

There are currently three devices under investigation with similar working principles. The Ultramed device (Fig. 1) consists of two small knives in the catheter tip, which can be moved over-the-wire, and cut segments of plaque which can then be aspirated and collected by vacuum and submitted for investigation (personal communication).

The Medtronic catheter consists of two cutting elements which rotate and move independently and also incorportates an over-the-wire system. The plaque material is trapped within the spirals of the catheter and can also be removed and studied.

The Simpson (6) atherectomy catheter (Fig. 2) utilizes a rotary cutting edge (600–2000 rpm) incorporated within a metal housing at its tip. A window in the housing is positioned alongside the stenosis and fixed by use of a low pressure

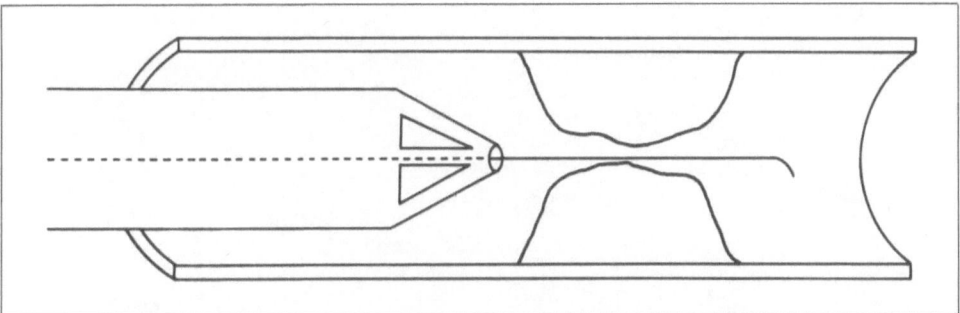

Fig. 1. Prototype model of the Ultramed atherectomy deivce, with two knives incorporated within the catheter tip

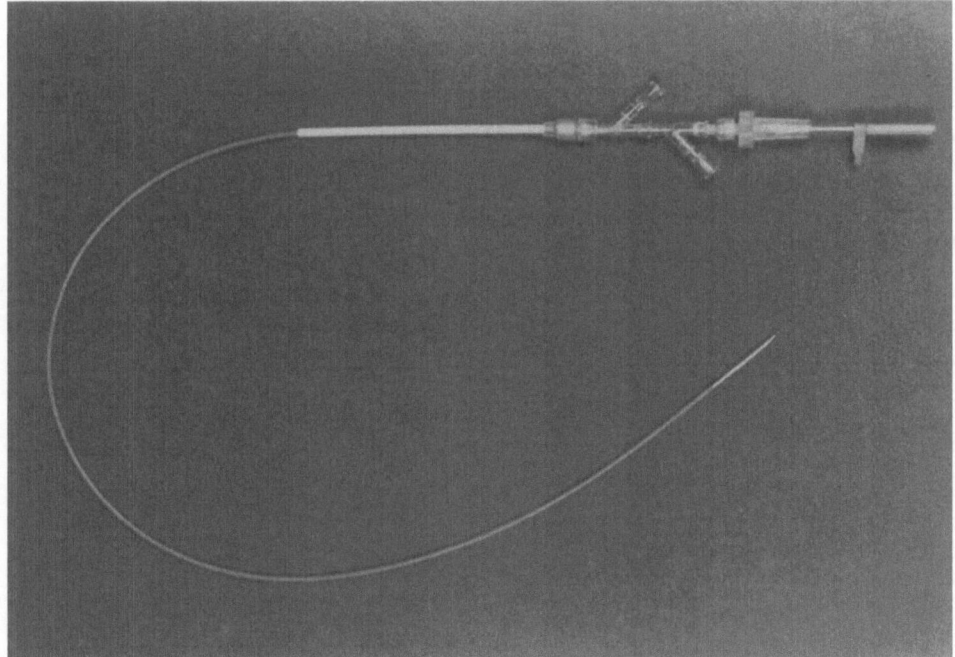

Fig. 2. The Simpson peripheral atherectomy catheter, whose rotary cutting edge is advanced by operator control and powered by a hand-held motor

(1–2 atm) balloon; thin slices of plaque are excised as the cutter is advanced and deposited within the housing; these can then be later removed (Fig. 3) and further investigated (histology, cell culture, immunohistological study). Initial work in the periphery has proved promising (7, 8) and the technique is currently undergoing study in the coronaries (9).

Our own group has performed peripheral atherectomy on a total of 40 patients with 72 stenoses or occlusions of the iliac (n = 5), superficial femoral (n = 62) and

3

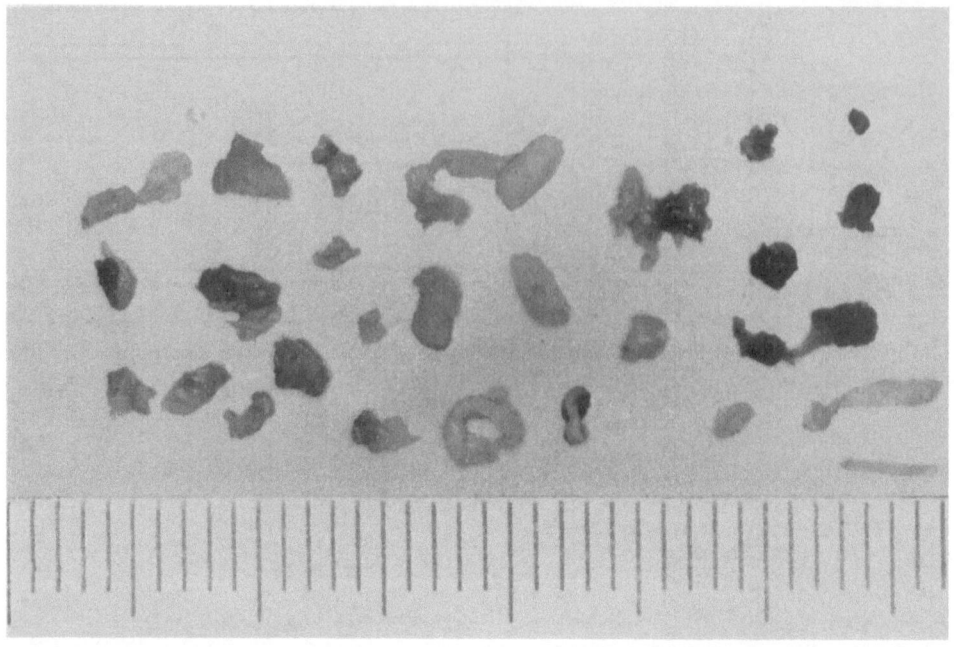

Fig. 3. Specimens of plaque material removed by atherectomy of a superficial femoral artery stenosis

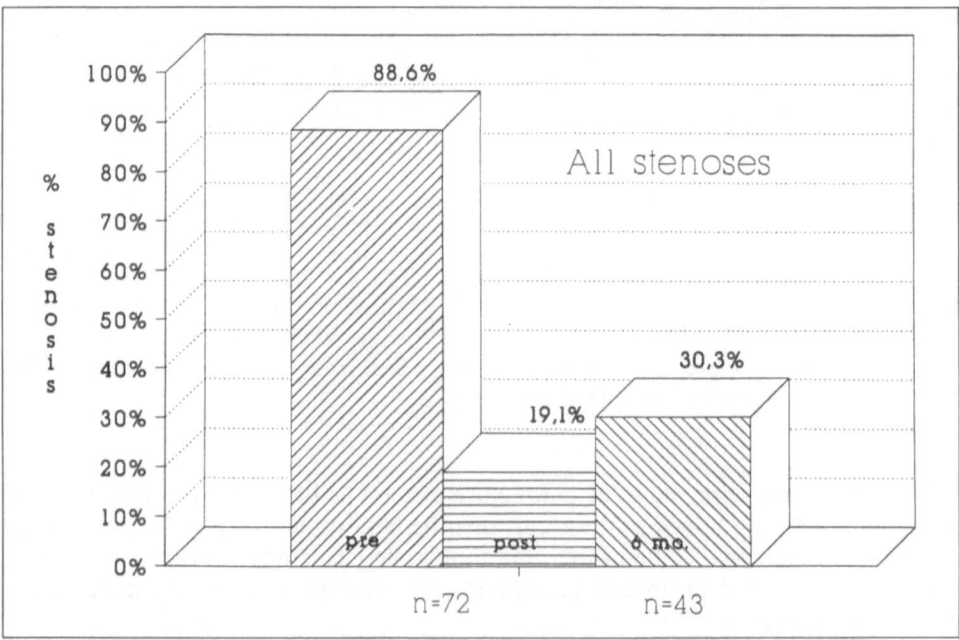

Fig. 4. Angiographic results in 72 lesions treated with the percutaneous Simpson atherectomy catheter pre- and postatherectomy and in 43 stenoses at 6 month control study

popliteal (n = 5) arteries. There was initial technical success in 91% of attempted lesions. The mean stenosis was reduced from $87.2 \pm 13.9\%$ to $16.6 \pm 15.5\%$; at 6 mo. follow-up, angiographic evaluation of 43 lesions showed a $35.7 \pm 30.9\%$ residual stenosis (Fig. 4), with angiographic re-stenosis found in only 5% of eccentric lesions, 27% of concentric lesions and 42% of total occlusions.

High energy angioplasty

Recanalization of occlusions is achieved by ablating plaque material with high energy such as laser, high frequency (10), spark erosion (11), or ultrasound (12). Whereas much experimental work remains to be done, several groups have used laser energy to recanalize stenosed and occluded peripheral arteries (13, 14, 15) and work in the coronaries is beginning (16); additional balloon angioplasty is necessary in most of these cases. Certainly a major limitation of laser angioplasty is the poor predictability of the amount of energy required. There are two possible laser action modes, vaporization which is a high energy mechanism and fragmentation which requires low energy. Furthermore, vaporization is highly dependent on the nature of plaque tissue (variation in several orders of magnitude) and since this cannot yet be predicted, laser energy requirement is necessarily not predictable.

In-depth details of laser energy application, as well as evaluation of the other interventional procedures outlined in Table 1 such as balloon valvuloplasty and catheter ablation, which are often not presented conjointly with angioplasty techniques, and of adjunctive procedures such as stent implantation and angioscopy will be addressed in detail by other authors in this book.

References

1. Facts about Coronary Artery Bypass Surgery. (1987) National Heart, Lung and Blood Institute, Publ 87:2891
2. Loop FD, Lytle BW, Cosgrove DM et al. (1986) Influence of the Internal-Mammary-Artery Graft on 10-year survival and other cardiac events. New Engl J Med 314:1–6
3. Kaltenbach M, Vallbracht C (1987) Rotationsangioplastik – Ein neues Katheterverfahren. Fortschr Med 105, 412–414
4. Ritchie JL, Hansen KK, Vracko R et al. Mechanical thrombolysis a new rotational catheter approach for acute thrombi. Circulation 73(5):1006–1012
5. Kensey, K.R. et al. (1987) Recanalization of obstructed arteries with a flexible, rotating tip catheter. Radiol 165:387–389
6. Simpson JB et al. (1985) Transluminal atherectomy: a new approach to the treatment of atherosclerotic vascular disease. Circulation 72 Suppl 2:III–146
7. Höfling B, von Pölnitz A, Backa D et al. (1988) Percutaneous atherectomy: a new technique for non-operative removal of obstructive plaques in peripheral vascular disease. Lancet: 384–386
8. Selmon MR, Robertson GC, Simpson JB (1988) Transluminal atherectomy: early results in the treatment of atherosclerosis. J Am Coll Cardiol 11 2:109A
9. Simpson JB, Robertson GC, Selmon MR (1988) Percutaneous coronary atherectomy. J Am Coll Cardiol 11 2:110A
10. Höher M, Hombach V, Arnold G et al. (1987) High frequency recanalization of thrombotically occluded vessels in experimental pigs. Circulation 76 Suppl 4:IV–28
11. Slager CJ, Phaff AC, Essed CE et al. (1987) Spark Erosion of atherosclerotic plaques. Z Kardiol 76 Suppl 6:67–71

12. Siegel RJ, Fishbein MC, Donmichael TA et al. (1987) Ultrasonic and electrohydraulic athero-sclerotic plaque dissolution. Circulation 76 Suppl:IV–46
13. Sanborn TA, Cumberland DC, Greenfield AJ et al. (1988) Percutaneous laser thermal angio-plasty: initial results and one-year follow-up in 129 femoropopliteal lesions. Radiology 168:121–5
14. Abela GS et al. (1988) Peripheral artery laser recanalization. J Am Coll Cardiol 11:107A
15. Fourrier JL et al. (1987) Human percutaneous laser angioplasty with sapphire tips: results and follow-up. Circulation 76:IV–231, 1987
16. Sanborn TA, Faxon DP, Kellett MA et al. (1987) Percutaneous coronary laser thermal angio-plasty. J Am Coll Cardiol 8:1437

1. Additional aspects to balloon angioplasty

Long wire technique for coronary angioplasty – the Frankfurt experience

C. Vallbracht, G. Kober, M. Kaltenbach

Center of Internal Medicine, Department of Cardiology, University Hospital, Frankfurt, FRG

In October 1977, four weeks after the first successful transluminal coronary angioplasty by Grüntzig (2) the second procedure was performed in Frankfurt using the original double lumen balloon catheter. In 1982, we began to use the steerable technique with a short guide wire as described by Simpson (7) which remarkably facilitated coronary angioplasty and led to an extension of its indication. In December 1983, Kaltenbach introduced the long wire technique (5) which has become routine in Frankfurt and some other European centers.

Technique

A special 3 meter long, 0.012 inch teflon coated guide wire, equipped with a ball shaped tip of 0.45mm diameter is introduced within the guiding catheter and the stenosis is first crossed without a balloon catheter (Fig. 1). To control and steer the wire, we developed a small plastic torquer which can be fixed to the wire from the side. The distal part of the long wire remains coiled up in a tube and does not hinder the procedure in any way. In particular, the torquability of the wire is unimpeded.

After the guide wire has been positioned in the peripheral vessel segment a balloon catheter can be advanced over the wire (Fig. 2); continuous pressure monitoring

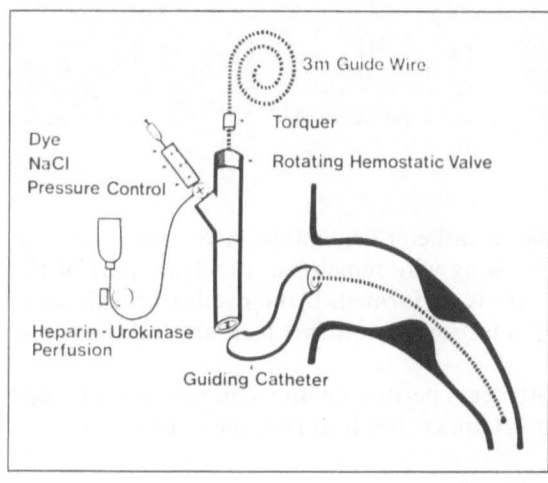

Fig. 1. Long wire technique: the stenosis is first crossed only with a 0.012 inch guide wire without a balloon catheter

7

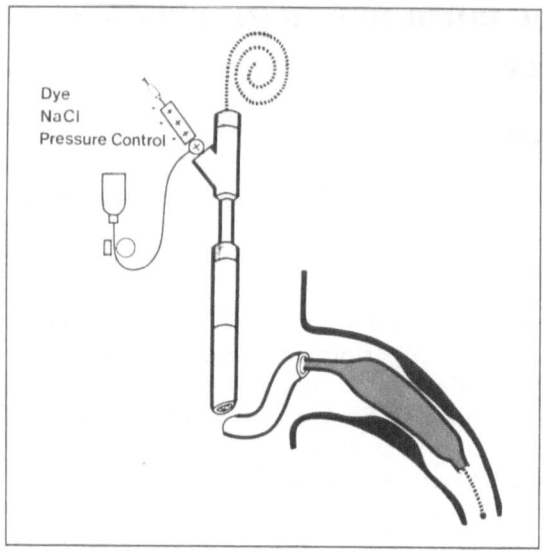

Fig. 2. When the guide wire has passed the stenosis, a balloon catheter can be advanced over the wire

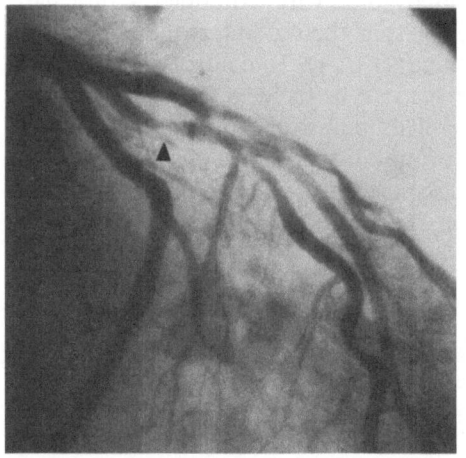

A

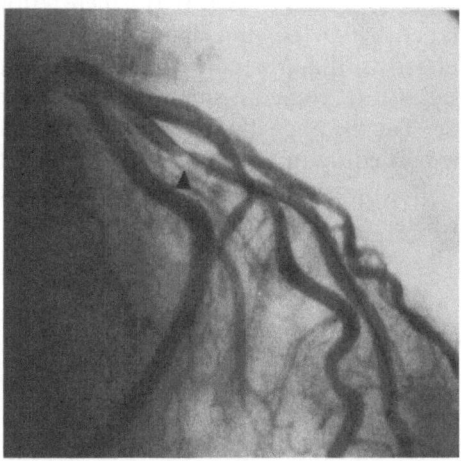

B

from the guiding catheter and the balloon catheter is possible. After dilatation, the balloon catheter is withdrawn while the long wire remains in the distal part of the coronary artery and a control angiogram is performed. If the result is satisfactory, the long wire is withdrawn and a last injection of contrast medium follows (Figs. 3a–e).

Using a Y-connector the guiding catheter is perfused with a combination of 2.000 units of heparin and 100.000 units of urokinase per h during the entire process of crossing and dilatation.

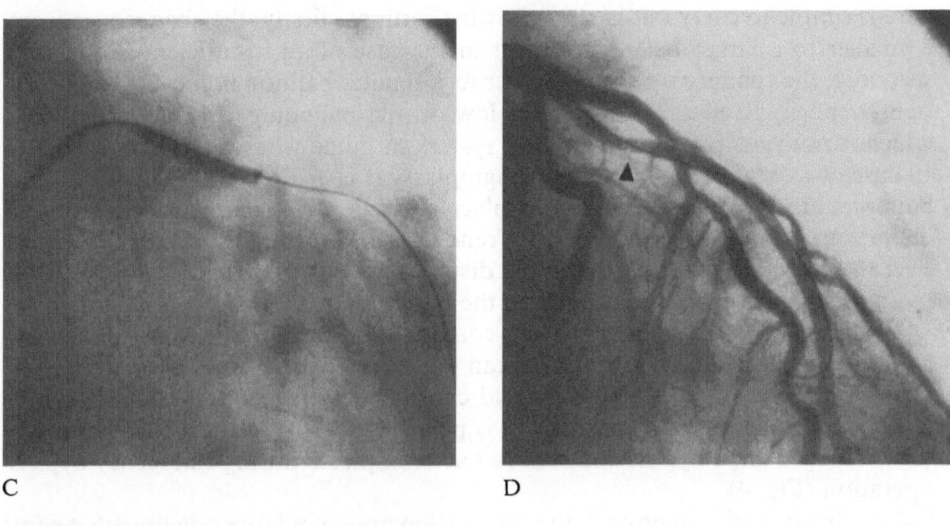

C   D

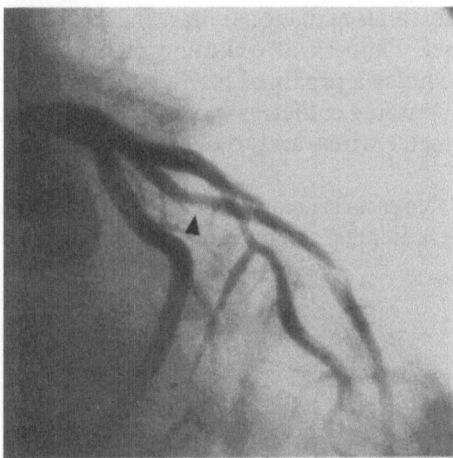

E

Fig. 3. (A) Stenosis in a big marginal branch. (B) The long wire has passed the stenosis, the control angiogram clearly shows the position of the wire. (C) A balloon catheter was introduced and inflated (D) Control angiogram after withdrawal of the balloon with the long wire remaining in place. (E) Final result after withdrawal of the wire

Special advantages

1) The guide wire is introduced without the balloon catheter allowing for excellent steerability and a very sensitive handling. Even the smallest resistance is directly transmitted and this guarantees the possibility of an immediate reaction. Therefore, precision and safety is considerably improved.
2) The long wire technique allows the balloon catheter to be exchanged without recrossing and repeat traumatization of the stenosis. Balloon catheters of different sizes and of different manufacturers can be used. Using the 0.012 inch guide

9

wire is simple to carry out in the following settings: firstly, the changeover from a smaller to a larger balloon catheter in the case of an insufficient result, and secondly, the changeover from a larger to a smaller balloon in the case of a very tight stenosis. Even a 2.0 mm super low-profile balloon catheter can be used, which is not possible with an add-on system of guide wires (extension wire).

3) In case of a total occlusion during angioplasty it is again possible to advance a balloon catheter over the wire into place. If under these circumstances repeat dilatations are not successful, a 4.5 French perfusion catheter can be advanced over the wire. The correct positioning distal to the occlusion can be documented by injection of contrast medium into the perfusion catheter.

Using an 8.5 or 9F guiding catheter, coronary perfusion (done by hand with the help of a conventional 5 ml syringe) can be started with arterial blood from the guiding catheter (up to 40 ml/min) and continued with blood from the patients femoral artery (up to 100 ml/min). It is possible to carry on perfusion until the distal and proximal bypass anastomoses are completed during emergency bypass operation (Fig. 4).

4) The localization of a stenosis in the bifurcation area of a large side branch, as for instance, in a stenosis involving the LAD and a large diagonal branch carries the danger of an occlusion of the second vessel. The risk of occlusion seems to be particulary high if the second branch also shows a proximal high-grade stenosis (6). Using only one brachial or femoral 9-F guiding catheter it is possible to cross both stenoses, one after the other, with 3-meter wires, and to dilate the stenoses sequentially (7).

5) In contrast to the monorail technique (1) pressure measurement through the balloon catheter, including intracoronary gradients and coronary capillary pressure, is preserved.

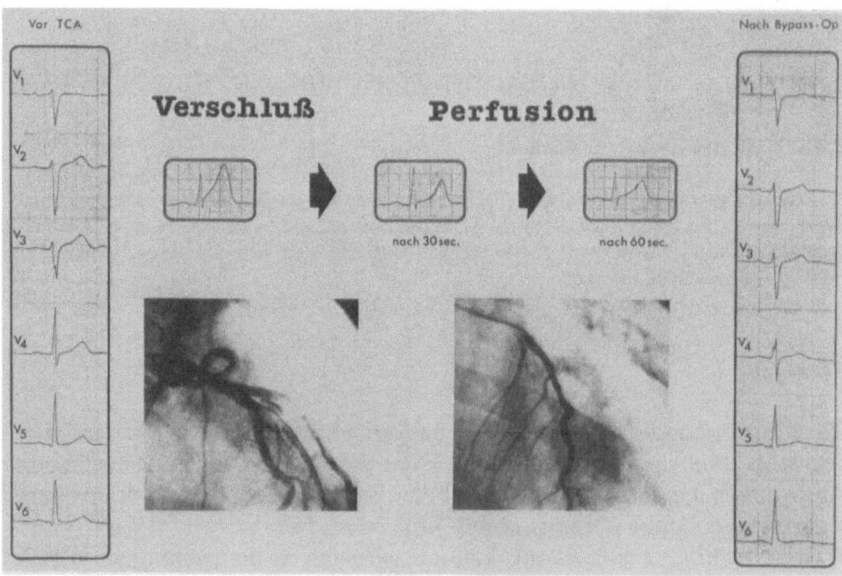

Fig. 4. Dissection after dilatation of a stenosis in the LAD with subsequent occlusion. Coronary perfusion over two hours could prevent a myocardial infarction

10

Results

Since its introduction in December 1983, the long-wire technique has been applied in Frankfurt in more than 1,500 patients. The acute success rate with respect to the stenoses was comparable to other techniques (90 %); the rate of severe complications with the need for emergency bypass operation was significantly reduced to less than 1 % in 1987. Exchange of balloon catheters was needed in 13 % of patients; either from a larger to a smaller balloon in case of very tight stenosis (5 %) or from a smaller to a larger balloon catheter in case of an insufficient acute result (8 %). In our experience the need for the double long-wire technique in case of a branching stenosis is a relatively rare event; in 20 patients with stenoses within a bifurcation of a large side branch two long wires were used. In two patients sequential dilatation because of occlusion of one vessel was necessary; in the majority of patients a dilatation over the second wire was not required. Total occlusions during angioplasty occurred in 4.5 % of the patients. With the long wire in place all occlusions could be recrossed and dilated with the same or a larger balloon catheter. In five patients repeat dilatation remained unsuccessful and a perfusion catheter was introduced.

Discussion

The long wire technique of Kaltenbach (5) has been shown to facilitate coronary angioplasty and to improve precision and safety of the procedure. Steerability of the wire and contrast display is unimpeeded because the guide wire is introduced without the balloon catheter. Any resistance to the tip is directly transmitted and therefore, immediate reaction is possible. In contrast to the monorail-technique (1) balloon catheters, not only of different sizes, but different manufacturers can be exchanged without recrossing the stenosis. Even a 2.0 mm super low-profile balloon catheter can be introduced over the 0.012 inch guide wire, which is not possible using an add on system of guide wires (extension wire system).

The occurrence of dissection with subsequent total occlusion during coronary angioplasty cannot be predicted. Therefore the possibility to recross the occlusion, either with a balloon or a perfusion catheter to restore blood flow is of considerable importance and may lead to a dramatic improvement (3). Coronary perfusion can be continued until surgical revascularization is completed. In contrast to the "kissing balloon" technique of Grüntzig which requires two guiding catheters, the double long wire technique can be performed with two long wires introduced through the same 9-F brachial or femoral guiding catheter (8). In our experience the need for a sequential dilatation because of an occlusion of the second vessel is a relatively rare event, so the second wire remains on "standby".

Heparin-urokinase perfusion and teflon coating of the guide wires is effective in reducing thrombus formation and fibrin coating of the guide wires (4). Their general use may be justified but further studies are required.

References

1. Bonzel T, Wollschläger H, Meinertz T et al. (1986) The steerable monorail catheter system – a new device for PTCA. Circulation 74 Suppl II:1829
2. Grüntzig A (1977) Coronary transluminal angioplasty. Circulation 84 Suppl:55
3. Hopf R, Kunkel B, Schneider M, Kaltenbach M (1985) Koronarperfusion bei akutem Gefäßverschluß im Rahmen der transluminalen Koronarangioplastik (PTCA). Z Kardiol 74:580
4. Kadel C, Jonczyk C, Kaltenbach M (1987) Thrombotic deposits on angioplasty guide wires. 5th Joint Meeting ESC, Santiage, Spain
5. Kaltenbach M (1984) The long wire technique – a new technique for steerable balloon catheter dilatation. Eur Heart J 5:1004
6. Meier B, Grüntzig AR, King SB III et al. (1984) Risk of side branch occlusion during coronary angioplasty. Am J Cardiol 53:10
7. Simpson JB, Baim DS, Robert EW and Harrison DC (1982) A new catheter system for coronary angioplasty. Am J Cardiol 49:1216
8. Vallbracht C, Kober G, Kaltenbach M (1987) Double long wire technique for percutaneous transluminal coronary angioplasty for narrowings at major bifurcations. Am J Cardiol 60:907

Advances in x-ray equipment – digital subtraction angiography with on-line quantification

Th. v. Arnim, M. Hengge, J. Prasil, B. Höfling

Department of Medicine I, University of Munich, Klinikum Großhadern, Munich, FRG

Quantification of coronary artery stenosis

In coronary artery disease the severity of a given luminal obstruction is dependent on the amount of reduction of the luminal area by fixed calcified stenosis and the degree of constriction of a normal segment of the vascular wall. Thus there are short-term and long-term variations in the degree of coronary stenosis (1, 6, 14, 16). Attempts have been made to quantify the anatomic and functional severity of coronary stenosis: apart from angiographic assessment (5, 9, 10, 15), assessment of flow with Doppler catheters, thallium imaging, PET scanning and intravascular ultrasound have been tried. The most widely used way of quantification is quantitative angiography, but it must be born in mind that angiography shows only the lumen opacified by contrast medium, while characteristics of the vessel wall can hardly, if ever, be discerned (12, 18).

Quantification of the progression of coronary atherosclerosis over a longer term in studies aimed at influencing the atheromatous process is obviously of great importance (2, 3, 4, 11, 17). Algorithms have been developed to objectively quantify the luminal narrowing by automatic edge detection in digitized magnified images taken from coronary angiography films (9, 10, 12, 15). This geometric quantification has problems with interpretation and reproducibility in eccentric stenoses, which are by no means rare. Therefore, a densitometric approach, which measures the degree of attenuation of the x-ray caused by the amount of contrast material within the vessel, is more independent of the geometry of the coronary obstruction (7, 12). If angiographic quantification of coronary artery diameters is to be used in practical clinical decision making in the angiographic laboratory, then a fast method of measurement is necessary (12). While methods which are dependent on digitization of film images have shown good reliability and reproducibility, the time lag for development of films and later quantification is obviously too great for implementation in acute clinical decision making. An on-line quantification of angiographic images, which is digitized directly during the angiographic procedure would therefore be advantageous (13). To overcome the problems of geometric diameter measurement and calculation of lumen area, the combination with a densitometric method would obviously enhance the reliability and usefulness of such measurements (8).

We describe here our first experience with new angiographic equipment (Digiton 3, Siemens AG, Erlangen, FRG) which allows digital image acquisition simultaneously with the usual angiographic films during coronary arteriography and further allows digital subtraction of these images followed by on-line geometric and densitometric quantification.

Experiences with Digitron 3

The practical approach of image acquisition and stenosis quantification is depicted in the series of examples in Fig. 1. The first step is to select an image of the angiographic series which is free of subtraction artifact and motion artifact and shows the stenosis with a minimum of geometric distortion and overlay. This can be done very easily and quickly in the angiographic laboratory on a videoscreen. In the next step of the program, a digitizing tablet is used and a normal reference part of the vessel defined, followed by defining a center line of the vessel with a digitizing pen. When this center line is drawn through the stenosis, the active part of the observer is completed and the computer program takes over. Starting from the reference point, the vessel wall is defined by an automatic edge-detection algorithm. The computer then defines the stenosis as the most narrowed part and compares the diameters with the diameter at the reference point. All these automatic calculations proceed very quickly. The result is immediately displayed on the video screen; it shows the outline of the vessel with the stenosis, the stenotic diameter and calculated area with geometric calculation. Simultaneously, the densitometric measurement which was obtained from densitometric information available for each pixel of the digitized image, is displayed. Thus a quick on-line quantification of the stenosis is possible and within the same procedure geometric and densitometric measurements are obtained. Obviously, with the comparison of images before and after PTCA as in our example, the angiographic success of an intervention can immediately be quantified.

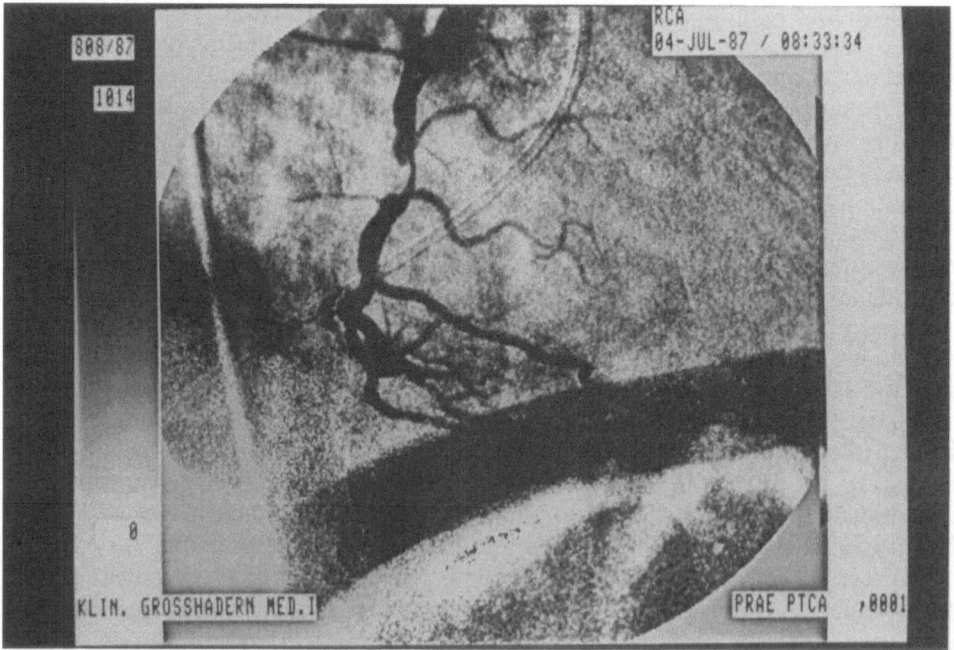

Fig. 1 a. Coronary angiogram of a right coronary artery taken with digital subtraction angiography. A high grade eccentric stenosis in the mid right coronary artery can be seen.

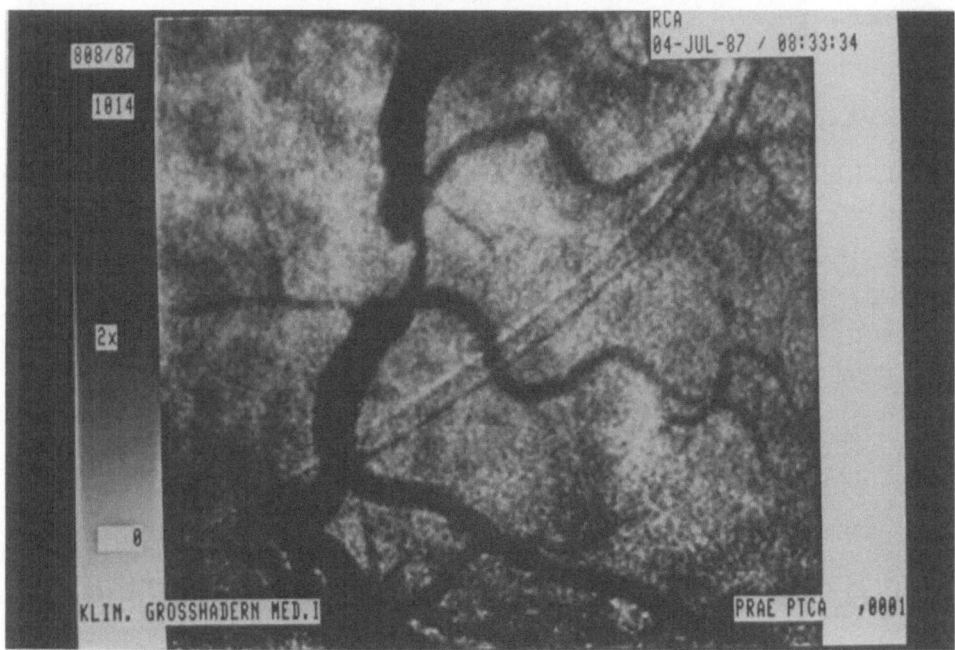

Fig. 1 b. In the first step of the evaluation, the digitized image is magnified by a zoom. Note the more coarsely grained image

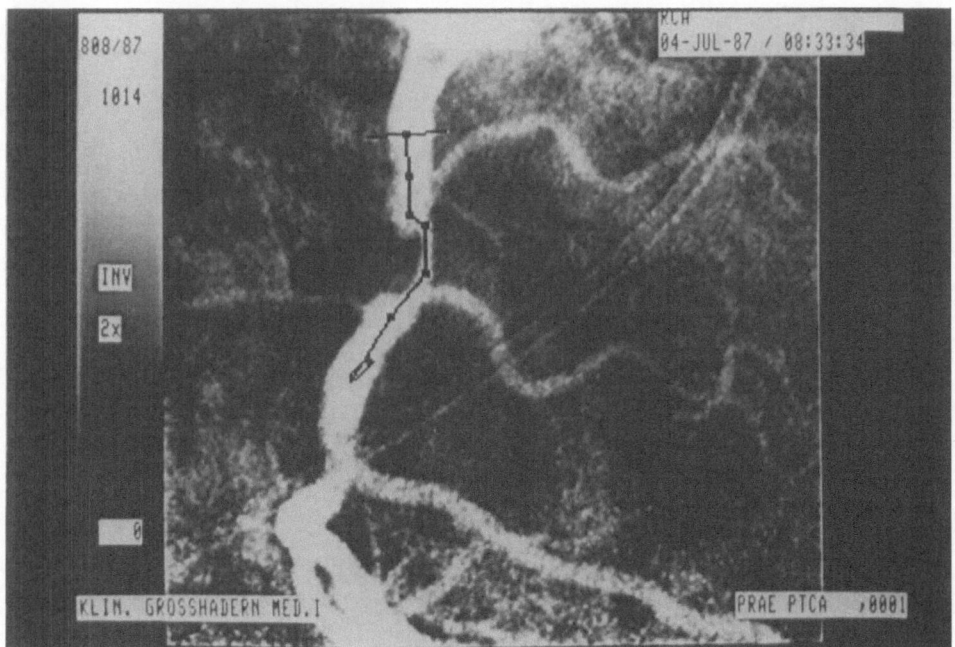

Fig. 1 c. After black and white have been reversed in the image, the process of quantification is started by defining a reference line and then defining a line within the vessel lumen on a digitizing tablet as a connection of several points. Each dot on the line is one quick press on the digitizing pen.

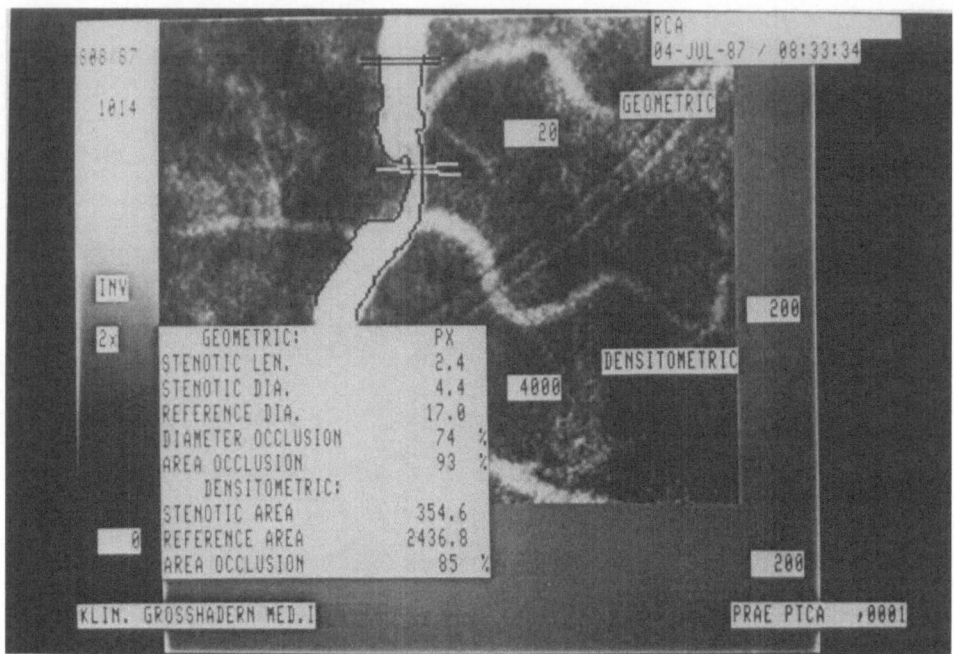

Fig. 1 d. After the digitizing pen has reached the post-stenotic normal portion of the vessel, the automatic quantification by the computer is immediately started and within less than 3 s the geometric and densitometric quantification is displayed on the screen. One can see where the reference line is and where the computer has defined the most severe stenosis

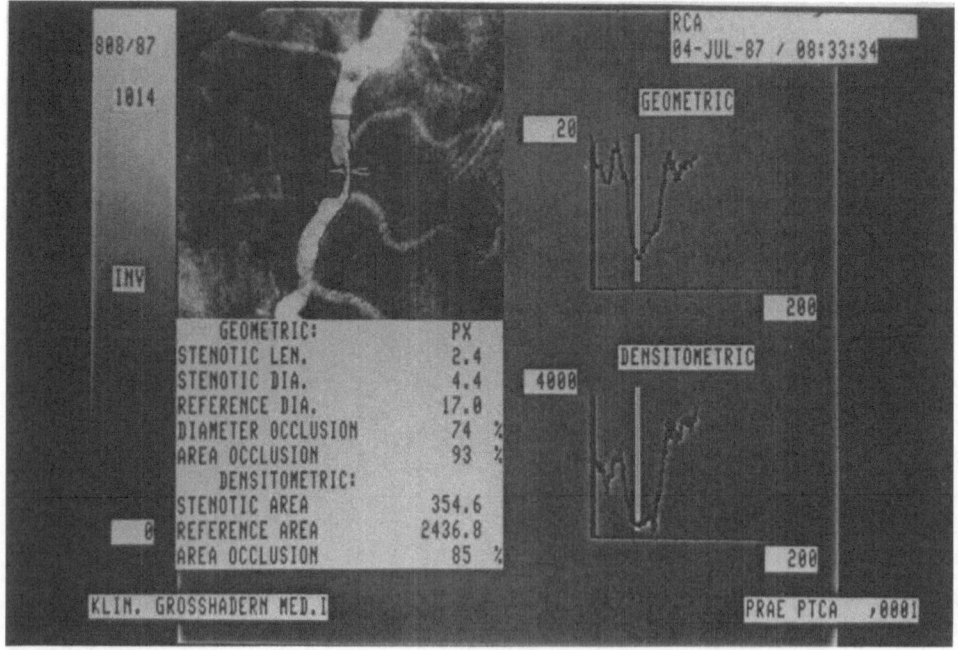

Fig. 1 e. The geometric and densitometric evaluation of the stenosis by the computer can be displayed in graphic form as the geometric diameter and densitometric area curves. The curves can be seen on the right of the picture and with use of the computer it is possible to reposition the marker lines for the reference part of the vessel and for the stenosis

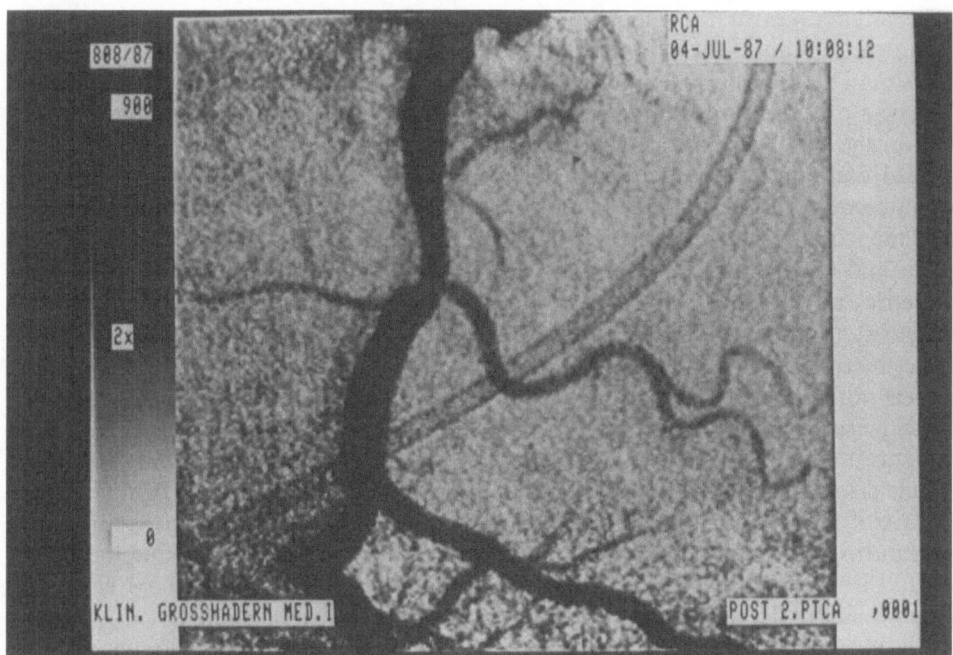

Fig. 2 a. Digital subtraction image of the same vessel as in Fig. 1 after two balloon dilatations

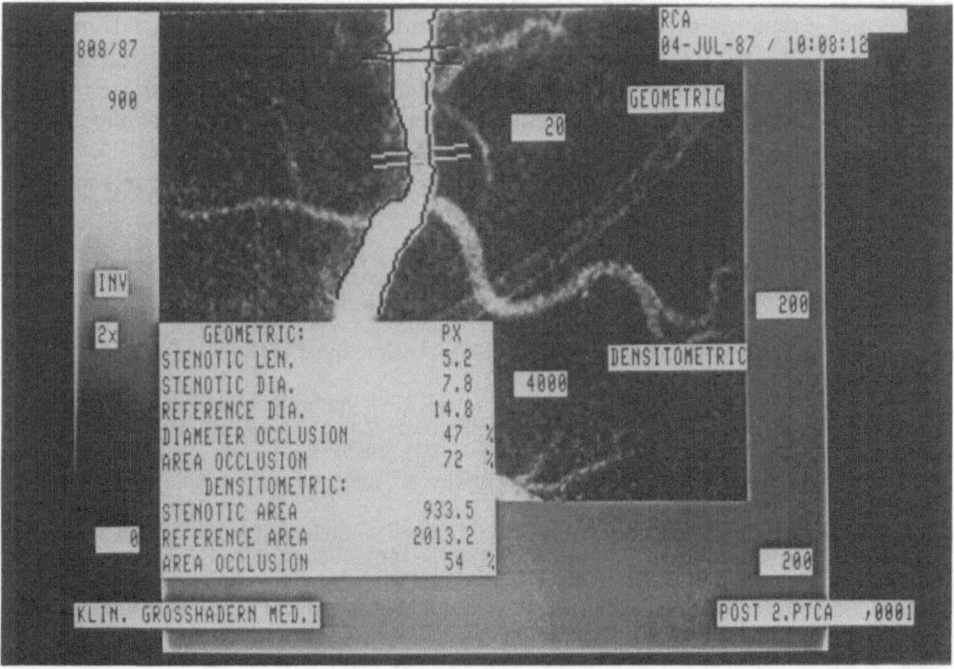

Fig. 2 b. Quantification of the stenosis after the balloon dilatation. This evaluation was done during the procedure and with still a relevant degree of stenosis persisting, further balloon dilatations were performed in this patient

The advantages of the Digitron system are obvious: the speed of the on-line quantification allows the examination of coronary stenosis during such procedures as PTCA. This may help in clinical decision making in some cases where the degree of success of a balloon dilatation is questionable. Another advantage besides the speed of the system is the easy application of the computer program. With a clearly outlined computer manual, personnel not specially trained in digital imaging or computer work can easily learn stenosis quantification. This evaluation is largely user independent and performed by automatic computer detection of the vascular outline and the stenosis. The third advantage of the system is the combination of a geometric and a densitometric measurement, which shows the angiographer the true complexity of the stenosis quantification. In our experience, geometric and densitometric measurements often show differing results, obviously due to the irregular geometry of coronary stenoses. With this approach, the Digitron system offers an honest picture of the possibilities of fast stenosis quantification, but also of the problems inherent in the great degree of physiological variability.

Some disadvantages of the present technology should also be mentioned, i.e., with a matrix of 512×512 pixels, an image of a complete coronary artery, as is normally taken during coronary angiography, gives too large a pixel size for fine measurements. With our greatest magnification from the image intensifier, we have calculated a pixel size of 0.2 mm. With narrow stenoses going down to diameters of 0.5 mm, a variation of ± 1 pixel at each side of the lumen would cause large percentage variations. Particularly in the case of pharmacologic intervention, where small diameter variations can be observed and may be of true physiological significance, a much smaller pixel size would be desirable for quantification. This can thus far only be achieved with later digitization of only a small portion of the filmed image. Thus, for fine measurements of coronary artery quantifications a direct digital imaging of a 512×512 matrix is probably too rough. In addition to this basic problem which comes from the direct digitization of the image and might be taken into account in exchange for the speed of an on-line system, we have had problems with calibration for metric analysis and reproducibility of the measurements. These observations have caused review and restructuring of the computer programs applied in this system.

References

1. Ambrose JA, Winters SL, Arora RR et al. (1286) Angiographic evolution of coronary artery morphology in unstable angina. JACC 7:472
2. Arntzenius AC, Kromhout D, Barth JD et al. (1985) Diet, lipoproteins, and the progression of coronary atherosclerosis: the Leiden intervention trial. N Engl J Med 312:805
3. Blankenhorn DH, Nessim SA, Johnson RL et al. (1987) Beneficial effects of combined colestipol-niacin therapy on coronary atherosclerosis and coronary venous bypass grafts. JAMA 27:3233
4. Brensike JF, Kelsey SF et al. (1984) Effects of therapy with cholestyramin on progression of coronary arteriosclerosis: results of the NHLBI Type II Coronary Intervention Study. Circulation 69:313
5. Brown BG, Bolson EL, Dodge HT (1982) Arteriographic assessment of coronary atherosclerosis: review of current methods, their limitations and clinical applications. Arteriosclerosis 2:2
6. Davies MJ, Thomas AC (1985) Plaque fissuring – the cause of acute myocardial infarction, sudden ischaemic death and crescendo angina. Br Heart J 53:363

7. Doriot PA, Pochon Y, Rasoamanambelo L et al. (1985) Densitometry of coronary arteries – an improved physical model. IEEE Computers in Cardiology, pp. 91–94
8. Editorial Review (1987) Computer measurements of coronary artery disease. Lancet 1499
9. Fleck E, Dirschinger J, Rudolph W (1985) Quantitative Koronarangiographie vor und nach PTCA. Restenosierungsrate, Analyse beeinflussender Faktoren. Herz 10:313
10. Gould KL, Kelley KO, Bolson EL (1982) Experimental validation of quantitative coronary arteriography for determining pressure-flow characteristics of coronary stenosis. Circulation 66:930
11. Levy RI, Brensike JF, Epstein SE et al. (1984) The influence of changes in lipid values induced by cholestyramine and diet on progression of coronary artery disease: results of the NHLBI Type II Coronary Intervention Study. Circulation 69:325
12. Mancini GBJ, Simon SB, McGillem MJ et al. (1987) Automated quantitative coronary arteriography: morphologic and physiologic validation in vivo of a rapid digital angiographic method. Circulation 75:454
13. Parker DL, Clayton PD (1985) The effects of motion on quantitative vessel measurements. Med Phys 12:698
14. Rafflenbeul W, Nellessen U, Galvao P et al. (1984) Progression and Regression der Koronarsklerose im angiographischen Bild. Z f Kardiol 73, Suppl 2:33
15. Reiber JHC, Serruys PW, Kooijman CJ et al. (1985) Assessment of short-, medium-, and longterm variations in arterial dimensions from compuiterassisted quantitation of coronary cineangiograms. Circulation 71:280
16. Ross R (1986) The pathogenesis of atherosclerosis – an update. N Engl J Med 314:488
17. v. Schacky C (1987) Prophylaxis of atherosclerosis with marine omega–3 fatty acid: a comprehensive strategy. Ann Int Med 107:890
18. White CW, Wright CB, Doty DB et al. (1984) Does visual interpretation of the coronary arteriogram predict the physiologic importance of a coronary stenosis? N Engl J Med 310:819

Myocardial release of lactate, hypoxanthine, and urate during and following percutaneous transluminal coronary angioplasty. Potential mechanism for the generation of free radicals

P.W. Serruys, T. Huizer, J. Bonnier*, R. Troquay*, H. Suryapranata, O. Leborgne, J. de Jong

Catheterization and Cardiochemical Laboratories, Thorax Center, Erasmus University, Rotterdam, The Netherlands
* Department of Cardiology, Catharina Hospital, Eindhoven, The Netherlands

Until recently the assessment of alteration in myocardial metabolism in man early after an abrupt occlusion of a major coronary artery has not been feasible. PTCA however, now provides a unique opportunity to study the time course of these metabolic changes during the transient interruption of coronary flow by the balloon occlusion sequence in patients with single-vessel disease and without angiographically demonstrable collateral circulation (1, 2). The need to detect any persisting metabolic or mechanical dysfunction becomes of even greater concern as the number of dilated vessels and the duration of balloon inflation tend to increase, thereby enhancing both the extent and the severity of ischemia. The risk exists that the damage induced by the intervention may exceed its benefit.

During and after ischemia, there is in the heart, as well as in other muscles, excessive ATP breakdown. This degradation of ATP causes an efflux of breakdown products, which are able to pass through the cell membrane into the blood before significant amounts of enzymes appear. The purine derivatives adenosine, inosine, hypoxanthine, xanthine, and urate are therefore thought to be early markers for ischemia (3, 4).

Recently high pressure liquid chromatography (HPLC) came into use for the determination of nucleosides and purine bases in whole blood (5, 6), facilitating the determination of purine derivatives, in particular hypoxanthine and urate. This new technical development prompted us to investigate the myocardial release of hypoxanthine and urate immediately after angioplasty. We studied the arterial-venous difference in urate, the endproduct of the reaction catalyzed by xanthine oxidoreductase, since the oxidase configuration of cardiac xanthine oxidoreductase has been implicated in the formation of oxyradicals which could damage the endothelium. This enzyme has been found in the heart of various species, however, its presence in human heart is still debated.

Patients and methods

All patients met the following criteria: a brief history of angina pectoris (less than one year), an isolated obstructive lesion in one coronary vessel (the left anterior descending) and an accessible stenosis of less than 1 cm in length. All patients were candidates for coronary artery bypass graft surgery because of disabling angina, but were selected for angioplasty rather than surgery because of their anatomy.

In the first group 15 patients were studied: 12 men, three women, aged from 38 to 74 years. Of these, four were in NYHA class II, 9 in class III, and 2 in class IV. In all, the ejection fraction was greater than 59% and none of them had wall motion abnormalities on their diagnostic resting left ventriculograms. Four transluminal dilatations were performed with a total duration of occlusion of 192 ± 40 s (mean $\pm$ SD). All patients in the study were successfully reperfused with four dilatations. The second study group of consisted 13 patients (Catharina Hospital, Eindhoven, The Netherlands). Urate was measured in arterial and coronary sinus blood plasma before, during, and after angioplasty.

PTCA technique

PTCA was performed according to the technique previously described. The inflation pressure ranged from 2-12 atmospheres, while the individual duration of occlusion ranged from 40 to 60 s. Coronary angiography with non ionic contrast medium (metrizamide) was performed before and at the end of the PTCA procedure.

Premedication consisted of aspirin and all patients selectively received 3 mg of isosorbide dinitrate into the left main coronary artery during control coronary arteriography, but the coronary flow measurements we report were not carried out within the period of the drug effect on the coronary circulation. Beta-blockers were not discontinued. During the procedure, heparin and low molecular weight dextran were administered intravenously.

Lactate, hypoxanthine and urate determination

Blood samples were obtained from the great cardiac vein and the left coronary artery at six consecutive measurement periods: before the PTCA procedure, 5-10 s after each transluminal occlusion, 5 min (group I) and 15 min (group II) after termination of the PTCA procedure. Five min were allowed between each dilatation for recovery.

Blood (1.5 ml) for lactate measurements was rapidly deproteinized with an equal volume of cold 8% perchloric acid and centrifuged. After centrifugation, the supernatant fluids were stored at $-20\,°C$. Lactate in the supernatant was analyzed enzymatically according to Apstein et al. (7) with the AutoAnalyzer (Technicon, Tarrytown, New York, USA). Standard curves were made with lithium lactate in 4% perchloric acid.

An isocratic high pressure liquid chromatographic system was used for the estimation of purine nucleosides and oxypurines in blood (6) (Fig. 1). Use was made of a

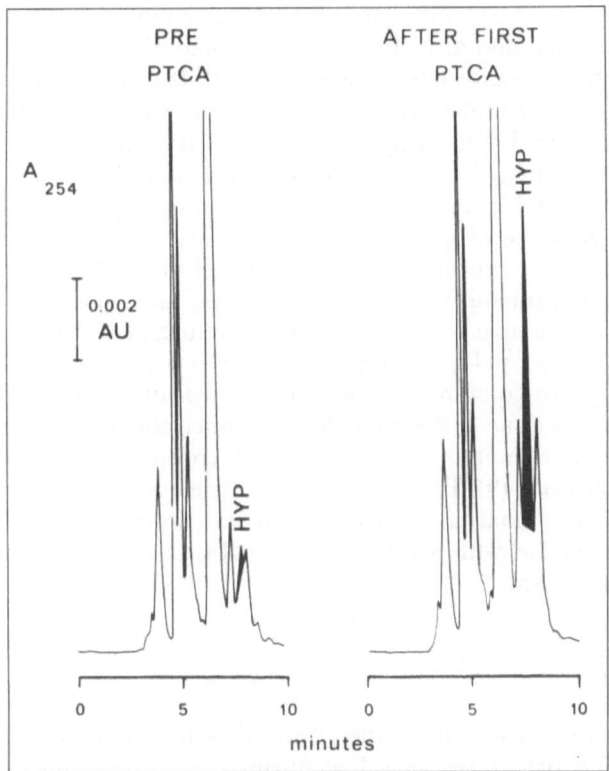

Fig. 1. Isocratic high pressure liquid chromatographic separation of nucleosides and purine bases from a patient before and after a single transluminal occlusion. hyp = hypoxanthine; AU = absorption units

reversed-phase column. Since nucleotides derived from erythrocytes affected the separation, these compounds had to be removed. We used the method of Chatterjee et al. (8), with some minor differences. For whole blood urate levels, 2 ml samples were mixed immediately after sampling with ice-cold perchloric acid to obtain the deproteinized extract. Extracts were brought to pH 5 with KOH and stored at $-20\,°C$ until urate quantification, according to a uricase method (enzyme provided by Sigma, St. Louis, Missouri, USA). In some samples urate was also quantified by HPLC. Samples were neutralized with 6 M $KOH/2M_2K_2CO_3$. Nucleotides (from the erythrocytes) were removed from the extract by adsorption on an AL_2O_3 column. Five ml 10 mH Tris-HCL was used to elute 1.5 ml sample through a column, containing 0.6 g AL_2O_3. Eluate was stored at $-15\,°C$ until analysis. HPLC determination of urate took place on a uBondapak c_{18} column (Millipore-Waters, Milford, Massachusetts, USA). A 100-ul sample was eluted with 1 % $K_2HPO_4 - 1$ % CH_3OH, pH 4.7, at a flow rate of 1.0 ml/min. The column was guarded by a Perisorb RP-18 pre-column (Merck, Darmstadt, FRG). The Waters-HPLC equipment consisted of: WISP 710B cooled autosampler, Model 6000 A pump, Model 490 multi wavelength detector, and Model 840 computer. Peaks were identified by retention times, internal standards, and enzyme shifts. The optimal wavelength for urate detection proved to be 290 nm since absorption is maximal and disturbance by other materials is minimal. Sample preparation and assay were derived from earlier work (6,10). To prepare plasma, blood was mixed in a heparinized tube with an equal volume of ice cold 154 nM NaCl, containing 40 µm dipyridamole (Boehringer, Ingelheim, FRG) and 20 µm EHNA (Wellcome, London, United Kingdom). These drugs were used to inhibit adenosine uptake and breakdown (11,12). Patient plasma samples were prepared and kept at $-80\,°C$. Deproteinization took place with an equal volume of 80% $HClO_4$; the supernatant fraction was neutralized with 2 M KOH/ 1 M K_2CO_3. HPLC-determination of urate in deproteinized, neutralized plasma took place on uBondapark C_{18} column. A 100-ul sample was eluted with a mixture of CH_3OH (100 ml) and KH_2PO_4 (10 g/l, 1000 ml), pH 5–7, at a flow rate of 0.6 ml/min. The column was guarded by a LC-18 guard-column (Superlco, Inc., Bellefonte, Pennsylvania, USA). Detection of urate was done at 254 and 290 nm, other conditions as described above. In 13 arterial and venous plasma samples of group 2, we also assayed for urate spectrophotometrically (9). The correlation coefficient between the two assay methods was 0.96. Statistical analysis was carried out with Student's t-test for paired variates, or where appropriate, with two-way analysis of variance, considering $p < 0.05$ as a significant difference.

Flow and resistance measurements

Great cardiac vein blood flow was measured by the continuous thermodilution method before and after the PTCA procedure, as well as during each transluminal occlusion. In the beginning of the investigation the location of the external thermistor in the great cardiac vein was verified by injection of 3 ml contrast material. Each recording of blood flow during coronary angioplasty began before balloon inflation and was interrupted at the moment of balloon deflation. Coronary vascular resistance (CVR) was calculated using the mean arterial pressure (MAP) and blood flow in the great cardiac vein (13):

$$CVR = MAP/FLOW \ (mmHg/ml/min)$$

Statistical analysis

Results are expressed as mean $\pm$ standard error of the mean. Comparison between pre-PTCA, post-PTCA and occlusion conditions were evaluated using analysis of variance for repeated measurements. When overall significance was found, multiple comparisons were significantly different at the 0.05 level.

Results

Coronary hemodynamic measurements

The results of the coronary hemodynamic observations are summarized in Fig. 2 and Table 1. During the initial dilatation the mean duration of balloon inflation was

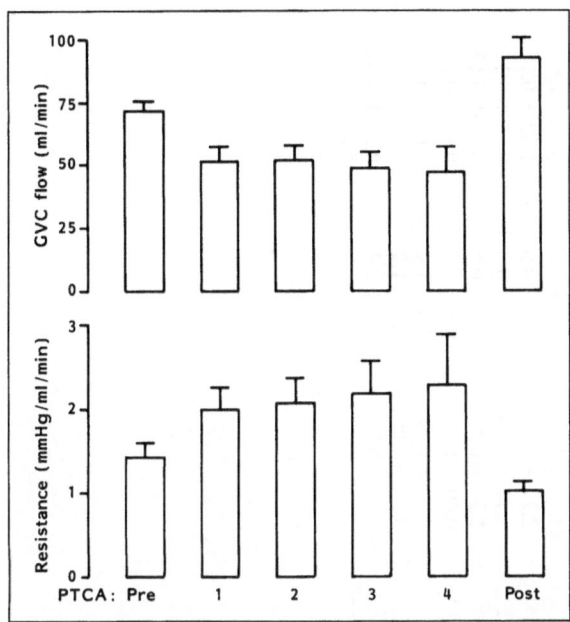

Fig. 2. Changes in great cardiac vein flow and resistance during four transluminal occlusions. GCV = great cardiac vein; pre = pre angioplasty; post = post angioplasty

44 ± 4 s. During the subsequent dilatations the duration of inflation was slightly increased to 49 ± 6 s. Occlusion pressure did not change throughout these occlusion times of 40 to 60 s and there was a high degree of reproducibility of the occlusion pressure during these successive occlusions (Table 1). The mean blood flow in the great cardiac vein before the first inflation was 72 ± 4 ml/min, falling to 47 ± 10 ml/min ($p < 0.003$) during the fourth inflation and rising slightly to 93 ± 8 ml/min ($p < 0.03$) after completion of the PTCA procedure (Table 1). Great cardiac vein coronary vascular resistance was 1.42 ± 0.18 mmHG/ml/min before balloon inflation, 2.3 ± 0.6 by the end of the fourth inflation ($p < 0.005$) and 1.02 ± 0.11 after completion of the PTCA procedure (Table 1).

Lactate, hypoxanthine and urate metabolism

The arteriovenous lactate measurements of the first study group, n = 15 are listed in Table 1 and shown in Fig. 3. The control measurements showed a difference of $+ 0.18$ mM, which decreased to -1.1 and -0.91 mM after the first and the second dilatations, respectively. After the third dilatation, the lactate difference was -0.60 mM, which was not significantly different from the values recorded after the first and the second dilatation. As a first approximation, the amount of lactate lost from the ischemic tissue during the four consecutive occlusions seems to be more or less constant and at least did not increase with time. During the four consecutive transluminal occlusions, an average rise in the great cardiac vein hypoxanthine from 3.0 ± 0.6 to 5.6 ± 1.1 µM ($p < 0.01$) was observed, which fell off after completion of

25

Table 1. Cornoary hemodynamics and metabolic disturbances during sequential transluminal occlusions (15 patients)

	before PTCA	first occlusion	second occlusion	third occlusion	fourth occlusion	after PTCA
Duration of occlusion (s)	–	44 ± 4*	54 ± 3	50 ± 4	49 ± 6	–
Occlusion pressure (mm Hg)	–	24 ± 4	23 ± 3	21 ± 2	25 ± 5	–
GCV flow (ml/min)	72 ± 4	51 ± 6[a]	52 ± 6[a]	48 ± 7[b]	47 ± 10[b]	93 ± 8[a]
Resistance (mm Hg/ml/min)	1.42 ± 0.18	2.0 ± 0.3[a]	2.1 ± 0.3[a]	2.2 ± 0.4[b]	2.3 ± 0.6[b]	1.02 ± 0.11
Arterial lactate (mM)	0.75 ± 0.15	0.67 ± 0.16	0.65 ± 0.12	0.71 ± 0.14	1.0 ± 0.3	0.64 ± 0.12
GCV lactate (mM)	0.59 ± 0.12	1.8 ± 0.4[b]	1.6 ± 0.3[c]	1.3 ± 0.3[b]	1.8 ± 0.6[a]	0.58 ± 0.13
Art-GCV lactate (mM)	0.18 ± 0.06	−1.1 ± 0.3[a]	−0.91 ± 0.18[c]	−0.60 ± 0.17[b]	−0.8 ± 0.4[b]	0.07 ± 0.03
Arterial hypoxanthine (µM)	3.4 ± 0.7	3.0 ± 0.7	3.3 ± 0.6	2.9 ± 0.8	3.0 ± 1.4	3.8 ± 0.7
GCV hypoxanthine (µM)	3.0 ± 0.6	5.2 ± 0.8[c]	7.8 ± 1.4[b]	4.2 ± 1.06	4.4 ± 1.2[a]	3.7 ± 0.7
Art-GCV hypoxanthine (µM)	0.3 ± 0.3	−2.2 ± 0.7[a]	−4.5 ± 1.4[b]	−1.4 ± 0.7	−1.5 ± 0.4	0.2 ± 0.44

GCV = great cardiac vein; Art = arterial.
* Mean ± SEM
[a] $p < 0.05$; [b] $p < 0.005$; [c] $p < 0.001$ versus before PTCA.

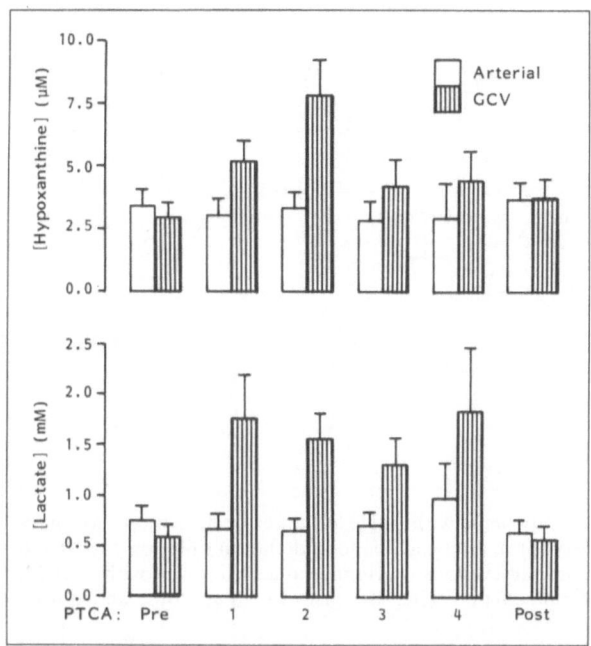

Fig. 3. Changes in arterial and venous concentration of hypoxanthine and lactate during transluminal occlusion. GCV = great cardiac vein; pre = pre angioplasty; post = post angioplasty

Table 2. Arterial and coronary venous urate levels before, immediately after four dilatations and during recovery

Angioplasty step	arterial (nmol/ml)	venous (nmol/ml)	p
Before	251 ± 18	259 ± 21	ns
Dilatation 1	248 ± 19	248 ± 22	ns
Dilatation 2	250 ± 21	249 ± 21	ns
Dilatation 3	243 ± 19	256 ± 21	<0.01
Dilatation 4	232 ± 21	254 ± 23	<0.02
Recovery	237 ± 20	244 ± 21	<0.05

Mean values are given $\pm$ SEM (n = 13)

the PTCA procedure. The arterial levels of these compounds remained constant during transluminal occlusion. The myocardial arterial – GCV difference of hypoxanthine changed from 0.3 ± 0.3 µM before angioplasty at rest to -2.4 ± 1.2 µM (p < 0.01) during sequential transluminal occlusions. Even if not statistically significant, a trend for hypoxanthine release to be reduced during occlusions three and four compared to occlusion one or two was observed. Significant production of hypoxanthine, calculated either as arterialvenous difference or extraction, only took place after the first two transluminal occlusions, while hypoxanthine release was absent five min after completion of the PTCA procedure.

27

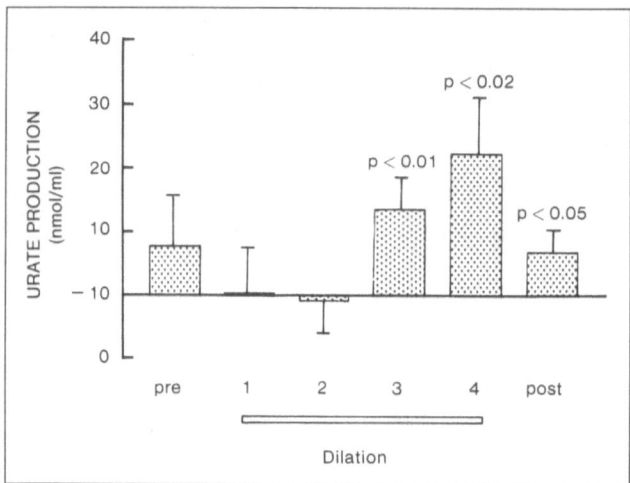

Fig. 4. Urate production by the hearts of 13 patients with single left anterior descending coronary artery stenosis, before coronary angioplasty (pre), after each balloon deflation (dilation 1 to 4) and after 15 min of recovery (post). Mean coronary venous – arterial values are given with 1 SEM. Significant urate production was found immediately after the last two dilatations, and during recovery

In the second study group (n = 13), we assayed the arterial and venous urate concentrations in plasma. In this study group, the arterio-venous difference was relatively small and we were unable to demonstrate urate production before coronary angioplasty (Table 2). After a third and fourth angioplasty attempt, urate production by the heart was significant (Fig. 4; $p < 0.01$ and $p < 0.02$ resp.). Even after 15 min of recovery, urate production remained significantly increased ($p < 0.05$; Table 2).

Discussion

Ischemia can be defined as a situation, where coronary blood flow cannot meet the tissue demand (14). As a consequence of the ensuing O2 deficiency, the balance between ATP production and usage is disturbed (15). ATP (and creatine phosphate) levels fall (3, 16), creatine, ADP, phosphate and hydrogen levels increase (17–19), glycolysis rate is enhanced (18, 19) and lactate levels rise. Shortly thereafter potassium, hydrogen and lactate are released into the coronary venous blood. ATP is converted to ADP and AMP, which is broken down to adenosisne, inosine, hypoxanthine, xanthine and urate (Fig. 5).

In the second study group, urate production became obvious after the third and fourth transluminal occlusion. Presumably, this is due to cardiac ATP breakdown, with a concomitant rise in hypoxanthine as a result of myocardial ischemia due to coronary occlusion by balloon inflation. Hypoxanthine serves as a substrate for xanthine oxidoreductase and our data suggest that the ischemic myocardium produces urate. Xanthine oxidoreductase activity is detectable in the heart of a number

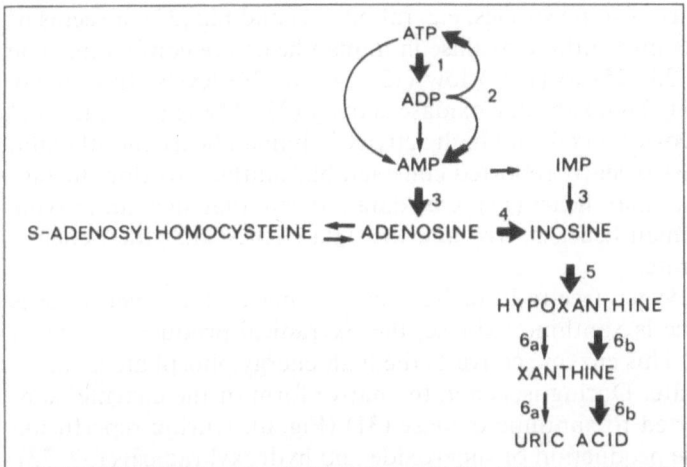

Fig. 5. Myocardial ATP catabolism. The main pathways are: 1) ATPase 2) adenylate kinase 3) 5'-nucleotidase 4) adenosine deaminase 5) nucleoside phosphorylase 6) xanthine oxidase (a)/dehydrogenase (b)

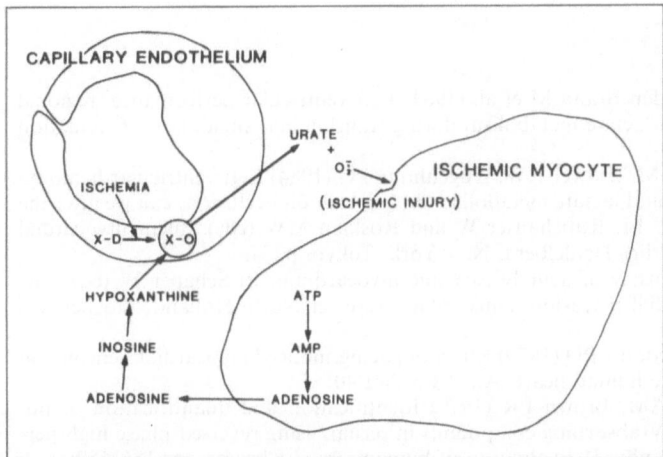

Fig. 6. Critical steps leading to the generation of superoxide from hypoxanthine in the ischemic heart. The degradation of adenine nucleotides in the ischemic heart. The degradation of adenine nucleotides in the ischemic myocyte leads to the accumulation of hypoxanthine which is degraded to uric acid in a reaction mediated by xanthine oxidase $(X-O)$. In the process, superoxide (O_{2-}) is produced which may induce damage in the ischemic myocyte. The xanthine activity is elevated in the capillary endothelium and increases as a consequence of the ischemia induced conversion of xanthine dehydrogenase $(X-D)$ to xanthine oxidase. (With permission of the authors Hears DJ et al. in: Acta Physiol Scand 1986, Suppl 548:65–78)

of species (20). In the heart of some species, e.g. rabbit (21) and pig (22), it seems to be absent. Literature data on xanthine oxidase in human heart are conflicting. The reports vary from high (23–25) to (very) low (12–14, 26–29) levels. In autopsy material some data indicate high xanthine oxidase activity (23). Using histochemical techniques, Jarasch and coworkers found high activity in human heart endothelium (24). Wajner and Harkness recently reported considerable xanthine oxidoreductase activity in biopsies from human heart (11). Our data indicate that such an enzyme could be active in the human heart in vivo and the data suggest that the ischemic myocardium produces urate.

In the last few years, oxygen free radicals have been implicated in atherogenesis (30). One potential source is xanthine oxidase, the oxyradical-producing form of xanthine oxidoreductase. This enzyme converts the high-energy phosphate metabolite (hypo)xanthine to urate. During ischemia the native form of the enzyme, xanthine reductase, is converted to xanthine oxidase (31) (Fig. 6). During reperfusion oxygen is available for the production of superoxide and hydroxyl radicals (32, 33), which are both strongly suspected to cause tissue damage (32, 34–36). We present evidence that the heart of a number of cardiac patients during and following angioplasty produces significant amounts of urate. Thus xanthine oxidoreductase may be active in the human heart in vivo.

References

1. Serruys PW, Wijns W, van den Brand M et al. (1984) Left ventricular performance, regional blood flow, wall motion and lactate metabolism during transluminal angioplasty. Circulation 70:25
2. Serruys PW, van den Brand M, Brower RW, Hugenholtz PG (1984) Left ventricular hemodynamics, regional blood flow and lactate metabolism during balloon occlusion: can we alter the sequence of ischemic events? In: Rutishauser W and Roskam MW (eds), Silent myocardial ischmia. Springer-Verlag. Berlin, Heidelberg, New York, Tokyo, p. 37
3. de Jong JW (1979) Biochemistry of acutely ischemic myocardium. In Schaper W (ed), The pathophysiology of myocardial perfusion. Amsterdam, Elsevier/North-Holland, Biochemical Press, p. 719
4. Remme WJ, de Jong JW, Verdouw PD (1979) Effect of pacing-induced myocardial ischemia on hypoxanthine efflux from the human heart. Am J Cardiol 40:55
5. Hartwick RA, Kristulovic AM, Brown PR (1979) Identification and quantification of nucleosides, bases and other UV-absorbing compounds in serum, using reversed-phase high-performance liquid chromatography. II Evaluation of human sera. J Chromatogr 186:659
6. Harmsen E, de Jong JW, Serruys PW (1981) Hypoxanthine production by ischemic heart demonstrated by high pressure liquid chromatography of blood purine nucleosides and oxypurines. Clin Chim Acta 115:73
7. Apstein CS, Puchner E and Brachfield N (1979) Improved automated lactate determination. Anal Biochem 38:20
8. Chatterjee SK, Bhattacharya M and Barlow JJ (1979) A simple, specific radiometric assay for 5'-nucleotidase. Anal Biochem 95:497
9. Scheibe B, Bernt E, Bergmeyer HU (1974) Uric acid. In: Bergmeyer HU (ed) Methods of enzymatic analysis. New York: Academic Press, pp. 1951–8
10. de Jong JW, Keijzer E, Uitendaal MP and Harmsen E (1980) Further purification of adenosine kinase from rat heart using affinity and ion-exchange chromatography. Anal Biochem 101:407
11. Edlund A, Berglund B, Van Dorne D, et al. (1985) Coronary flow regulation in patients with ischemic heart disease: release of purines and prostacyclin and the effect of inhibitors of prostaglandin formation. Circulation 71:1113

12. Ontyd J, Schrader J (1984) Measurement of adenosine, inosine and hypoxanthine in human plasma. J Chromatogr 307:404
13. Metha J, Pepine CJ (1978) Effect of sublingual nitroglycerin on regional flow in patients with and without coronary disease. Circulation 58:803
14. Manning AS, Hearse DJ, Dennis SC et al. (1980) Myocardial ischemia: an isolated, globally perfused rat heart model for metabolic and pharmacological studies. Eur J Cardiol 11:1
15. Wilson DF, Owen CS, Erecinska M (1979) Quantitative dependence of mitochondrial oxidative phosphorylation on oxygen concentration. A new mathematical model. Arch Biochem Biophys 195:494
16. Danforth WH, Naegle S, Bing RJ (1960) Effects of ischemia and reoxygenation on glycolytic reactions and adenosine triphosphate in heart muscle. Circ Res 8:965
17. Garlick BP, Radda GK, Seeley PJ (1979) Studies of acidosis in the ischemic heart by phosphorous nuclear magnetic resonance. Biochem J 184:547
18. Hearse DJ (1979) Oxygen deprivation and early myocardial contractile failure. Reassessment of the possible role of adenosine triphosphate. Am J Cardiol 44:1115
19. Hearse DJ, Crome R, Yellon DM, Wyse R (1983) Metabolic and flow correlates of myocardial ischemia. Cardiovasc Res 17:452
20. Schouten B, de Jong JW (1987) Age-dependent increase in xanthine oxidoreductase differs in various heart cell types. Circ Res 61:604−7
21. Downey JM, Chambers DE, Miura T et al. (1986) Allopurinol fails to limit infarct size in a xanthine oxidase deficient species. Circulation 74 Suppl 2:372
22. Podzuweit T, Braun W, Müller A, Schaper W (1986). Arrhythmias and innfarction in the ischemic pig leart are not mediated by xanthine oxidase-derived free oxygen radicals. Circulation 74 Suppl 2:346
23. Krenitsky TA, Tuttle JV, Cattau EL, Wang P (1974) A comparison of the distribution and electron acceptor specificities of xanthine and aldehyde oxidase. Comp Biochem Physiol 49B:687
24. Jarasch ED, Bruder G, Held HW (1986) Significance of xanthine oxidase in capillary endothelial cells. Acta Physiol Scand 548 Suppl 1:39
25. Wajner M, Harkness RA (1988) Distribution of xanthine dehydrogenase and oxidase activities in human and rabbit tissues. Biochem Soc Trans, in press
26. Eddy LJ, Stewart JR, Jones HP et al. (1987) Free radical-producing enzyme, xanthine oxidase, is undetectable in human hearts. Am J Physiol 253:H709
27. Ramboer CRH (1969) A sensitive and nonradioactive assay for serum and tissue xanthine oxidase. J Lab Clin Med 74:828
28. Muxfeldt M, Schaper W (1987) The activity of xanthine oxidase in hearts of pigs, guinea pigs, rats, and humans. Basic Res Cardiol 82:486
29. Watts RWE, Watts JEM, Seegmiller JE (1965) Xanthine oxidase activity in human tissues and its inhibition by allopurinol. J Lab Clin Med 66:688
30. Hearse DJ, Manning AS, Downey JM, Yellon DM (1986) Xanthine oxidase: a critical mediator of myocardial injury during ischemia and reperfusion? Acta Physiol Scand 548:Suppl:65
31. McCord JM (1984) Are free radicals a major culprit? In Hearse DJ, Yellon DM (eds). Therapeutic approaches to myocardial infarct size limitation. New York, Raven Press, p. 209
32. Chambers DE, Parks DA, Patterson G, et al. (1985) Xanthine oxidase as a source of free radical damage in myocardial ischemia. J Moll Cell Cardiol 17:145
33. Van dr Vusse GJ (1985) Pharmacological intervention in acute myocardial ischemia and reperfusion. Trends Pharmacol Sci 6:76
34. England MD, Cavarocchi NC, O'Brien JF, et al. (1986) Influence of antioxidants (mannitol and allopurinol) on free radical generation during and after cardiopulmonary bypass. Circulation 74 Suppl 3:134
35. Peterson DA, Asinger RW, Elsperger KJ et al. (1985) Reactive oxygen species may cause myocardial reperfusion injury. Biochem Biophys Res Commun 127:87
36. Zweier JL, Flaherty JT, Weisfeldt ML (1987) Direct measurements of free radical generation following reperfusion of ischemic myocardium. Proc Natl Acad Sci (USA) 84:140−7

Adenosine production during balloon-induced ischemia

H. Bardenheuer, B. Höfling, A. Fabry

Department of Anesthesiology, University of Munich, Klinikum Großhadern, FRG

It is well established that myocardial metabolites play a significant role in the local adjustment of coronary blood flow (5, 19). Beside others (7, 19), vasoactive adenosine has been described to be a major factor involved in the metabolic control of coronary flow. Experimental studies have demonstrated that inadequate supply of oxygen to the heart, e.g. during ischemia, leads to enhanced formation of adenosine which in turn increases coronary flow to meet the enhanced oxygen requirement (6, 11, 22). According to these results adenosine is proposed to be involved in a feed-back controlled system in which the ratio between supply and demand of oxygen is the major trigger mechanism for enhanced production of adenosine by the heart (1, 5, 25).

More recently, the coronary endothelium has been characterized to be a potential sink for myocardial adenosine. For instance, endothelial cells can rapidly incorporate adenosine, either applied from the luminal (vascular) or the abluminal site (16). In addition, the endothelium contains all enzymes necessary for the degradation of nucleosides (16, 18). Thus, adenosine, once taken up into the coronary endothelium, is rapidly transformed to vasoinactive metabolites due to enzymatic degradation.

In 1976, Grüntzig (12) first described the method of percutaneous transluminal coronary angioplasty (PTCA), which has been clinically proven to be an alternative tool for the therapy of coronary artery stenosis (8, 14). This technique offers an excellent tool to investigate the mechanisms involved in the regulation of coronary blood flow under conditions of regional myocardial ischemia. Therefore, using PTCA, the present study was undertaken to characterize the role of adenosine for metabolic flow regulation in the human heart. Concerning the activity of the endothelium in adenosine metabolism, the particular interest of the present study was focused to determine whether endogenously formed adenosine is produced in sufficient amount to attain intravascular and interstitial concentrations that can be responsible for the changes in coronary blood flow.

Patients and methods

18 male patients (mean age 56 ± 8 years) with 90% proximal stenoses of the left coronary artery underwent PTCA during angina-free intervals. The balloon catheter was placed in the technique first described by Grüntzig (12). In addition, a coronary sinus catheter was advanced via the subclavian vein, the position of which was verified by fluoroscopy and control of blood gases.

33

During PTCA, left coronary arteries were consecutively occluded for 30, 60, and 90 s (± 5 s each). The balloon pressure ranged from 6 to 10 bars. Arterial and coronary sinus blood samples were taken before PTCA, during balloon inflation, and in short term intervals during reperfusion. Lactate and nucleoside concentrations were deteremined in each patient in a randomized sequence. While lactate was enzymatically determined (4), adenosine and hypoxanthine were separated using high performance liquid chromatography (HPLC) (Waters Assoc., Milford, Massachusetts, USA). In brief, during the first separation the fractions of adenosine and hypoxanthine were collected and enzymatically transformed to inosine using either the adenosine deaminase (E.C.: 3.5.4.4) or the nucleoside phosphorylase (E.C.: 2.4.2.1), respectively. Thereafter the fractions were evaporated to dryness, re-chromatographed, and quantitated at 254 nm (LC spectrophotometer, Lambda Max Model 481, Waters Assoc.). To prevent nucleoside uptake by red blood cells, blood was collected in syringes containing ice-cold dipyridamole solution (5×10^{-5} M; vol:vol $= 1:1$). Including all analytical steps recovery of plasma adenosine was $86.8 \pm 3.1\%$ (SD; n $= 7$).

In a second group of patients (n $= 4$) coronary sinus adenosine was measured under resting conditions and following intravenous infusion of dipyridamole (45 mg). Simultaneously, coronary blood flow was determined using the thermodilution technique.

Results

Figures 1 and 2 show the changes in the concentration and the extraction of coronary sinus lactate when the balloon is inflated for 30, 60, and 90s, respectively. Under

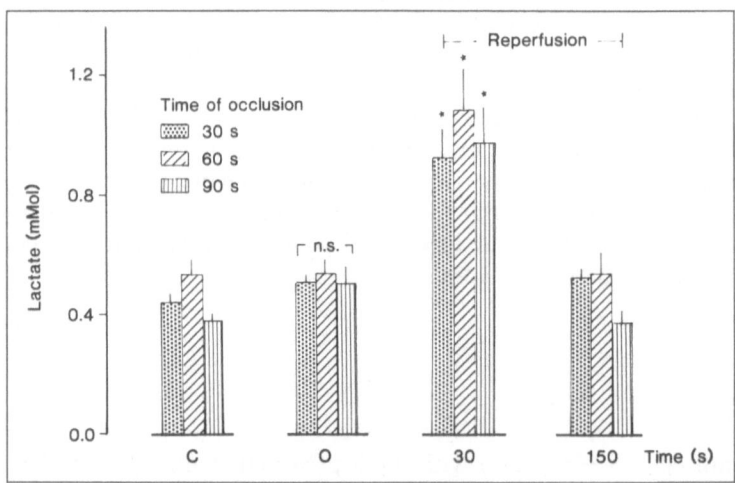

Fig. 1. Coronary sinus concentrations of lactate under control (C), during coronary occlusion (O), and during reperfusion in patients (n $= 18$) with proximal stenosis of left coronary artery undergoing PTCA. $\star$ = p < 0.05 (significantly different from respective occlusion); n.s. = not significantly different from respective control

34

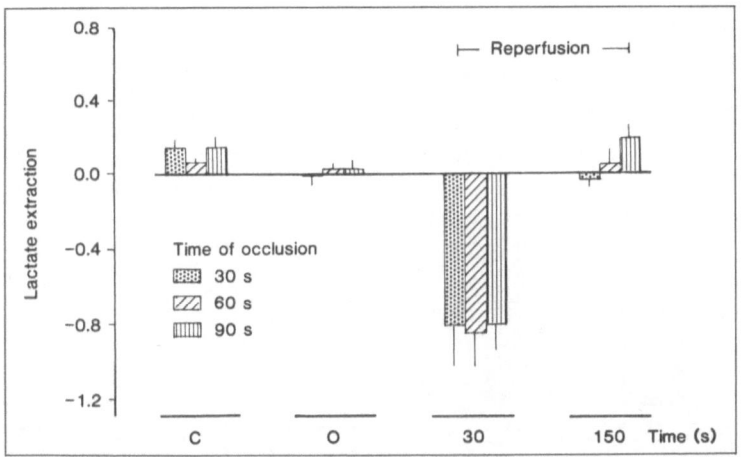

Fig. 2. Changes in lactate extraction after 30, 60 and 90 s lasting coronary occlusions in patients undergoing PTCA. Lactate extraction is calculated as (La-Lcs)/La (a: arterial; cs: coronary sinus)

control conditions (C) lactate is in the range of 0.5 mmol/l and extracted by the heart. Only minor increases in lactate can be observed during coronary occlusion (O) (1.2-fold after 30 s vs 1.4-fold following 90 s). However, during reperfusion, coronary sinus lactate is transiently increased, exhibiting the largest changes at 30 s of reperfusion. As indicated by the tremendous changes in lactate extraction under these conditions, anerobic glycolysis is greatly stimulated during regional ischemia, and lactate washed out from cardiac tissue into the vascular space along an intra- to extracellular concentration gradient.

Fig. 3 summarizes the changes of coronary sinus adenosine before PTCA (C), during balloon inflation (O), and during reperfusion. Under resting conditions aortic and coronary sinus adenosine are 109 and 176 nMol, respectively. These numbers indicate that adenosine is continuously produced and released by the human heart under resting conditions. During PTCA adenosine exhibits a similar transient pattern in the time course of its concentration changes peaking at 30 s of reperfusion. However, there are major differences in comparison to lactate. During coronary occlusion the changes in adenosine are significantly different from the respective control values ($p < 0.05$) and directly proportional to the duration of regional myocardial ischemia (1.5-fold after 30 s vs 2.5-fold after 60 s). In addition, the differences between both metabolites are also evident during reperfusion, when the production of adenosine is 2.4- and 3.9-fold increased following 30 and 90 s of balloon inflation. Thus, in contrast to lactate, the formation of adenosine closely parallels the degree of cardiac ischemia. Similar changes were obtained in the case of hypoxanthine as for adenosine (data not shown). The influence of calcium channel blockers on cardiac metabolite production is shown in Fig. 4. During coronary occlusion (60 s) the adenosine is increased by +90% in the absence of nifedipine. In comparison, lactate is enhanced by only 25% under these conditions. Following intracoronary infusion of nifedipine (0.2 mg), the adenosine concentration is drastically lowered, while coronary sinus lactate concentration remains almost unaffected.

35

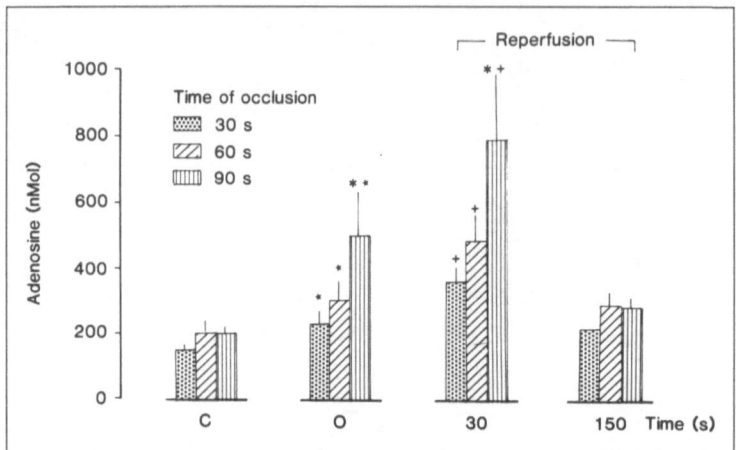

Fig. 3. Influence of regional myocardial ischemia on coronary sinus adenosine concentrations. Purine compounds are determined under control (C), during coronary occlusion (O) for 30, 60 and 90 s, and during reperfusion (mean ± SE). ★ = p < 0.05 (significant different from respective control) + = p < 0.05 (significant different from respective occlusion) * = p < 0.05 (significant different from respective value after 30 s balloon dilatation)

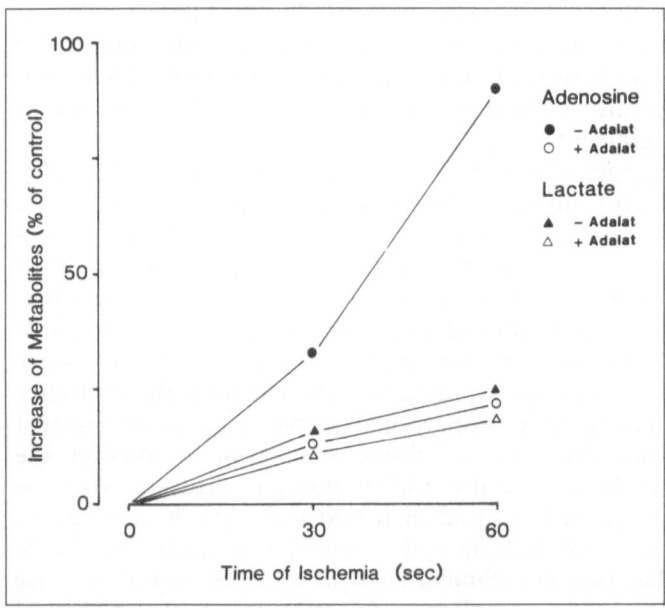

Fig. 4. Effect of nifedipine (0.2 mg) on the increase in cardiac metabolites (% of control) following 30 and 60 s lasting coronary occlusions (n = 6).

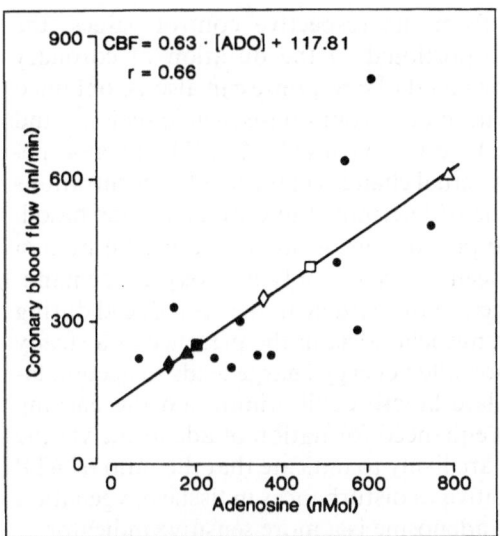

Fig. 5. Relationship between coronary sinus adenosine concentration and coronary blood flow under conditions of intravenous infusion of dipyridamole (45 mg) (closed points). The changes in coronary sinus adenosine under control conditions (closed symbols) and during reperfusion (open symbols) are included for comparison (values are taken from Fig. 3). On the basis of this comparison, the measured concentrations of adenosine can account for a 2–4 fold increase in coronary blood flow.

In a separate group of patients (n = 4) coronary blood flow was enhanced by intravenous infusion of dipyridamole (45 mg). Dipyridamole was chosen, because this substance has been demonstrated to specifically act via enhanced adenosine production by the heart (3). With dipyridamole present, coronary blood flow was three- to four-fold increased, which was associated with a proportional increase in coronary sinus adenosine (see Fig. 5, closed points). The close relationship between coronary flow and adenosine can be described by the equation CBF = 0.63 x (ADO) + 117.8 (r = 0.66). When the adenosine antagonist theophylline (170 mg) was additionally infused, the dipyridamole-induced increase in flow was almost fully reversed (data not shown). The adenosine concentrations before PTCA (closed symbols: rhomb = 30 s, rectangle = 60 s, triangle = 90 s) and the respective concentrations during reperfusion (resp. open symbols) are included in this graph for comparison.

Discussion

The results of the present study demonstrate that brief periods of coronary occlusion are associated with significant changes in the production of adenosine and lactate. Although both metabolites exhibit an almost identical pattern in the concentration changes following balloon deflation, only adenosine is significantly and proportionally altered, when coronary arteries are occluded for 30, 60, and 90 s. Thus, these results point to substantial differences in the sensitivity of adenosine and lactate indicating the impairment of tissue oxygenation. While lactate concentrations during balloon inflation are not different from the respective control values, the adenosine concentrations are directly proportional to the duration of coronary occlusion ($p < 0.05$). Similar changes in the metabolic response can also be obtained during reperfusion. Because of dilution with blood from non-ischemic regions, and because of reuptake of released adenosine by erythrocytes (17, 21, 27) and endothelial cells (2, 16, 18), it is most likely that the actual changes in the local concentrations are by far underestimated, when adenosine is determined in coronary sinus blood.

Thus, this study demonstrates that the production of adenosine by the human heart is closely coupled to the ratio between oxygen supply and oxygen demand. Conditions like inadequate supply of oxygen to the cardiac tissue, as induced during PTCA, result in reduced ATP synthesis in mitochondria in the presence of a steady ATP use (6, 26). Any disturbance of this so-called energy charge leads to accumulation of ADP, which will shift the adenylate kinase equilibrium, and the ensuing increased production of AMP will lead to enhanced formation of adenosine via the 5'-nucleotidase reaction. The present data are likely to indicate that the ratio of ATP production vs ATP utilization is more sensitive to disturbances in tissue oxygenation than the rate of anerobic glycolysis. Thus, adenosine is a more sensitive indicator of adequate tissue oxygenation than lactate. This even more, because the formation and removal of lactate are significantly influenced by conditions, that all can be present during PTCA, like blood fatty acids, acidosis and hypoglycemia (29).

From the viewpoint of control theory, adenosine production is imbedded in a close-loop system, in which tissue pO_2 is assumed to be the regulated variable. Assuming that the adenosine production is closely linked to the supply-to-demand ratio of oxygen, any improvement of this ratio should result in a reduction of the adenosine formation. In the present study, nifedipine was used to prove the prediction of a close relationship between tissue oxygenation and metabolite production.

As shown in Fig. 4, coronary sinus adenosine was significantly lower when nifedipine was present during PTCA. Thus, the adenosine data strongly support previous findings in which nifedipine was demonstrated to improve the ischemic tolerance of the heart as indicated by a prolongation of the balloon inflation time and a later appearance of ST-segment changes (9).

Two mechanisms are likely to be responsible for the beneficial effect of calcium antagonists. First, these substances are known to relax vascular smooth muscle. Because all patients included exhibited a chronic proximal coronary lesion of $> 90\%$, one can suppose that this lesion severity is associated with a considerable development of collateral vessels (20). Rentrop et al. have demonstrated that a lesion exhibiting a diametric narrowing of $> 70\%$ may represent a threshold value for the development of collaterals in human hearts which are demonstrable by angiography during occlusion. Assuming calcium channel blockers improve tissue oxygenation by increasing the collateral flow (28), they are likely to reduce the area at risk of cardiac tissue during acute coronary occlusion. Secondly, calcium antagonists exert a direct protective influence on myocardial cells due to the inhibitory influence on calcium entry into the ischemic tissue (10). As a result these substances significantly reduce the appearance of reperfusion arrhythmias as observed under experimental (28) and clinical conditions (9). Karsch et al. (13) have shown that the end-diastolic pressure and the irregularity in wall motion were significantly reduced in the presence of calcium antagonists. Therefore one can conclude that calcium channel blockers improve tissue oxygenation by both the increase of oxygen delivery and the reduction of oxygen demand, consequently leading to a reduced production of adenosine by the heart.

A major concern regarding metabolic flow regulation is directed to the question of whether endogenously formed adenosine is produced in sufficient amounts to reach an intravascular and interstitial concentration, which could explain the obtained changes in coronary blood flow. Simon et al. (24) reported a two- to three-fold increase in coronary blood flow following a 30 s balloon inflation period. When dipyridamole was intravenously applied in patients under resting conditions, the concentrations of coronary sinus adenosine were altered in close proportion to the changes in coronary blood flow. These clinical data support experimental results demonstrating that the dipyridamole-induced changes in blood flow are mediated by adenosine (3, 15). This explanation is even more likely, because the adenosine antagonist theophylline could almost completely abolish the flow increase following infusion of dipyridamole. Assuming the regression line represents the adenosine-mediated changes in coronary blood flow (see Fig. 5), it is obvious that the concentrations of coronary sinus adenosine obtained during regional ischemia (open symbols) are sufficient to account for a two to fourfold increase in coronary blood flow.

In summary, the present study demonstrates that adenosine is produced by the human heart in close proportion to the extent of regional myocardial ischemia. Under these conditions the concentrations reached in coronary sinus blood are sufficient to account for a great portion of the coronary vasodilation during reperfusion. Because of substantial uptake and inactivation by red blood cells and cells lining the vascular wall one has to consider that the actual concentrations at the site of the smooth muscle cells are by far underestimated, when adenosine is determined in coronary sinus blood. In addition, adenosine seems to be a more sensitive parameter to signal adequate tissue oxygenation than lactate. The results in the presence of nifedipine support the proposed hypothesis that the production of adenosine closely corresponds to the impairment of tissue oxygenation. With respect to the metabolic results of this study calcium channel blockers might be highly recommended in patients undergoing PTCA, because these substances most likely increase patient safety and allow a prolongation of balloon inflation time.

References

1. Bardenheuer H, Schrader J (1986) Supply-to-demand ratio for oxygen determines formation of adenosine by the heart. Am J Physiol 250:173
2. Bardenheuer H, Whelton BK, Sparks HV (1987) Cellular compartmentation of adenosine in the heart. In: Gerlach E, Becker BF (eds). Topics and perspectives in adenosine research, Springer Verlag, Berlin, Heidelberg, pp. 480–485
3. Becker BF, Bardenheuer H, Overhage de Reyes I, Gerlach E (1985) Effects of theophylline on dipyridamole-induced coronary venous adenosine release and coronary dilation. In: Stefanovich V, Rudolphi K, Schubert P (eds). Adenosine:receptors and modulation of cell function IRL, Oxford, pp. 441–449
4. Bergmeyer HU (1974) Methoden der enzymatischen Analyse. Weinheim FRG. Verlag Chemie
5. Berne RM (1980) The role of adenosine in the regulation of coronary blood flow. Circ Res 47:807

6. Berne RM (1963) Cardiac nucleotides in hypoxia:possible role in regulation of coronary blood flow. Am J Physiol 204:317

7. Cobbe SM, Poole-Wilson PA (1982) Continuous coronary sinus and arterial pH-monitoring during pacing-induced ischemia in coronary artery disease. Br Heart J 47:369

8. Detre K, Holubkov R, Kesley S et al. (1988) Percutaneous transluminal coronary angioplasty in 1985-1986 and 1977-1981. N Engl J Med 318:265

9. Erbel R, Henkel B, Schreiner G et al. (1986) Clinical, electrocardiographic, and hemodynamic changes during coronary angioplasty. Influence of nitroglycerine and nifedipine. In: Coronary angioplasty: a controlled model for ischemia. Serruys PW, Meester GT (eds), Martinus Nijhoff Publishers, pp. 39-53

10. Fleckenstein A, Döring HJ, Leder O The significance of high-energy phosphate exhaustion in the etiology of isoproterenol-induced cardiac ulcerosis and its prevention by iproveratril, compound D or precylamin. In: Lamasch M, Royer R (eds) International Symposium on Drugs and Metabolism of Myocardium and Striated Muscle. Nance, pp. 11-22

11. Gerlach E, Deuticke B, Dreisbach RH (1963) Der Nukleotid-Abbau im Herzmuskel bei Sauerstoffmangel und seine mögliche Bedeutung für die Coronardurchblutung. Naturwissenschaften 50:228

12. Grüntzig A (1976) Perkutane Dilatation von Coronarstenosen – Beschreibung eines neuen Kathetersystems. Klin Wochenschr 54:543

13. Karsch KR, Mauser M, Spiel L (1985) Wirkungsmechanismen von intrakoronarem, sublingualem und intravenösem Nifedipine bei Patienten mit instabiler Angina pectoris. In: Meyer J, Erbel R. (eds) Intravenöse und intrakoronare Anwendung von Adalat. Springer Verlag Berlin Heidelberg, pp. 114-124

14. Kober G, Vallbracht C, Kaltenbach M (1987) Early and late results after percutaneous transluminal coronary angioplasty compared with bypass operation. In: B. Höfling (ed) Current problems in PTCA. Steinkopff Verlag Darmstadt, Springer New York pp. 21-26

15. Miura M, Tominaga S, Hashimoto K (1967) Potentiation of reactive hyperemia in the coronary and femoral circulation by the selective use of 2,6-bis-(diaethanolamono)-4,8-dipiperidinopyrimido- (5,4-d)-pyrimidine. Arzneim Forsch 17:976

16. Nees S, Gerlach E (1982) Adenine nucleotide and adenosine metabolism in cultured coronary endothelial cells:formation and release of adenine compounds and possible functional implications. In: Berne RM, Rubio R (eds) Regulatory function of adenosine Nijhoff, Boston, pp. 347-355

17. Ontyd J, Schrader J (1984) Measurement of adenosine, inosine, and hypoxanthine in human plasma. J Chromatogr 307:404

18. Pearson JD, Carleton JS, Hutchings A, Gordon JL (1978) Uptake and metabolism of adenosine by pig endothelial and smooth muscle cells in culture. Biochem J 170:265

19. Poole-Wilson PA, Webb SC (1986) Role of potassium in the genesis of arrhythmias during ischemia. Evidence from coronary angioplasty. In: Coronary angioplasty: a controlled model for ischemia. Serruys PW, Meester GT (eds) Martinus Nijhoff Publishers. pp. 95-103

20. Rentrop KP, Thornton JC, Feit F et al. (1988) Determinants and protective potential of coronary arterial collaterals as assessed by an angioplasty model. Am J Cardiol 61:677

21. Schrader J, Berne RM, Rubio R. (1972) Uptake and metabolism of adenosine by human erythrocyte ghosts. Am J Physiol 223:159

22. Schrader J, Haddy FJ, Gerlach E (1977) Release of adenosine, inosine and hypoxanthine from the isolated guinea pig heart during hypoxia, flow-autoregulation and reactive hyperemia. Pfluegers Arch 369:1

23. Serruys PW, Wijns W, van den Brand M et al. (1984) Left ventricular performance, regional blood flow, and lactate metabolism during transluminal angioplasty. Circulation 1:25

24. Simon R, Amende I, Herrmann G et al. (1986) Effect of prolonged balloon inflations on hemodynamics and coronary flow with respect to balloon position in patients undergoing coronary angioplasty. In: Coronary angioplasty: A controlled model for ischemia. Serruys PW, Meester GT (eds) Martinus Nijhoff Publishers. pp. 63-76

25. Sparks HV, Bardenheuer H (1986) Regulation of adenosine formation by the heart. Circ Res 58 (2):193

26. Taegtmeyer H, Roberts AFC, Raine AEG (1985) Energy metabolism in reperfused heart muscle: metabolic correlates to return of function. JACC 6:846

27. Van Belle VM (1969) Uptake and deamination of adenosine by blood: species differences effect of pH ions, temperature and metabolic inhibitors. Biochim Biophys Acta 192:124
28. Vatner SF, Patrick TA, Knight DR et al. (1988) Effects of calcium channel blocker on responses of blood flow, function, arrhythmias and extent of infarction following reperfusion in conscious baboons. Circ Res 62:105
29. Verdouw PW, Stam H (1980) Lactate. Physiologic, methodologic and pathologic approach. In: Moret PR et al. (eds), Springer Verlag Berlin. pp. 207–223
30. Wendt VE, Sundermeyer JF, den Bakker PB, Bing RJ (1962) The relationship between coronary flow, myocardial oxygen consumption and cardiac work as influenced by persantin. Am J Cardiol 9:449

Can one predict reversibility of regional ventricular dysfunction?

P. Schanzenbächer, K. Kochsiek

Medizinische Universitätsklinik, Würzburg, FRG

Introduction

Patients with coronary artery disease frequently show left ventricular dysfunction at rest. It is an important challenge for the clinician to identify those patients with left ventricular asynergy that is potentially reversible with successful revascularization, and distinguish them from those with irreversibly damaged myocardium that has been replaced by scar tissue.

In 1935, Tennant and Wiggers (1) analyzed the effects of brief periods of myocardial ischemia on cardiac contraction. They showed that within 60 s of coronary artery occlusion the active systolic shortening changed to passive systolic lengthening. After a brief period of myocardial ischemia, restoration of coronary blood flow led to rapid and complete recovery of normal contraction.

Based on these and many subsequent experimental and clinical observations (2) it has been believed for many years that, depending on the duration and severity of myocardial ischemia, there may be two distinct outcomes:

1) With total coronary occlusion for longer than approximately 20 min in the absence of substantial collateral flow, the subendocardial myocardium becomes irreversibly damaged, resulting in necrosis and failure of return of function despite reperfusion.
2) With briefer periods of myocardial ischemia, depression of myocardial function is transient and restoration of myocardial blood flow results in normalization of left ventricular contraction.

During the past decade this concept has been challenged. Two pathophysiologic conditions have been identified in which major discrepancies occur between myocardial function and the manifestation of ischemia. These conditions are called myocardial stunning and myocardial hibernation.

Myocardial stunning

Myocardial stunning means prolonged postischemic left ventricular dysfunction without myocardial necrosis (3). Several experimental studies have shown that the rate of improvement of contractile function is inversely proportional to the duration of coronary occlusion. In the dog, after a period of total occlusion shorter than 20 min, the function of a previously ischemic myocardium may remain depressed for several days.

Table 1. Assessment of myocardial viability

I. *Inotropic contractile reserve*
   A. Postextrasystolic potentiation
   B. Infusion of a sympathomimetic amine
   C. Nitroglycerin

II. *Perfusion-metabolism mismatch*
   A. N13 Ammonia
   B. Fluorine 18 deoxyglucose

III. *Clinical predictors*
   A. Absence of Q-waves
   B. Presence of collaterals

Ellis et al. (4) studied the time course of contractile function in the central ischemic zone and the peripheral ischemic zone in dogs after permanent or 90 min of coronary occlusion followed by reperfusion. In the central ischemic zone, active thickening did not occur until 72 h of reperfusion and remained depressed at 14 days. In animals with permanent occlusion, no systolic thickening was observed at two weeks. In the peripheral ischemic zone, recovery of systolic wall thickening occurred earlier at six h and recovery at two weeks appeared nearly complete.

Myocardial stunning may also occur with ischemia in the absence of total coronary occlusion. Ischemia maintained for several hours by subtotal coronary occlusion can also cause left ventricular dysfunction that persists for days after release of the occlusion and restoration of myocardial blood flow (5).

Myocardial hibernation

Myocardial hibernation refers to a condition of permanently impaired LV function as a result of a chronic reduction of myocardial perfusion (6). In this situation myocardial blood flow is still sufficient to maintain the viability of tissue. Whereas stunned myocardium results from a discrete episode of ischemia, hibernating myocardium results from weeks or months of chronic ischemia. It is possible that the impairment of contractile function serves as a protective mechanism in that it reduces the oxygen demands of the hypoperfused myocardium.

Inotropic contractile reserve

Viability of myocardial tissue in an area of reduced contractility can be assessed by postextrasystolic potentiation during left ventriculography. Popio et al. (7) analyzed ejection fraction and regional wall motion in 31 patients before and after aortocoronary bypass surgery. Of seven patients whose ejection fraction improved postoperatively, six had shown postextrasystolic potentiation compared with only 10 of 24 patients without such improvement. Regional wall motion analysis also showed a significant association between postextrasystolic potentiation and postoperative improvement in wall motion. Of 26 zones judged to have an increased vascular supply after operation, 11 showed increased motion postoperatively. All 11 zones had shown postextrasystolic potentiation, compared with only five of 15 zones with increased vascular supply but without increased postoperative wall motion.

Nesto et al. (8) showed that an increase in ejection fraction after a positive inotropic intervention such as epinephrine infusion is a valuable predictor of short- and long-term results after revascularization in patients with depressed left ventricular function. An increase in ejection fraction of 10%, and more after stimulation, correlated well with a postoperative improvement in ejection fraction and a better five- year survival.

Perfusion-metabolism mismatch

Thallium 201 perfusion scanning can be useful in detecting reversible left ventricular asynergy in individual patients. The finding of a reversible, exercise-induced perfusion defect in an area of myocardium that exhibits impaired wall motion suggests that the myocardial dysfunction might be related to impaired perfusion rather than myocardial necrosis (9).

Recently, it has been shown that reversibility of cardiac wall motion abnormalities can be predicted by positron emission tomography. N13-ammonia is an indicator of myocardial blood flow and fluorine-18-deoxyglucose (FDG) is an indicator of exogenous glucose uptake which reflects myocardial metabolic viability (10). Extraction of glucose is increased in ischemic myocardium primarily due to anerobic metabolism.

Whereas myocardial infarction is characterized by a reduction in both N13-ammonia and FDG activities, ischemic segments show a discordant increase in FDG activities relative to N13-ammonia. According to these criteria Tillisch et al. (11) were able to predict reversibility of abnormal contraction in 35 of 41 LV segments in 17 patients who underwent aorto-coronary bypass surgery. This represents an 85% predictive accuracy.

Fudo et al. (12) reported two types of mismatch between myocardial blood flow and glucose metabolism in patients with anterior myocardial infarction. The peripheral type showed increased uptake of FDG in the border zone between normal and infarcted myocardium, especially in the exercise-induced areas. The diffuse type showed increased uptake of FDG in the infarcted region characterized by hypoperfusion both at rest and during exercise. This was due to probably ischemic, but metabolically active myocardium. It is likely that myocardial function will benefit from reperfusion interventions.

Presence of collaterals and absence of Q-waves

In order to identify a subset of patients with reversible left ventricular dysfunction by application of easily obtainable clinical data, we studied seven patients with chronic LAD occlusion and anterior wall asynergy before and up to seven months after recanalization by angioplasty. In all patients, the LAD was perfused in a retrograde fashion by well-developed collaterals originating from the right coronary

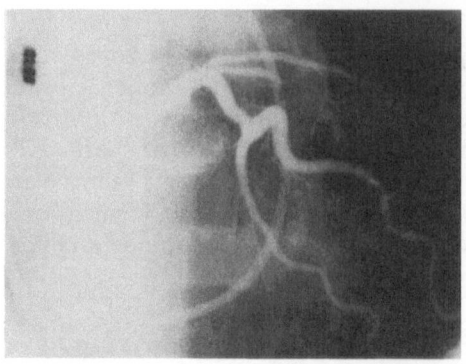

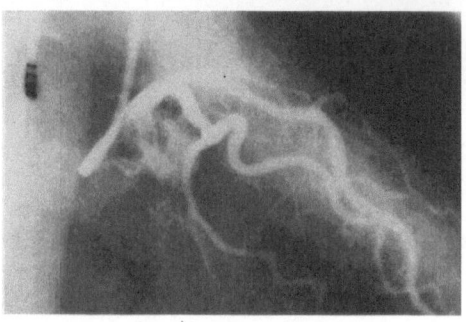

Fig. 1. Coronary angiogram showing proximal LAD occlusion (top). After successful recanalization by angioplasty, the LAD is patent without evidence of restenosis on follow up 4 months later (bottom)

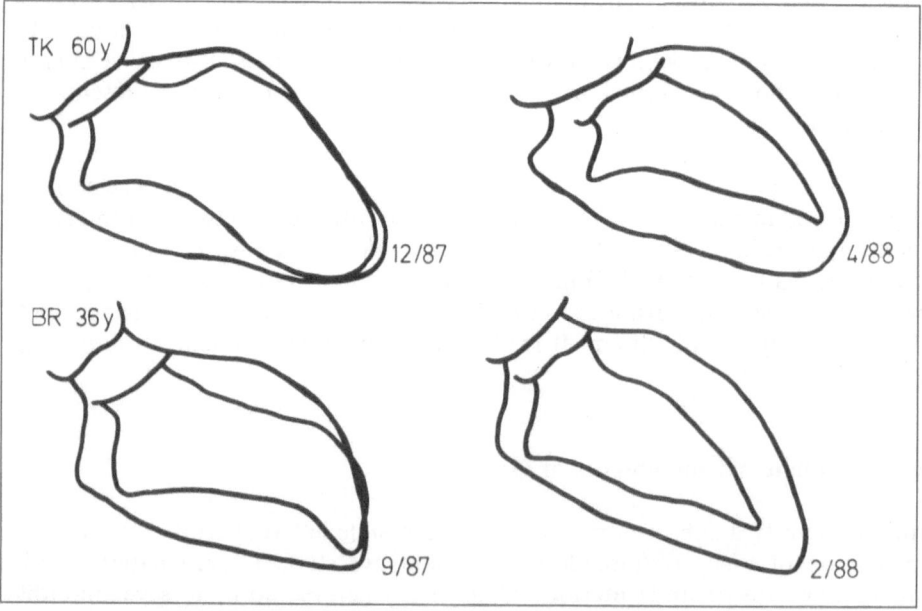

Fig. 2. Left ventricular endsystolic and enddiastolic contours prior to angioplasty (left) and on follow up (right). Top: same patient as in figure 1. A second selected case is shown on the bottom

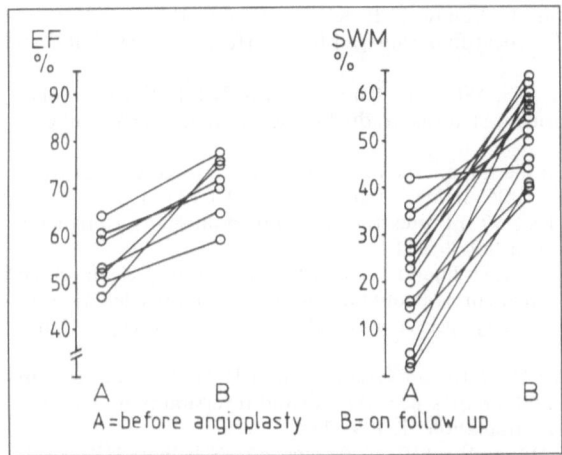

Fig. 3. Ejection fraction (EF) and segmental wall motion (SWM) before angioplasty and on follow up. Percent of systolic shortening in two anterior segments are shown for each patient

artery. None of the patients had a Q-wave infarction and the R-waves were maintained in the precordial leads. All patients suffered from persistent angina. Regional wall motion analysis revealed anterior akinesis in two patients and hypokinesis in five patients.

Figure 1 shows the coronary angiogram of an index case before and after recanalization. Figure 2 shows the end-systolic and end-diastolic contours of the left ventricle prior to angioplasty and on follow up in the same patient; contraction had completely normalized in the previously akinetic anterior segments.

In all seven patients the global ejection fraction increased after angioplasty (from 55 ± 6 to $71 \pm 7\%$, $p < 0.01$). The same was true for segmental wall motion as assessed by the chord method (13). Percent of shortening increased from 22 ± 13 to $52 \pm 8\%$ ($p < 0.01$, Fig. 3).

In conclusion, the absence of Q-waves and the presence of well-developed collaterals in an asynergistic area seem to be valuable predictors of reversibility of abnormal contraction after successful recanalization of chronic occlusions. This is in agreement with previous reports. Banka et al. (14) found that the presence of coronary collaterals and absence of pathologic Q-waves in the corresponding left ventricular zones were associated with a higher incidence of residual contractile ability of asynergistic segments.

References

1. Tennant R, Wiggers CJ (1935) The effect of coronary occlusion on myocardial contraction. Am J Physiol 112:351–361
2. Blumgart HL, Gilligan DR, Schlesinger MJ (1941) Experimental studies on the effect of temporary occlusion of the coronary arteries. Am Heart J 22:374–389
3. Braunwald E, Kloner RA (1982) The stunned myocardium: prolonged, postischemic left ventricular dysfunction. Circulation 66:1146–1149

4. Ellis SG, Henschke CI, Sandor T, Wynne J, Braunwald E, Kloner RA (1983) Time course of functional and biochemical recovery of myocardium salvaged by reperfusion. J Am Coll Cardiol 1:1047–1055
5. Matsuzaki M, Gallagher KP, Kemper WS, White F, Ross J Jr (1983) Sustained regional dysfunction produced by prolonged coronary stenosis:gradual recovery after reperfusion. Circulation 68:170–182
6. Rahimtoola SH (1985) A perspective on the three large multicenter randomized clinical trials of coronary bypass surgery for chronic stable angina. Circulation 72 (IV):123–135
7. Popio KA, Gorlin R, Betel D, Levine JA (1977) Postextrasystolic potentiation as a predictor of potential myocardial viability. Am J Cardiol 39:944–953
8. Nesto RW, Cohn LH, Collins JJ Jr., Wynne J, Holman L, Cohn PF (1982) Inotropic contractile reserve: a useful predictor of increased 5 year survival and improved postoperative left ventricular function in patients with coronary artery disease and reduced ejection fraction. Am J Cardiol 50:39–44
9. Bodenheimer MM, Banka VS, Fooshee C, Hermann GA, Helfant RH (1978) Relationship between regional myocardial perfusion and the presence, severity and reversibility of asynergy in patients with coronary heart disease. Circulation 58:789–795
10. Marshall RC, Tillisch JH, Phelps ME, Huang SC, Carson R, Henze E, Schelhart HR (1983) Identification and differentiation of resting myocardial ischemia and infarction in met with PET. Circulation 67:766–778
11. Tillisch J, Brunken R, Marshall R, Schwaiger M, Mandelkern M, Phelps M, Schelbert H (1986) Reversibility of cardiac wall-motion abnormalities predicted by PET. N Engl J Med 314:884–888
12. Fudo T, Kambara H, Hashimoto T, Hayashi M, Nohara R, Tamaki N, Yone Kura Y, Jenda M, Konishi J, Kawai C (1988) F–18 deoxyglucose and stress N13 ammonia PET in anterior wall healed myocardial infarction. Am J Cardiol 61:1191–1197
13. Carroll RJ, Verani MS, Falsetti HL (1974) The effect of collateral circulation on segmental left ventricular contraction. Circulation 50:709–713
14. Banka VS, Bodenheimer MM, Helfant RH (1974) Determinants of reversible asynergy. Effect of pathologic Q-waves, coronary collaterals, and anatomic location. Circulation 50:714–719

2. Current assessment of balloon valvuloplasty

Quantitative and qualitative morphological changes during intraoperative balloon valvuloplasty

K. R. Karsch

University of Tübingen, Tübingen, FRG

Introduction

In 1985, a new therapeutic approach to patients with calcified aortic stenosis was proposed – percutaneous transluminal aortic valvuloplasty (PTAV) (10). Dilatation of stenosed and calcified aortic valves, however, is not a new idea stemming from interventional cardiologists as a result of the success of balloon dilatation of coronary artery stenoses (7), but has been used since the beginning of heart surgery (11). The only detectable difference between both approaches is the instruments used for this maneuver; surgical dilatation of the aortic valve has incorporated the bare finger approach of Swann et. al (19), as well as widely varying instruments including the tripronged steel implement (1, 11). In 1956, the failure of this intervention on the early postoperative course of these patients led to a generally accepted discontinuation of its use for the routine treatment of calcific aortic stenosis (2).

Although these unsatisfactory results both on short- and long-term follow-up led to the opinion that dilatation of the stenotic aortic valve is not possible, PTAV affords the non-operative reduction of the gradient across a stenotic valve in patients otherwise unsuitable for open heart surgery, i.e., patients with very high risk, patients older than 80 years or with a second, severe systemic disease (16). Because of the inherent clinical importance and the obvious lack of large intraoperative study on the efficacy of this method under visual control, we performed PTAV in the operating room in a large series of patients in order to assess the morphological changes and the improvement of valve area in acquired calcific aortic stenosis.

Material and method

PTAV was performed in 25 consecutive patients undergoing aortic valve replacement for acquired calcific aortic stenosis. Mean age was 58.9 years, ranging from 43 to 69 years; there were 17 men and eight women. The mean peak aortic pressure gradient was 88.28 mm Hg (range 62 to 138 mm Hg). Mean valve opening area pre-operatively was 0.6 ± 0.3 cm^2 using the modified Gorlin equation for calcuation of valve area. Thirteen patients had an additional grade I and II aortic regurgitation as diagnosed during left heart catheterization by angiographic criteria according to the New York Heart Association. Seven patients underwent additional aorto-coronary bypass grafting due to severe concomittant coronary artery disease. Calculation of the aortic valve diameter to assess the appropriate balloon size for PTAV was performed from the angiogram in the 30 RAO and 60 LAO projection and corrected for magnification. Additionally, the size of the annulus was measured echocardiographically preoperatively in 18 of these patients.

After sternotomy, the aortic valve was exposed using the transverse aortotomy. The annulus was stabilized using three to four sutures. Pre-intervention, the morphological criteria such as the status of the commissures, extent of calcification and subjectively determined leaflet mobility were recorded. For photographic documentation, a camera with a fixed focus was placed at a certain distance and multiple color photographs of the valve were taken. The angle between valve orifice and camera was fixed between 85° and 95° to avoid angulation problems. In 20 patients a Mansfield Balloon (3 cm long) was used, seven balloons with a 21 mm diameter, six with a 23 mm diameter and seven with a 25 mm diameter (Mansfield Balloons, Meditech, Inc. Watertown, Washington, USA). In the other five patients, a Trefoil balloon (Schneider, Zürich, Switzerland) was used, in four patients a 3×12 balloon and in one patient a 3×15 balloon. The balloons were extended in all patients to the maximal diameter using pressures between 3.5 and 5 atm. Dilatation time was at least 15 s at maximum inflation. After dilatation, the morphologic changes and leaflet mobility were subjectively recorded and rephotographed under identical conditions. Extreme care was used in detection of calcific debris, midleaflet tears, and valve ring disruption after dilatation.

In an attempt to quantify the balloon-induced changes of the aortic valve area, the pre- and postprocedural photographs were magnified and the static valve orifice area (Fmin) and the total valve area were determined by planimetry. Besides the determination of the static orifice size, the actual change was calculated and also expressed as percent change of the total valve area.

Results

The individual changes of the static orifice area are depicted in Fig. 1 and summarized in Table 1. A considerable increase of F min. was achieved in three patients with an increase of more than two cm^2 from pre- to post-PTAV. All three patients had a tricuspid valve. Although extensive leaflet calcification was present, the commissures were fused but not bridged by calcium deposits or ridges. In all three patients, the orifice was in the center of the valve. PTAV resulted in nearly complete separation of the commissures as demonstrated in Fig. 2. The inflation of the balloon separated the commissures and forced the leaflet into an open position. After dilatation incomplete reapproximation could be observed; the increase of the orifice area, however, proved that the additional fraction of calcium deposits on the leaflets is an important second mechanism for successful PTAV in patients with calcific aortic stenosis.

In six patients an increase of the static orifice area between one to less than two cm^2 was observed. Four of these patients had a tricuspid and two a bicuspid calcific valve with fused commissures. In comparison with the patients in whom an increase of Fmin of more than two cm^2 was found, in these patients not only sclerotic changes and masses of calcium deposits on the mural surface of the leaflet were found but also considerable calcification of the fused commisures was present. Although the commissures were covered by calcium nodules, they could be identified by gross examination. Balloon dilatation resulted in partial separation of the com-

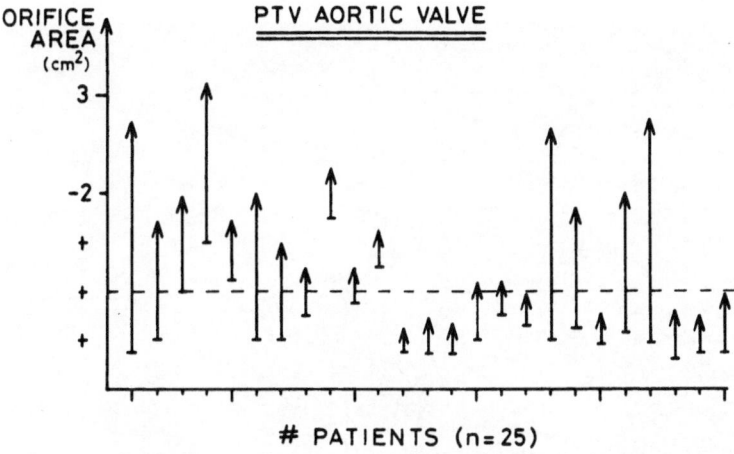

Fig. 1. Quantitative changes pre to post PTAV in cm^2 in all 25 patients.

Table 1. Changes in the static orific area (Fmin) in 25 patients undergoing intraoperative balloon valvuloplasty. The majority of patients (n = 16) had an increase in the static orific area of less than 1 cm^2.

PTV aortic valve		
Results		
– increase ΔFmin	>2 cm^2	: 3
	>1 – < 2 cm^2	: 6
	< 1 cm^2	:16
– with ΔFmin < 1 cm^2	> 0.5 cm^2	: 9
	< 0.5 cm^2	: 7

missures only. In three of these patients the fused commisural ridge broke nearly complete, but reapproximation of the leaflets occured readily after deflation of the balloon. The increase in leaflet mobility was modest, probably due to the extensive calcification of the leaflets and the commissures. In the majority of patients, the increase of the static orifice area Fmin was minimal with less than 1 cm^2. In eight of these patients just a fishmouth-like, small central oval orifice was open, in the other eight patients the orifice was eccentric. The commissures were represented by calcified ridges. In these patients, balloon dilatation did spread the calcified leaflets but did not result in a splitting of the commisural ridges (Fig. 3). After deflation reapproximation occured almost immediately. Leaflet mobility was only moderately increased probably because no major dent in the calcified masses of the mural aspects of the leaflets was found on gross examination. In two of these patients liberation of calcific debris was observed. Midleaflet tears or valve ring disruption did not occur in any patient.

51

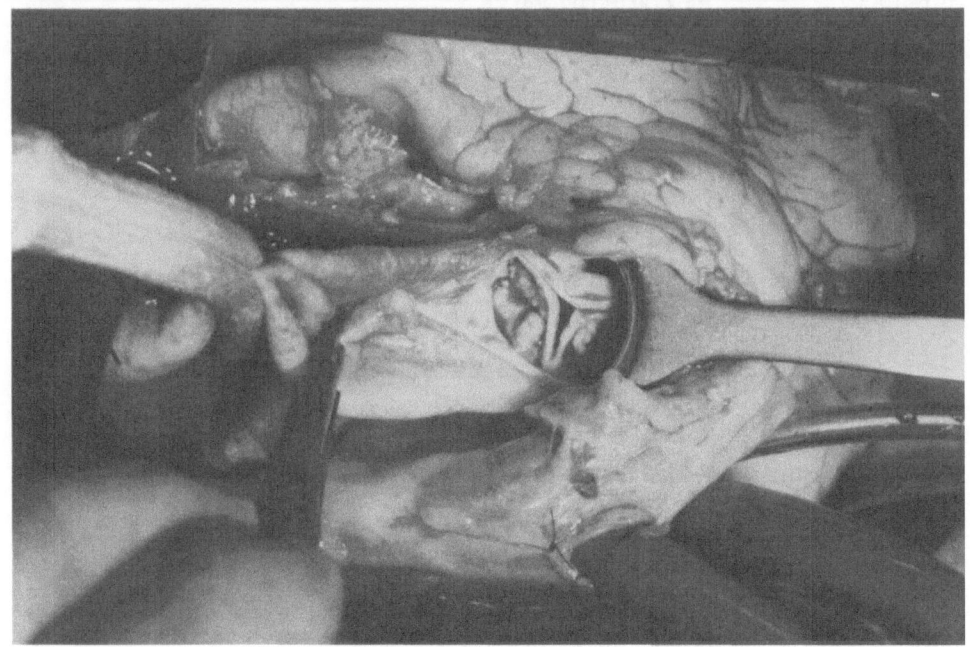

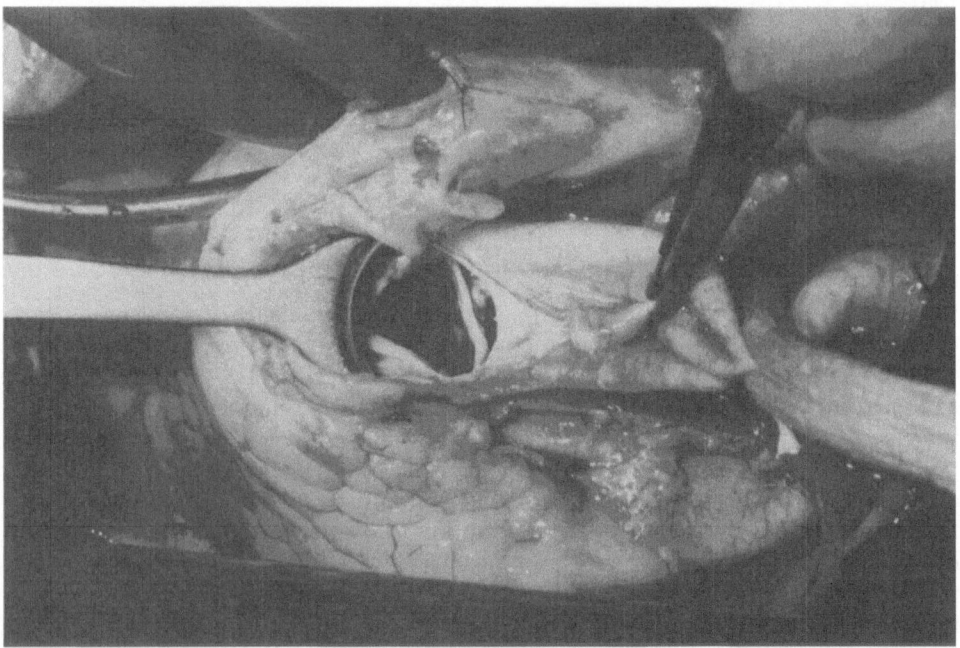

Fig. 2. a) Tricuspid calcific valve with two fused commissures before and **b)** after valvuloplasty. Improvement of static valve area was more than 2 cm². No obvious reapproximation occurred. Due to fractures of the calcific masses on the leaflets, mobility was considered increased

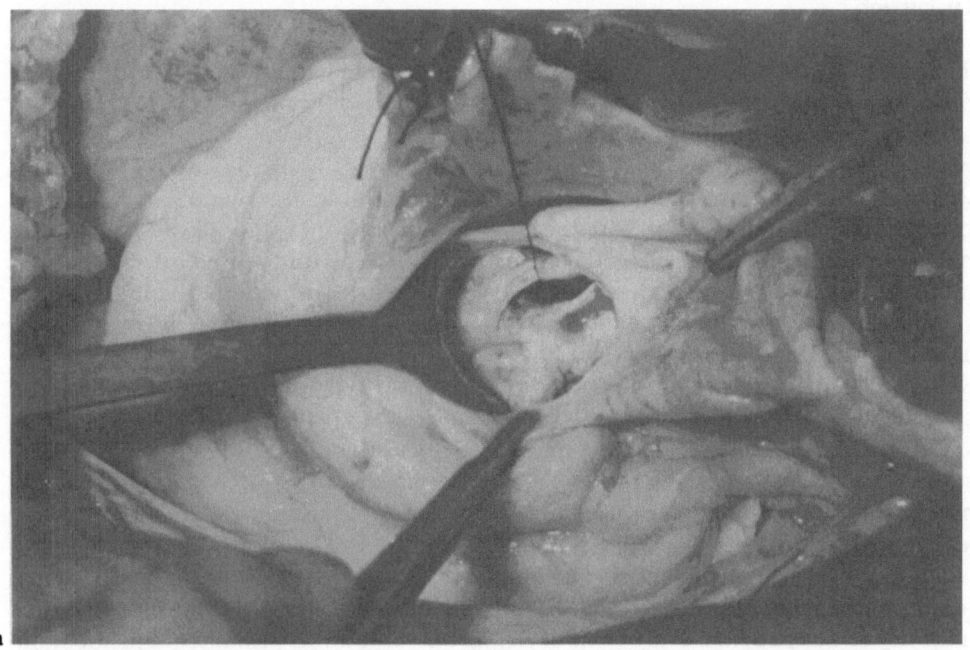

a

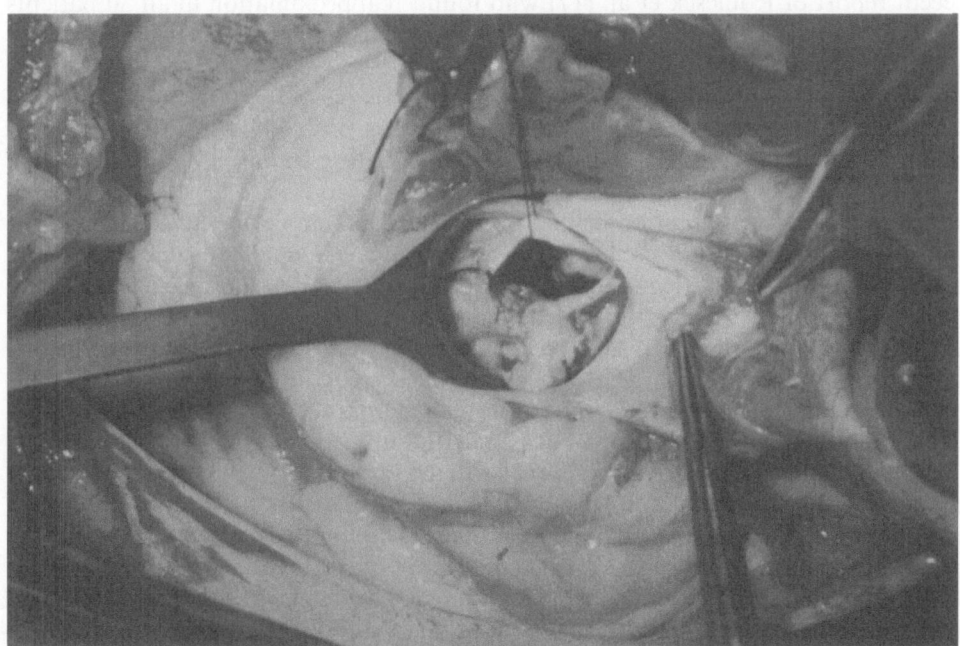

b

Fig. 3. a) Bicuspid "fish mouth"-like calcific aortic valve before and **b)** after balloon valvuloplasty. The orifice area is moderately enlarged and leaflet mobility (suture) is also moderately increased. Additionally, a calcific ridge between the commissures of the left sinus can be observed.

Discussion

The initial short term results of balloon valvuloplasty in patients with aortic stenoses proposed by Cribier et al. (5) and Mc Kay (14) proposed the method as an alternative to aortic valve replacement. Although the technique of valve dilatation in young patients with congenital aortic stenosis has been used by cardiovascular surgeons with considerable success and the impact of transluminal valvuloplasty in these patients is tremendous (12, 15); the anatomical and morphological situation in patients with acquired and calcific stenosis is obviously quite different. Studies on intraoperative and postmortem balloon valvuloplasty in acquired calcific aortic stenosis are surprisingly rare considering the clinical widespread use of this method as a routine procedure even in patients with low operative risk (16, 21). In 1987, Safian et al. (18) published the results of balloon valvuloplasty on 33 postmortem specimen and six intraoperative dilatations in calcific aortic stenosis. In all patients valve orifice dimensions and leaflet mobility increased. Balloon dilatation resulted in separation of fused commissures in correspondence with our results and leaflet mobility was accordingly increased due to fractures of nodular calcifications of the leaflet surface. Reapproximation after deflation of the balloon was not observed which might be due to the effect of long periods of formalin fixation on the postmortem specimens. Reapproximation after deflation of the balloon occured in the majority of our patients. The extent of reapproximation was primarily dependent on the success of separation of the commissures and at least in our series not on the incidence of fractures of the calcific masses on the leaflet. This is substantiated by a recent report of Robicsek et al. (17) who found reapproximation in all 30 patients after intraoperative balloon valvuloplasty in patients with aortic stenoses. In comparison to the results of Robicsek who in his series in 19 patients found no change in orifice area using quantitative methods most of our patients demonstrated an effect on orifice area after PTV. This difference is probably due to the different methods in determination of the static valve area before and after dilatation, which is limited by certain restrictions.

On one hand determination of the orifice area even under magnification as used in our study is difficult in patients with a fishmouth-like oval orifice and extensive calcification since identification of the correct borders may be complicated by additional subvalvular calcification which was present in the majority of patients with extensive calcification (6,13). The second major drawback is the calculation of static orifice area and the more or less subjective measurement of leaflet mobility used as a measurement for the normally pulsating flow across the valve. The biologic relevance of the observed effects remains open to question and especially in patients with an increase of orifice area more than two cm^2, a significant regurgitation might occur. Besides the methodological problems of the quantitative and qualitative parameters on orifice area and leaflet mobility the findings of our study and the report of Robicsek et al. suggest that the effect of balloon valvuloplasty in patients with acquired calcific aortic stenosis is limited. Although orifice area and leaflet mobility could be considerably increased in one third of the patients, morphology remained nearly unchanged in the other two third of the population. It is well-known that arteriosclerotic valvular disease produces stiff and calcified leaflets which are further immobilized by calcific masses and may even lead to obliteration of the commissures (2). Such severely calcified and distorted valves are most unsuitable for dilatation. In patients, however, in whom a tricuspid valve has fused but not calcified commissures although the leaflets are calcified, balloon valvuloplasty may result in a considerable improvement even for a longer postinterventional period. In such Mönckeberg-type stenosis the commissures can be separated resulting in a considerable increase of orifice area and improvement of leaflet mobility. In view of the very small anatomical changes achieved in two thirds of our patients and in the study of Robicsek et al. indication for balloon valvuloplasty in calcific aortic stenosis has to be revisited. Although the clinical and hemodynamic improvement in most patients is remarkable, the very small change in orifice area predicts a high recurrance rate during the early postinterventional period in the majority of these patients. In view of our results we can not agree with the statement of Isner et al. (9) that valvuloplasty is indicated in all patients with documented stenosis and no more than I + aortic regurgitation. The method which is clearly an alternative treatment in patients who are truely inoperable should not be misused for adventures which had been shown to be unacceptable some thirty years ago. In patients older than 70 years the mortality of aortic valve replacement is 12.1% to 14.3% (3, 8, 19, 20). Percutaneous transluminal balloon valvuloplasty may be indicated in patients with class IV heart failure as an intermediate short-term method to improve the clinical status and recompensate the patient by an increase of global left ventricular function even with small changes in orifice area.

Conclusion

Balloon valvuloplasty resulted in a considerable increase of orifice area in one third of all patients with calcific aortic stenosis. In the majority (two thirds) of patients the change in orifice area as well as in leaflet mobility was minimal. Thus, application of PTV should be limited to patients who are in class IV heart failure and in whom the surgeon cannot perform aortic valve replacement with an acceptable chance of operative survival.

References

1. Bailey CP, Bolton HE, Jamison WL, Nichols HT (1954) Commissurotomy for rheumatic aortic stenosis. Surgery 9:22
2. Bailey CP, Bolton HE, Nichols HT et al. (1956) The surgical treatment of aortic stenosis. J Thorac Surg 31:375
3. Bessone LN, Pupello DF, Blank RH et al. (1977) Valve replacement in patients over 70 years. Ann Thorac Surg 24:417
4. Cribier A, Savin T, Saou N et al. (1986) Percutaneous transluminal valvuloplasty of acquired aortic stenosis in elderly patients: an alternative to valve replacement. Lancet 1:63
5. Cribier A, Savin T, Saoudi N et al. (1986) Percutaneous balloon valvuloplasty (PBV) in adult aortic stenosis: an alternative to surgery for valve replacement. Circulation 74 (Suppl 2), 365
6. Gorlin R, Matthews MB, Mc Millan JKR et al. (1954) Physiological and clinical observations in aortic valvular disease. Bull N Engl Med Center 16:13
7. Grüntzig AR, Senning A, Siegenthaler WE (1979) Non-operative dilatation of coronary artery stenosis: percutaneous transluminal coronary angioplasty. N Engl J Med 301:61

8. Hochberg MS, Morrow AG, Michaelis LL et al. (1977) Aortic valve replacement in the elderly. Arch Surg 112:1475
9. Isner JM, Salem DN, Desnoyers MR et al. (1987) Treatment of calcified aortic stenosis by balloon angioplasty. Am J Cardiol 59:313
10. Labadi Z, Jiunn-Ren W, Wall JT (1984) Percutaneous balloon aortic valvuloplasty: results in 23 patients. Am J Cardiol 53:194
11. Larzelere HB, Bailey CP (1953) New instrument for cardiac valvular commissurotomy. J Thorac Surg 25:78
12. Lawson RM, Bonchek LI, Menashe V, Starr A (1976) Late results of surgery for left ventricular outflow tract obstruction in children. J Thorac Cardiovasc Surg 71:334
13. Lewis JF, Shumway NE, Niazi SA, Benjamin RB (1956) Aortic valvulotomy under direct vision during hypothermia. J Thorac Surg 32:481
14. Mc Kay RG, Safian RD, Lock JE et al. (1986) Balloon dilatation of calcific aortic stenosis in elderly patients: postmortem, intraoperative and percutaneous valvuloplasty studies. Circulation 74:119
15. Presbitero P, Somerville J, Revel-Chion R, Ross D (1982) Open aortic valvulotomy for congenital aortic stenosis: late results. Br Heart J 47:26
16. Roberts WC (1987) Good-bye to thoracotomy for cardiac valvuloplasty. Am J Cardiol 59:198
17. Robicsek F, Harbold NB, Daugherty HK, Cook JW, Selle JG, Hess PJ, Gallagher JJ (1988) Balloon valvuloplasty in calcified aortic stenosis: a cause for caution and alarm. Ann Thorac Surg 45, pp. 515–525
18. Safian RD, Mandell VS, Thurer RE, Hutchins GM, Schnitt SJ, Grossman W, Mc Kay RG (1987) Postmortem and intraoperative balloon valvuloplasty of calcific aortic stenosis in elderly patients: mechanism of successful dilatation. JACC Vol 9 No 3: pp. 655–60
19. Swann WK, Bradsher JT, Rodriguez-Arroyo J (1954) The surgical treatment of aortic stenosis. South Med J 47:1067
20. Teply JF, Grunkemeier GL, Starr A (1981) Cardiac valve replacement in patients over 75 years of age. Thorac Cardiovasc Surg 29:47
21. Vahanian A, Guerinon J, Michel PL et al. (1986) Experimental balloon valvuloplasty of calcified aortic stenosis in the elderly. Circulation 74:(Suppl 2) 365

What can we learn from classical operative techniques for valvular balloon dilatation?

B. Reichart, J. Odell, U. v. Oppell, H. Reichenspurner, S. Vosloo,
P. J. Commerford*, A. Horak*, M. de Moor**

Departments of Cardiothoracic Surgery, Cardiology* and Paediatrics**, Groote Schuur and Red Cross War Memorial Children's Hospital, University of Cape Town, Medical School, South Africa

In light of the rapidly increasing use of percutaneous transluminal coronary angioplasty, valvular balloon dilatation has recently been recommended in paediatric and adult cases as an alternative to various classical operative techniques (1, 2). Interventional cardiology seems to avoid traumatic surgery, and valvular balloon dilatation might have a lower mortality and morbidity rate, and repeat dilatations are thought to be easier to perform. In Table 1, an attempt is made to compare these postulated benefits with those of "classic" cardiac surgical techniques which, in general, provide well established and documented results.

The following review of our own short- and long-term results should be understood as an attempt to critically summarize the outcome in surgical patients with mitral stenosis, and left and right ventricular outflow tract obstruction. The ultimate aim should be a list of indications for the two, as we see them, complimentary approaches: interventional cardiology and cardiac surgery.

Historical background

Surgeons started valvular dilatation as early as 1923, when Cutler (3) described dilatation of a stenotic mitral valve by means of a transventricular inserted instrument. In 1925, Souttar (4) introduced his finger through the left appendage and digitally enlarged the mitral orifice. Primbram (5) dilatated the mitral valve, in 1928.

Probably because of the largely unsuccessful outcome and the attitude of many surgeons at the time that good exposure was necessary to do an operation, further developments stagnated for approximately 20 years. Surgical dilatation of the mitral valve was revived in the late 1940s and early 1950s by Bailey and Harken who both

Table 1. Comparison of postulated advantages of interventional cardiological techniques with those of cardiac surgery.

Postulated advantages	
Of interventional cardiology	Of cardiac surgery
– avoidance of surgery	– "Straight forward" results
– lower mortality	– open heart procedures allow final decision-making
– repeat procedures relatively easy	– non-lethal complication rate lower
	– long-term (10–20 yrs) results available

57

standardized their "finger fracture" techniques (6,7); Dubost (8) devised a transatrially inserted instrument, which was soon thereafter replaced by a more convenient transventricular one, described by Logan et al. (9) – an instrument which is still in use after a modification by Tubbs (10).

In the late 1940s and early 1950s Sellors (11) and Brock (12) had independently pioneered "blind" surgical treatment of the pulmonary valve; the latter applied his techniques also to the aortic position (13).

All these surgical interventions were of course so called "closed-heart" procedures, with the heart exposed via a thoracotomy but allowing no direct view of the diseased valves. This was changed for the first time in 1956, by applying the method of hypothermia (14, 15); the "open-heart" era had begun. These procedures were made easier, when a clinically reliable extracorporeal circulation system became available (16, 17). It soon, however, became clear that some of the stenotic valvular diseases were not amenable to repair procedures. The results were especially disappointing after maneuvers with heavily calcified and malformed aortic valves. Removal and replacement with a prosthesis became the treatment of choice soon thereafter – as was the case in patients with irreparable stenotic mitral valves (18).

1988 – Possibilities of cardiac surgery for stenotic valvular lesions and ventricular outflow tract obstructions

Percutaneous balloon dilatation is attempted for right and left ventricular outflow tract obstruction and in patients with mitral stenosis. In contradistinction, cardiac surgery offers a variety of techniques individually tailored to the specific pathological lesions present.

Closed heart ("blind") surgery

It is the closed heart ("blind") surgery that is actually challenged by percutaneous interventional procedures.

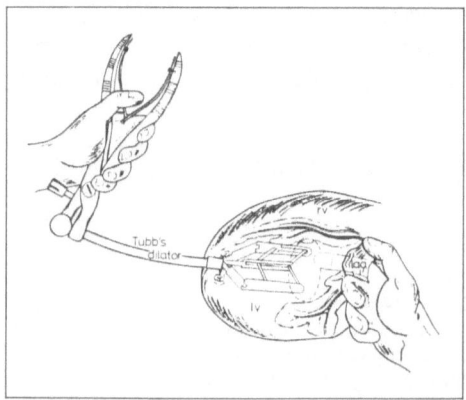

Fig. 1. Schematic drawing of closed mitral valvotomy (abbreviations: rv = right ventricle; lv = left ventricle; laa = left atrial appendage; figures 1, 4a to c with permission of M. Antunes, Coimbra, Portugal)

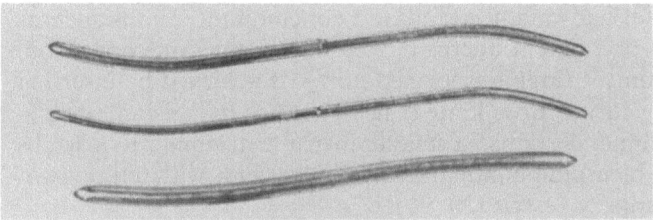

Fig. 2. Three different sizes of Hegar dilators as used for closed aortic and pulmonary valvular dilatation

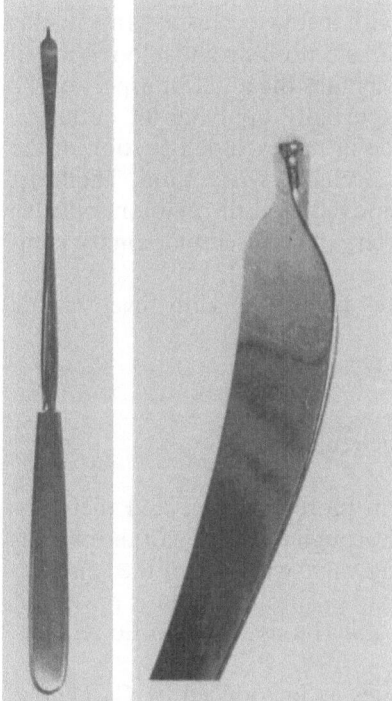

Fig. 3. The Brock knife, as used in cases of valvular and infundibular right ventricular outflow tract obstruction

For classical mitral commissurotomy using the transventricular dilator, the chest is entered via a small left-sided antero-lateral incision. The pericardium is opened anterior to the phrenic nerve. The right index finger of the surgeon is inserted through the left atrial appendage and the mitral valve assessed digitally to determine the mobility of the leaflets and the presence or absence of reflux. The dilator is then gently inserted into the left ventricular cavity and across the orifice of the stenosed mitral valve, guided by the right index finger and opened (Fig. 1). A screw allows for a controlled dilatation of 3 to 4 cm.

Closed aortic valvotomies may be achieved by increasing sizes of straight Hegar dilators, pushed through the stenosed area (Fig. 2) (19). The blunt tipped metal dilators are inserted through a stab wound in the left ventricular apex. The technique is applied during the neonatal and infant period and concomitant lesions such as coarctation may be repaired or a patent ductus ligated during the same operation.

Classic pulmonary valvotomy – rarely performed now – is achieved by inserting Hegar dilators or the slightly curved Broc knife (Fig. 3) via a stab incision made in the right ventricular wall. Klinner described a smaller instrument similar to a Tubbs dilator with which he dilated bicuspid pulmonary valves in patients with tetralogy of Fallot and hypoplastic pulmonary vessels (20, 21).

Open heart surgery without the help of extracorporeal circulation

These procedures are done at normothermia and with inflow occlusion. In valvular pulmonary stenosis, the chest is opened via a median sternotomy and a longitudinal incision of the pericardium is made. The surgeon excludes the anterior aspect of the main pulmonary artery from the circulation by partially applying an occlusion clamp. A longitudinal incision of 3 to 4 cm is made in the excluded portion of the artery. Superior and inferior venae cavae are then occluded with snares. The heart is allowed to beat empty, the occlusion clamp is removed, and the pulmonary valve visualized through the opened main pulmonary artery. The fused pulmonary commissures are then incised precisely (22).

The same technique may be applied in neonates presenting with severe aortic stenosis (23).

Open heart surgery with the help of extracorporeal circulation

Heart lung machines allow the surgeon to perform more extensive and therefore more time consuming valvular repair work. After thorough inspection of the pathology, he may decide to replace an irreparable looking valve with one of the common mechanical or biological prostheses. In the pulmonary position, antibiotic preserved homografts are recommended; similar techniques may be used for aortic replacement (24–26).

For open mitral commissurotomy (and techniques as introduced by Carpentier (27)) the chest is opened via a median sternotomy. After heparinization, the patient is attached to the extracorporeal circulation and after cross-clamping the aorta, cardioplegic solution is given. The left atrium is entered from the right side (and not via the left-sided appendage where clots usually are located). Open mitral valve techniques include sharp commissurotomy (Fig. 4a), freeing of fused chordae, incision of papillary muscles (Fig. 4b), removal of abundant fibrotic, calcific tissue at the coaptation area (Fig. 4c) and transection of short, rigid secondary chordae in order to further mobilize the mitral leaflets. Pathologic lesions which cause mitral incompetence may also be repaired, again according to the techniques of Carpentier (27).

Left-ventricular outflow tract obstruction may be caused not only by stenosed aortic valves, but also by sub- or supra-valvular lesions. Sub-aortic stenosis may be due to a discrete membrane which can be easily resected, a narrow fibrotic left-ventricular outflow tract tunnel, making complex Konno-Koncz enlargement neces-

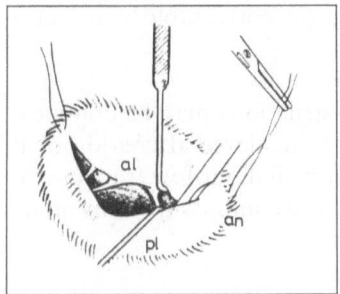

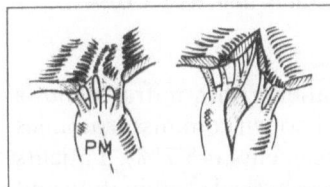

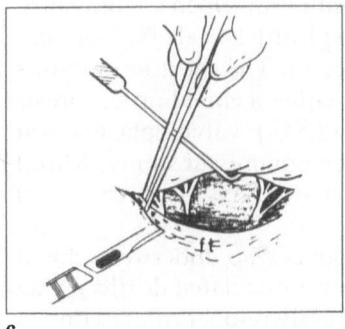

Fig. 4 a, b, c. Techniques of open mitral commissurotomy: (a) Commissurotomy with the help of a scalpel (abbreviations: al, pl = anterior, posterior leaflet; an = annulus of the mitral valve). (b) Splitting of papillary muscle (PM). (c) Removal of abundant fibrous tissue (ft) on top of the posterior mitral leaflet

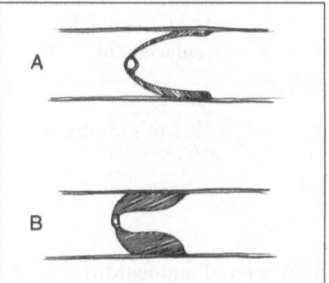

Fig. 5. Schematic drawing of an "ideal" valvular pulmonary stenosis (a) suitable for balloon dilatation. In comparison, dysplastic pulmonary valves (b) may be unsuitable for dilatation

61

sary (28, 29), or a hypertrophic obstructive cardiomyopathy, correctable by myectomy according to Morrow (30).

Supra-aortic lesions necessitate patch enlargement.

In similar fashion, right ventricular outflow tract obstructions may be complex, and significant right ventricular pressure relief may only be achieved after additional infundibular muscle resection or insertion of a large pericardial outflow tract patch. A dysplastic pulmonary valve usually requires excision since commissurotomy alone does not relieve the pressure gradient (Fig. 5).

Surgery in patients with pure mitral stenosis at Groote Schuur and Red Cross Children's Hospital

From September 1984 until June 1988, a total of 151 patients with mitral stenosis were treated; there were 42 closed valvotomies (27.8%), 40 open commissurotomies (plus additional techniques; 26.5%) and 69 valve replacements (45.7%). Patients were considered suitable for closed interventions whenever physical examination and echocardiography demonstrated fully mobile leaflets, without signs of regurgitation and calcification and there was no history of thromboembolism. Open commissurotomy was recommended when decreased mobility of the leaflets, calcification, mitral incompetence, or a history of embolization was present. The short term results are presented in Table 2. None of the patients died after either a closed procedure or mitral valve replacement, but one died after open repair (2.5%). Valvuloplasty failed three times after closed valvotomy and twice after open commissurotomy. Mitral valve replacement was then necessary immediately, after two days, at three (twice) and at six post-operative months, respectively.

Results are available from another group of 654 patients who underwent closed valvotomy over a 12-year period (31). There were 20 operation related deaths giving an operative mortality of 2.9%. Four patients required early re-operation (within a month of the initial procedure) because of excessive mitral regurgitation produced at the time of the closed valvotomy. Approximately one fourth of the patients were clinically considered to have pulmonary hypertension; 9% were in NYHA class II, 86% in class III, and 5% in class IV. The overall cumulative survival at six years was 90% and 78% at 12 years. Initial and long-term results were poor in patients with NYHA Class IV while pulmonary hypertension had no influence on outcome.

Table 2. Short-term results of 151 patients with pure mitral stenosis who received their operation between September 1984 and June 1988.

Procedure	Closed	Open valvotomy	Mitral valve replacement
number	42	40	69
age (mean, range, years)	25.3 (12–42)	31.9 (7–68)	38.3 (4 months– 68)
30-day mortality	0%	1 (=2.5%)	0% ***
repeat valvular failure	3* (=7%)	2** (=5%)	---

* immediate, after 2 days, 6 months
** both at 3 months
*** add. interventions and lesions: Revascularization 4×, subacute bacterial endocarditis 2×

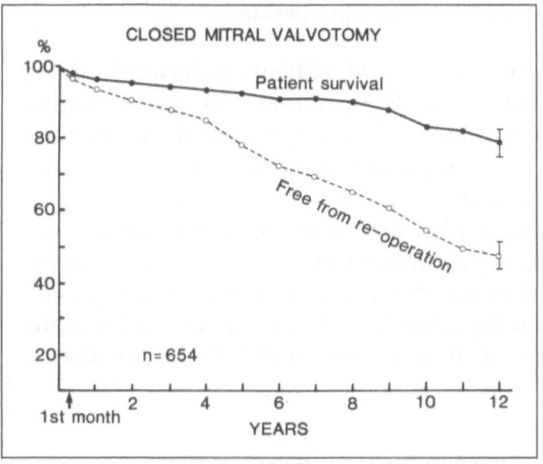

Fig. 6. Long-term results of 654 patients who received closed mitral valvotomy: Upper curve indicates cumulative survival, lower curve freedom from reoperation

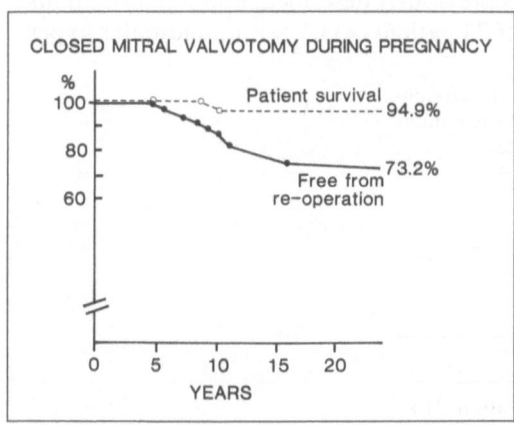

Fig. 7. Patient survival and freedom from reoperation of 39 women who had altogether 41 closed valvotomies during their pregnancies

Importantly, clinical assessment of mobility and suitability for valvotomy was an independent predictor for successful outcome.

In another study (32) 39 women who underwent 41 closed mitral valvotomies during pregnancy were reviewed. There were no deaths and thirty-six (87.8%) babies were delivered successfully. Two late deaths occurred, one as a result of pneumonia and meningitis, the other because of heart failure (Fig. 7). Nine women needed futher surgical procedures for restenosis 5 to 17 (mean 10.2) years postoperatively; repeat closed valvotomy was necessary in three patients (two during subsequent pregnancies), open commissurotomy once and valve replacement on five occasions. All patients survived repeat procedures.

The safety of mitral replacement after previous repair procedure is confirmed by results accumulated during the interval September 1984 until June 1988; 48 patients required repeat operation after a mean of 15.7 years; one patient (2%) died. The previous repairs included two open and 46 closed valvotomies; four patients had two closed interventions.

Surgery in patients with left ventricular outflow tract obstruction

During the interval September 1984 until June 1988, 86 patients underwent surgery for left-ventricular outflow tract obstruction (Table 3). In one-fifth, reconstruction of complex congenital malformations was attempted (surgery included three Konno-Koncz procedures and six myectomies). In this young age group (mean 12.7 years; range two months to 24 years) a high 30-day mortality of 17.7% was observed.

In 80% valvular replacement was necessary because of severe calcific aortic stenosis. Twenty-one patients had additional revascularization, nine an aortic root enlargement; subacute bacterial endocarditis was present in six cases. In one patient, an aberrant right-sided Kent bundle was transected, in another a ventricular septal defect closed. In this older age group (mean 40, range 4-82 years) the 30-day mortality was 5.8%.

Surgery in patients with right ventricular outflow tract obstruction

The period of observation was the same as previously described. Pulmonary commissurotomy alone was sufficient in only 8 of 24 patients (33.5%); infundibular hyper-

Table 3. Thirty-day mortality of 86 patients with left-ventricular outflow tract obstruction who received their interventions between September 1984 and June 1988.

Reconstructive surgery of LVO		
− subvalvular stenosis	2/12	
− valvular stenosis	0/1	3/17 (= 17.7%)
− supravalvular stenosis	1/4	
Aortic valve replacement *	4/69(= 5.8%)	
Grand total	86	

* add. interventions and lesions: Revascularization 21 ×, root-enlargement 9 ×, subacute bacterial endocarditis 6 ×; WPW, VSD 1 each

Table 4. Surgery for isolated right-ventricular outflow tract obstruction between September 1984 and June 1988. The mean age of the patients at the time of the operation was 9.3 years (range 1 month to 36 years). There was no operative mortality.

Pulm. valvotomy alone	8 (= 33.5%)
Pulm. valvot. + outflow tract patch	7 (= 29%)
Excision of dysplastic pulm. valve + outflow tract patch	7 (= 29%)
Outflow tract patch alone	2 (= 8.5%)
Grand total	24 (= 100%)
add. procedures:	(14/24 = 58%)
ASD, PFO closure	12
PDA closure	1
Wooler plasty	1

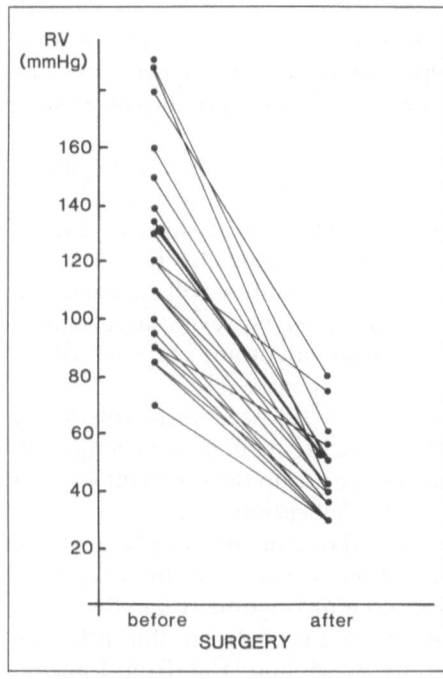

RV
(mmHg)

160
140
120
100
80
60
40
20

before   after
SURGERY

Fig. 8. Decrease of the right-ventricular systolic pressure of patients who had correction of right-ventricular outflow tract obstructions at Groote Schuur and Red Cross Children's hospital (mean value in bold)

trophy necessitated muscular resection in all other 16 cases; a dysplastic pulmonary valve was removed seven times. In more than half of the patients (58%), additional procedures were done, closure of an atrial septal defect, a patent ductus, and in one patient a Wooler annuloplasty (Table 4). There were no deaths and the decrease of the systolic right ventricular pressure is shown in Fig. 8.

Conclusion

Surgery for mitral stenosis

Most of the European and North American cardio-surgical groups prefer open repairs for their patients with mitral stenosis, since these techniques produce better overall results – specifically a lesser degree of restenosis or incompetence (33, 34). Gross et al. (35) report a reoperation rate of only 6% within a 10-year period; Carpentier (27) notes a 90% freedom from further intervention after eight years.

This concept is attractive. Intuitively one would expect better results with open mitral valve repair since a variety of interventions are possible, including splitting papillary muscles, removing abundant sclerotic or calcific valvular tissue, and cutting off rigid secondary chordae. A point often overlooked is that the visualized valve may look worse than anticipated and valve replacement rather than repair is undertaken. It is often not possible to determine from the literature how frequently this occurs and what proportion of patients referred for open valvotomy end up with valve replacement. Surgeons may argue that replacement is desirable, but in some circumstances, particularly in South Africa, replacing the valve often replaces one disease with another. Fine intraoperative judgment and understanding of existing socio-economic circumstances are needed.

In disagreement therefore, and especially in the context of a South African patient population, we still believe that closed mitral valvotomies have a definite place in 1988, foremost in patients with pliable, non-calcific pure mitral stenosis. Closed maneuvers are safe, quick, effective and last but not least, cost-effective interventions. In the near future, however, percutaneous balloon dilatation will eventually be the preferred procedure, with probably similar results. It is, however, important to us that clear indications (the same as for closed mitral valvotomy) be adhered to, thus learning from the lessons of the past.

This statement confirms the basic conclusions of the "closed mitral valvotomy pioneer" Harken, whose series started in 1949: Consistent, beneficial long-term results up to 20 years were only found in a younger age group (less than 40 years at surgery) without signs of mitral incompetence and calcification (36).

According to our own experience, a 10-year survival rate of 80% can be expected with a freedom from mitral valve reintervention of 50%. The latter figure appears disappointingly low; acute rheumatic fever, however, is an ongoing risk in the South African patient population and recurrence of the disease is common, thus affecting otherwise good operative results. In a recent study by Molajo et al. from England (37), 91% and 80% of patients required no further operation at four and eight year intervals, respectively – a long-term result considerably better than our own (four and eight year freedom from operation of 86% and 65%, respectively).

Surgery for left-ventricular outflow tract obstruction

Aortic valve replacement is necessary in the majority of adult cases with calcific aortic stenosis – 80% of our patients. Percutaneous balloon dilatation, which recently is receiving much attention, yields short-term success in only 50% of cases (see contribution of Erdmann et al. in this book). In a recent article, Robicsek and co-workers are even less optimistic (38). They investigated the validity of balloon valvuloplasty carried out in the operative theater under direct vision, prior to aortic valve replacement. By visual inspection, as well as measurements, dilatation procedures rendered a minimal or moderate enlargement of the valvular orifice in only 11 of 30 treated patients; in the remainder, no difference was found.

It can thus be concluded, that percutaneous balloon dilatation of aortic stenosis should only be offered to the very sick or elderly patients, in order to try to decrease valvular gradient. In a few cases, aortic valve replacement is then unnecessary; in most it is postponed (39, 40).

In a younger age group, congenital malformations at sub-, supra- or valvular levels may cause severe left-ventricular outflow tract obstructions. Sometimes only complex repairs carrying a considerable operative mortality can be offered. In a few cases of subvalvular membrane and supravalvular stenosis, an attempt at percutaneous balloon dilatation may be justified.

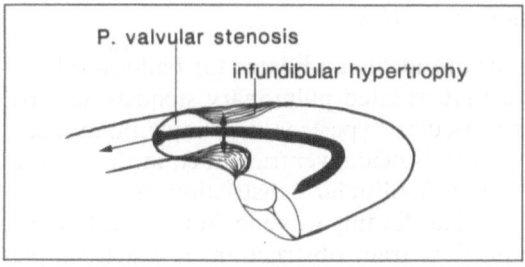

a

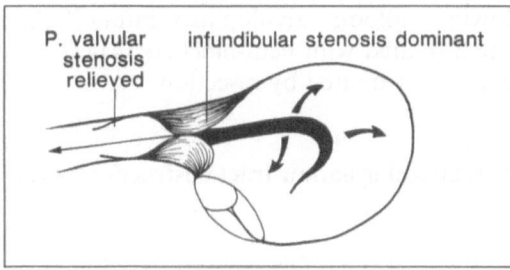

b

Fig. 9. Schematic drawing of the development of a "suicide ventricle"; the relief of the pulmonary valvular stenosis alone leads to increased constriction of the right-ventricular infundibulum. The right-ventricular pressure remains unchanged unless the infundibular stenosis is relieved by resection and concomitant patch insertion

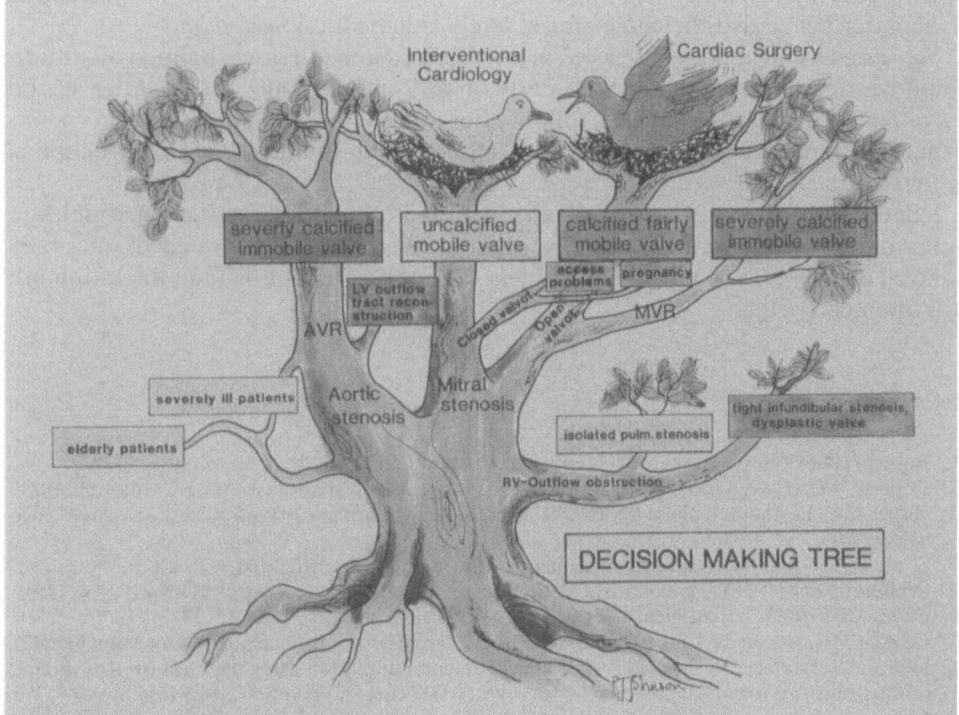

Fig. 10. The decision making tree (see text)

67

Patients with pulmonary valvular stenosis are ideal candidates for balloon dilatation. One should however keep in mind that isolated pulmonary stenosis may be complicated by additional infundibular muscular hypertrophy. Simple pulmonary commissurotomy could then create a so called "suicidal ventricular condition" – the relief of valvular narrowing aggravates the infundibular constriction, maintaining the high right-ventricular pressures (Fig. 9). This finding was encountered in 4 of our 24 cases (17%) with right ventricular outflow tract obstruction in which simple commissurotomy was first attempted. Additional infundibulectomy in combination with an ample outflow tract patch resulted in a definite pressure decrease. Rao et al., however, have shown recently that following balloon valvuloplasty infundibular stenosis may decrease over six months when treated with beta-blockers (41).

Dysplastic pulmonary valves are probably best treated by resection.

Treatment of mitral stenosis, left and right ventricular outlow tract obstructions – the decision making

In patients with mitral stenosis but uncalcified, fully mobile leaflets, percutaneous balloon dilatation is advised. Presently, closed mitral valvotomy seems to be only indicated when access problems exist or during pregnancy. In cases with slightly calcified, but still mobile leaflets, sometimes complicated by mitral incompetence, an open procedure is advised, leaving then the option for either repair or replacement – the latter being also the choice for severely calcified lesions.

Valve replacement is mostly necessary in calcified aortic lesions. Balloon dilatation could be tried in the young or the elderly or very sick patients – in the latter, aortic valve replacement would mostly follow after an interval of "cooling off".

Surgical repair of complex congenital left ventricular outflow tract obstruction is preferred.

Dilatation of the pulmonary valve is ideal; additional lesions such as dysplastic pulmonary valves or infundibular obstructions must however be watched, since they are well proven to be amenable to surgery, and the results of balloon dilatation are still at an early stage.

References

1. Bull C (1986) Interventional catheterization in infants and children. Br Heart J 56:197
2. Roberts WC (1987) Goodbye to thoracotomy for cardiac valvotomy. Am J Cardiol 59:198
3. Cutler CE, Levine SA, Beck CS (1924) The surgical treatment of mitral stenosis. Arch Surg 9:689
4. Souttar HS (1925) The surgical treatment of mitral stenosis. Brit Med J 2:603
5. Primbram BO (1926) Die operative Behandlung der Mitralstenose. Arch Klin Chir 142:458
6. Bailey CP (1949) The surgical treatment of mitral stenosis. Dis Chest 15:377
7. Harken DE, Dexter L, Ellis LB et al. (1951) The surgery of mitral stenosis. Ann Surg 134:722
8. Dubost C, Blondeau P, Piwnica A (1962) Instrumental dilatation using the transatrial approach in the treatment of mitral stenosis: A survey of 1000 cases. J Thorac Cardiovasc Surg 44:392
9. Logan A, Turner R (1959) Surgical treatment of mitral stenosis with particular reference to the transventricular approach with a mechanical dilator. Lancet 2:874

10. Tubbs OS (1962) Transventricular mitral valvotomy. NT Geneesk 106:335
11. Sellors TH (1948) Surgery of pulmonary stenosis; a case in which the pulmonary valve was successfully divided. Lancet 1:988
12. Brock RC (1949) The surgery of pulmonary stenosis. Brit Med J 2:399
13. Brock RC (1954) Valvotomy for aortic stenosis. Brit Heart J 16:468
14. Ellis FJ, Shumway NE, Niazi SA et al. (1956) Aortic valvotomy under direct vision during hypothermia. J Thorac Cardiovasc Surg 32:481
15. Bailey CP, discussion in 14
16. Gibbon JH (1954) Application of a mechanical heart and lung apparatus to cardiac surgery. Minn Med 37:171
17. Lillehei WC, discussion in 14
18. Starr A, Edwards ML (1961) Mitral valve replacement. Clinical experience with a ball valve prosthesis. Ann Surg 154:726
19. Duncan K, Sullivan I, Robinson RP et al. (1987) Transventricular aortic valvotomy for critical aortic stenosis in infants. J. Thorac Cardiovasc Surg 93:546
20. Klinner W, Reichart B (1978) Die Anomalien des rechtsventrikulären Ausflußtrakts. In: Herz und herznahe Gefäße. Borst HG, Klinner W, Senning A (eds), Springer Verlag, Heidelberg, New York, p. 290
21. Reichart B, Kreuzer E, Felgenauer N, Klinner W (1978) Correction of tetralogy of Fallot patients after previous Brock procedure. Congressbook, 27th meeting of the European Society of Cardiovascular Surgery, Lyon, p. 239
22. Klinner W, Reichart B (1978) Anomalien des rechtsventrikulären Ausflußtrakts. In: Herz und herznahe Gefäße. Borst HG, Klinner W, Senning A (eds), Springer Verlag, Heidelberg, New York, p.319
23. Sink JD, Smallhorn JF, MacCartney FJ et al. (1984) Management of critical aortic stenosis in infancy. J Thorac Cardiovasc Surg 897:82
24. Duran CG, Gunning AJ (1962) Method for placing a total homologous aortic valve in the subcoronary position. Lancet 2:488
25. Ross DN (1962) Homograft replacement of the aortic valve. Lancet 2:487
26. Barratt-Boyes BG (1964) Homograft aortic valve replacement in aortic incompetence and stenosis. Thorax 19:131
27. Carpentier A (1983) Cardiac valve surgery – the "French correction". J Thorac Cardiovasc Surg 86:323
28. Konno S, Imai Y, Jida Y et al. (1975) A new method for prosthetic valve replacement in congenital aortic stenosis associated with hypoplasia of the aortic ring. J Thorac Cardiovasc Surg 70:909
29. Rastan H, Abu-Aishah N, Rastan D et al. (1978) Results of atrioventriculoplasty in 21 consecutive patients with left-ventricular outflow tract obstruction. J Thorac Cardiovasc Surg 75:659
30. Morrow AG, Brockenbrough EC (1961) Surgical treatment of idiopathic hypertrophic subaortic stenosis: Technique and hemodynamic results of subaortic ventriculotomies. Ann Surg 154:181
31. Commerford PJ, Hastle T, Beck W (1982) Closed mitral valvotomy: Actuarial analysis of results in 654 patients over 12 years and analysis of preoperative predictors of long-term survival. J Thorac Cardiovasc Surg 33:473
32. Vosloo S, Reichart B (1987) The feasibility of closed mitral valvotomy in pregnancy. J Thorac Cardiovasc Surg 93:675
33. Spencer FC (1988) Results of closed mitral commissurotomy. Ann Thorac Surg 45:355
34. Bonchek LI (1981) Current status of mitral commissurotomy: Indications, techniques, and results. Am J Cardiol 47:821
35. Gross RI, Cunningham JN, Snively et al. (1981) Long-term results of radical mitral commissurotomy: Ten year follow-up of 202 patients. Am J Cardiol 47:821
36. Ellis LB, Singh JB, Morales DD (1973) Fifteen to twenty year study of one thousand patients undergoing closed mitral valvuloplasty. Circulation 48:357
37. Molajo AO, Bennett DH, Bray CL et al. (1982) Actuarial analysis of late results after closed mitral valvotomy. Ann Thorac Surg 45:364
38. Robicsek F, Harbold NB, Daugherty et al. (1988) Balloon valvuloplasty in calcified aortic stenosis: A cause for caution and alarm. Ann Thorac Surg 45:515

39. Block PC (1988) Aortic valvuloplasty – a valid alternative. N Engl J Med 319:169
40. Safian RD, Berman AD, Diver DJ et al. (1988) Balloon aortic valvuloplasty for congenital cyanotic heart defects. Am Heart J 115:1105
41. Rao PS, Fawzy ME, Solymar et al. (1988) Longterm results of balloon pulmonary valvuloplasty. Am Heart J 115:1291

Percutaneous balloon valvuloplasty of aortic stenosis in 110 consecutive patients

E. Erdmann, W. v. Scheidt, K. Werdan, M. Hörmann

Department of Medicine I, University of Munich, Klinikum Großhadern, Munich, FRG

Introduction

Aortic valve replacement in symptomatic aortic valvular stenosis is the treatment of choice. However, there are many absolute or relative contraindications to open heart surgery: pulmonary congestion with pneumonia, fever and leukocytosis, respiratory insufficiency, cardiogenic shock, other serious diseases with organ failure, advanced age along with poor physical condition, bleeding disorders, etc. Recently, several groups have published encouraging results in patients with calcific aortic stenosis undergoing balloon valvuloplasty rather than aortic valve replacement surgery (1–13). Marked immediate improvement in hemodynamics and symptoms was noted almost universally. In view of the operative and perioperative risks involved in elderly patients undergoing surgery (14–16), an alternative treatment should be seriously considered. We therefore report our experience with balloon valvuloplasty of aortic stenosis in 110 consecutive patients. The purpose of this communication is to assess the immediate results and some follow up data in order to judge the efficacy of this relatively new method in interventional cardiology.

Methods

Between September 1986, and July 1988, we performed aortic valvuloplasty in 110 patients with valvular aortic stenosis. Two patients were excluded in whom we were unable to place the balloon catheter. The characteristics of the 110 patients are summarized in Table 1.

Indications for balloon valvuloplasty

Generally, balloon valvuloplasty was offered to patients considered as poor candidates for cardiac surgery (age over 75, pulmonary disease, other serious and limiting diseases, left ventricular ejection fraction < 35%). Twelve patients presented in cardiogenic shock and were treated as emergency candidates. Fourteen patients who would have been eligible for aortic valve replacement surgery and so advised by us, refused surgery and were treated by valvuloplasty. Among the first 20 patients, we recommended balloon valvuloplasty in six patients although they were good candidates for open heart surgery. Twenty-two patients were > 80 years old and were primarily considered for balloon valvuloplasty. An aortic insufficiency of grade 1 + or 2 + was not considered a contraindication to valvuloplasty.

Table 1. Baseline characteristics of 110 patients who underwent aortic valvuloplasty

Characteristic	Value
Age (years)	70 ± 12
(range)	25–88
male : female	49 : 61
calcific : non calcific	107 : 3
Symptoms:	
a. heart failure IV NYHA	66
b. syncope	21
c. angina pectoris	11
d. emergency procedure	12
follow up (months)	10 ± 6
(range)	1–23

Aortic valvuloplasty procedure

All patients (except emergency candidates) gave informed written consent for the procedure after an explanation of the potential risks and complications. Balloon valvuloplasty was performed in all cases by the retrograde approach via the femoral artery. Since the ninth patient, a 16.5 F introducer sheath (11) was used. Monofoil or trefoil catheters (Mansfield Scientific or Schneider Medintag) 20–23 mm (3 × 12 mm) were used as a rule. In a few cases other balloons were used if the procedure failed with the above mentioned balloons. After measuring cardiac output and transvalvular gradients, valvuloplasty was performed by applying 2.5–9 bar for 10–30 s. This procedure was repeated up to 11 times until the calculated aortic valve area increased by at least 50%. In case of complications, the procedure was stopped immediately. At the end of the procedure, cardiac output, transvalvular gradient and pulmonary artery pressures were measured and an aortogram was performed. The catheters were then removed and groin compression applied for 1–3 h until no further bleeding was detected.

Follow-up

Follow-up data for a mean (± SD) of 10 ± 6 months (range 1–23) were available for all patients discharged from the hospital. Invasive reinvestigations were performed in 35 patients; in 12, because of restenosis, repeat valvuloplasty was performed. Restenosis was considered to have occurred if the aortic valve area had decreased by more than 50% of the initial increase. Doppler echocardiography was performed in all nine patients presenting in 1988, with regular follow-up every three months.

Numerical data are presented as mean ± one standard deviation.

Results

Hemodynamic measurements

Balloon valvuloplasty was performed in 110 patients. One patient in cardiogenic shock died during the procedure (after the second dilatation). In the remaining

Table 2. Hemodynamic data in 109 patients surviving aortic valvuloplasty

	before dilatation	after
1. peak systolic pressure gradient (mm Hg)	90 $\pm$ 31	39 $\pm$ 22
2. AVA (cm^2)	0.40 $\pm$ 0.12	0.76 $\pm$ 0.29
3. cardiac output (l/min.)	4.32 $\pm$ 1.10	4.25 $\pm$ 0.97
4. LVEDP (mm Hg)	23 $\pm$ 11	21 $\pm$ 9
5. mean pulmonary artery pressure (mm Hg)	28 $\pm$ 14	25 $\pm$ 13

Table 3. Complications in 110 patients undergoing aortic valvuloplasty

1. death during dilatation	1
2. in-hospital deaths	5
3. emergency operation	3
aortic insufficiency	1
cardiac tamponade	2
4. surgical repair of a. fem.	14
5. cerebral complications	3
6. asystole	2
7. AV-block III°	1
8. aortic regurgitation of minor importance	22
9. left bundle branch block	4
10. ventricular fibrillation	3

109 patients, peak systolic pressure gradients were reduced from 90 $\pm$ 31 to 39 $\pm$ 22 mmHg, the aortic valve areas increased from 0.4 $\pm$ 0.12 to 0.76 $\pm$ 0.29 cm^2, the cardiac output stayed constant (before dilatation 4.32 $\pm$ 1.10, after 4.25 $\pm$ 0.97 l/min), LVEDP was 23 $\pm$ 11 mmHg and stayed constant immediately after valvuloplasty at 21 $\pm$ 9 mm Hg, mean pulmonary artery pressure was 28 $\pm$ 14 before and 25 $\pm$ 13 after the procedure (Table 2).

Complications

One 82 year old patient who presented in cardiogenic shock and was therefore treated by emergency valvuloplasty died during the procedure. Five additional patients (mean age 82 years) died during the hospital stay (one with acute aortic regurgitation, one with ventricular arrhythmia on the third day after dilatation, one with uremia one week after dilatation, and one with pneumonia 10 days after an unsuccessful procedure). Three patients required acute cardiac surgery (one with acute aortic regurgitation and two because of ventricular perforation and acute cardiac tamponade). All three patients survived aortic valve replacement. In 14 patients the femoral artery required surgical repair; in two, this complication contributed significantly to the in-hospital deaths because of prolonged mechanical ventilation after general anesthesia. The other complications were reversible: cerebral ischemia or embolization in three, asystole, III degree AV-Block, left bundle branch block and ventricular fibrillation (Table 3). In 22 patients, as compared with prevalvuloplasty aortography, aortic insufficiency had newly appeared or slightly increased without apparent hemodynamic importance.

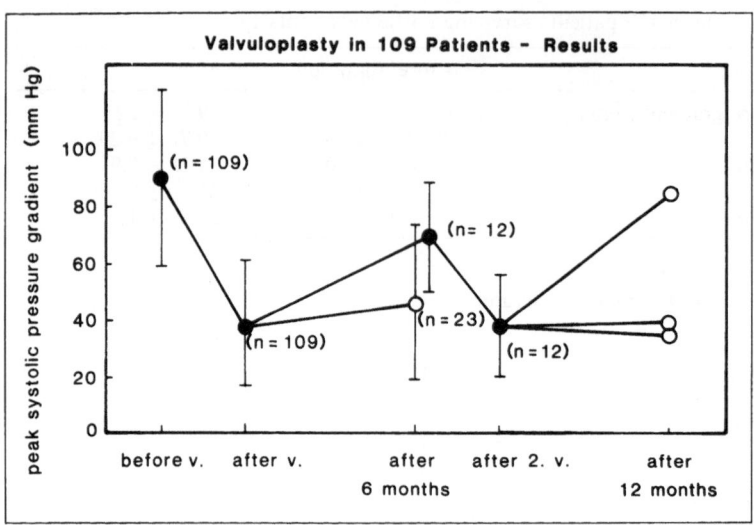

Fig. 1. Immediate and late results in 109 patients undergoing balloon valvuloplasty of aortic stenosis. This figure shows the invasively measured peak systolic gradients after valvuloplasty, after a mean of six months follow up and after the second valvuloplasty in those patients with restenosis and symptoms

Follow-up

Ninety patients were discharged from the hospital and were followed for 10 ± 6 months (range $1-23$ months). 14 patients underwent cardiac surgery during hospital stay, six died. Four patients died during the follow-up because of various medical reasons (carcinoma, stroke, heart failure, pneumonia). Thirty-five patients could be reinvestigated invasively after 6 ± 4 months. In 23 more or less asymptomatic patients, the peak systolic gradient had increased only slightly to 46 ± 27 mm Hg (Fig. 1). In 12 patients either because of symptoms or because of the restenosis, a second successful valvuloplasty was performed (systolic gradient was lowered from 69 ± 19 mm Hg to 38 ± 18). In three patients, a second invasive reinvestigation revealed a restenosis in one asymptomatic patient (pressure gradient of 86 mm Hg). He was then successfully treated by aortic valve replacement.

Eleven patients underwent aortic valve replacement surgery at 9 ± 3 months after valvuloplasty. Two of these had been considered unacceptable risks before valvuloplasty. None of these patients died perioperatively.

Six patients could be followed by Doppler-echocardiography. A significant restenosis of the aortic valve area was noted in all of them within four to six months (systolic pressure gradient 26 ± 6 to 78 ± 25 mm Hg). These patients have not been restudied invasively because they are still relatively asymptomatic.

Concomitant coronary heart disease

Significant coronary artery stenosis ($> 70\%$ or left main stem $> 50\%$) was detected in 14 of 82 patients in whom the coronaries were studied: two with left main stem disease; six with three-vessel disease; two with two-vessel disease and six with one-

74

vessel disease. In these patients, dilatation time did not exceed 10 s; in the 85-year-old with left main stem 70% stenosis, only one dilatation of the valve was performed, reducing the pressure gradient from 72 to 43 mm Hg, not optimal but an acceptable result. None of these patients experienced an infarction or unstable angina. Because of this finding, routine coronary angiography is no longer performed.

Discussion

The prognosis of medically treated patients with symptomatic aortic stenosis is very poor. Once heart failure is the leading problem, one year survival rates are below 50% (17, 18). Therefore, rapid removal of severe outflow obstruction to relieve the left ventricle of the intolerable afterload is necessary in this situation. Of course, surgical aortic valve replacement is the therapy of choice. However, there are some problems with the surgical approach:

1) patients with decompensated aortic stenosis (heart failure NYHA IV) are often in a poor condition with LVEF < 40% and have pneumonia;
2) elderly patients often have additional serious diseases (e.g., coronary heart disease, pulmonary or renal insufficiency, etc.);
3) perioperative mortality in advanced age may be between 16% and 31% (15, 16).

Because of this, balloon valvuloplasty has some advantages:

1) it can be performed rapidly, even under emergency conditions by a team experienced in left heart catheterization;
2) it immediately relieves outflow obstruction in most patients;
3) complications are tolerable in view of the age group treated (22 of our 110 patients were octogenarians) and in view of the severity of the disease (see Table 1). Nevertheless, ongoing experience and newer, smaller diameter catheters will help to decrease the complication rate;
4) short-term results are good (most of our patients could be discharged from the hospital as free or almost free of symptoms after a mean of 9 ± 8 days, range $1-37$ (n = 90).

However, the main limitation of balloon valvuloplasty as therapy for aortic stenosis is restenosis (13). As also found by other groups, restenosis occurred in about 50% of our patients within six months. Apparently, the calcification of the aortic valve in some elderly patients is a progressive disease (19), which cannot be stopped by dilatation of the valvular apparatus. Valvuloplasty is severely limited by the occurrence of restenosis. As yet, we do not know the reasons for this. As the successful dilatation of the stenosed aortic valve may result from microfractures within the leaflets (9), the restenosis might be caused by reconsolidation of the calcific orifice. This hypothetical explanation needs further investigation. The characteristics of the patients without restenosis after six months were not significantly different from those with restenosis. Only 10 of our patients had aortic valve areas above 1 cm- after dilatation. Restenosis among these patients was as frequent as among the others. Repeated dilatation is possible and was successfully performed 12 times. Our impression was that the second dilatation is easier and more rapidly performed. The results

Table 4. Indication for balloon valvuloplasty of aortic stenosis

1. decompensated condition (cardiogenic shock)
2. before urgent non cardiac surgery
3. in patients with unacceptable risks for surgery (pneumonia, other serious disease)
4. in the very old patient
5. if it cannot be decided, whether the poor condition of the patient (cachexia) can be improved by aortic valve replacement.

are similar as compared with the initial procedure (Fig. 1). However, restenosis may nevertheless recur.

The technique for balloon valvuloplasty is not difficult. Independent of the type of balloon used, most groups report similar results in respect to aortic valve area, decrease of pressure gradient, cardiac output, restenosis rate, etc. (1–13).

Thus, we think that balloon valvuloplasty is a palliative procedure (Table 4) suited for patients with limited life expectancy or unacceptable perioperative risks. However, our positive experience with patients in cardiogenic shock indicates that primary balloon valvuloplasty in this condition is the therapy of choice – followed by cardiac surgery days or weeks later. Furthermore, the preoperative discovery of severe aortic valvular stenosis in a patient undergoing urgent non-cardiac surgery was the indication for balloon valvuloplasty four times. All patients survived abdominal surgery after previous successful dilatation of the aortic stenosis.

Rarely patients are seen in a cachectic, moribund condition with a low ejection fraction, low cardiac output and also a low systolic pressure gradient. In this situation, the decision for aortic valve replacement surgery is not easy because of the high perioperative and late mortality (15, 16). In these patients, a good recovery after balloon valvuloplasty helps in the decision process for cardiac surgery.

In conclusion, we feel that balloon valvuloplasty in patients with severe aortic stenosis, although a palliative treatment, has its place in interventional cardiology because the resulting decrease in afterload affords immediate hemodynamic improvement and palliation of symptoms in the great majority of patients. Restenosis occurs but can be treated by repeat valvuloplasty or – if possible - by cardiac surgery.

References

1. Cribier A, Saodi N, Berland J et al. (1986) Percutaneous transluminal valvuloplasty of acquired aortic stenosis in elderly patients: an alternative to valve replacement? Lancet 11:63
2. Cribier A, Savin T, Berland J et al. (1987) Percutaneous transluminal balloon valvuloplasty of adult aortic stenosis: report of 92 cases. JACC 9:381
3. Isner JM, Salem DN, Desnoyers MR et al. (1987) Treatment of calcific aortic stenosis by balloon valvuloplasty. Am J Cardiol 59:313
4. Schneider JF, Wilson M, Gallant TE (1987) Percutaneous balloon aortic valvuloplasty for aortic stenosis in elderly patients at high risk for surgery. Ann Intern Med 106:696
5. McKay RG, Safian RD, Lock JE et al. (1987) Assessment of left ventricular and aortic valve function after aortic balloon valvuloplasty in adult patietns with critical aortic stenosis. Circulation 75:192
6. Jackson G, Thomas S, Monaghan M et al. (1987) Inoperable aortic stenosis in the elderly: benefit from percutaneous transluminal valvuloplasty. Brit Med J 294:83

7. Holmes DR, Nishimura RA, Reeder GS (1987) Aortic and mitral balloon valvuloplasty: emergence of a new percutaneous technique. Int J Cardiol 16:227
8. Buchler JR, Braga SLN, Assis SF et al. (1987) Balloon valvuloplasty in calcific aortic stenosis: a therapeutic alternative. Int J Cardiol 16:263
9. Safian RD, Mandell VS, Thurer RE et al. (1987) Postmortem and intraoperative balloon valvuloplasty of calcific aortic stenosis in elderly patients: mechanism of successful dilatation. J Am Coll Cardiol 9:655
10. Scherer HE, Hörmann E, Engel HJ (1987) Ballondilatation verkalkter Aortenstenosen. Dtsch med Wschr 112:1694
11. Erdmann E, Höfling B (1987) Perkutane transfemorale Valvuloplastie der verkalkten und nicht verkalkten Aortenklappe. Dtsch med Wschr 112:1067
12. Erdmann E, Werdan K, v. Scheidt W, Hörmann M (1988) Ballondilatation der verkalkten Aortenklappenstenose. Münch med Wschr 130:51
13. Safian RD, Berman AD, Diver DJ et al. (1988) Balloon aortic valvuloplasty in 179 consecutive patients. N Engl J Med 319:125
14. de Vivie ER, Eisenschenk A, Neuhaus KL et al. (1986) Klappenersatz bei Patienten über 70 Jahre. Z Kardiol 75:379
15. Edmunds Jr LH, Stephenson LW, Edie RE et al. (1988) Open heart surgery in octogenarians. N Engl J Med 319:131
16. Magovern JA, Pennock JL, Campbell DB, et al. (1987) Aortic valve replacement and combined aortic valve replacement and coronary artery bypass grafting: predicting high risk groups. J Am Coll Cardiol 9:38
17. Mathews AW, Barritt DDW, Keen GE, Belsey RH. (1974) Preoperative mortality in aortic stenosis. Brit Heart J 36:101
18. Horstkotte D, Loogen F (1987) Erworbene Klappenfehler. Urban und Schwarzenberg, München, Wien Baltimore
19. Robicsek F, Harbold NB, Daugherty HK et al. (1988) Balloon valvuloplasty in calcified aortic stenosis: a cause of caution and alarm. Ann Thorac Surg 1988 45:515

Balloon aortic valvuloplasty in adults: report of 78 consecutive patients

H. E. Scherer

Department of Medicine (Cardiology), Zentralkrankenhaus "Links der Weser", Bremen, FRG

Since the first reports of percutaneous balloon valvuloplasty in calcific aortic stenosis in 1986 (5, 11), this method has attracted rapid worldwide interest because of the rather large number of elderly patients with symptomatic aortic stenosis. Until recently, septuagenarians or even octogenarians recieved medical therapy, despite the well known poor prognosis in the spontaneous course of this disease (12, 17). Several groups began to evaluate the feasibility of this technique and its results in terms of hemodynamic and symptomatic improvement as well as possible improved prognosis (2, 6, 13). To date more than 2 000 BAV procedures have been performed, mainly in France and the United States. Early studies suggest that marked immediate symptomatic and hemodynamic improvement can be achieved, while the restenosis rate seems to be relatively high in short term follow-up (7).

Methods

Between November 1986, and June 1988, 78 patients, (33 men and 45 women), with a mean age of 73.5 ± 10 years (25 to 88) underwent one or two retrograde valvuloplasty attempts at our institution (Table 1). All but two patients were in the NYHA functional class III or IV, 15 of the 49 patients with class III symptoms had at least one episode of left ventricular failure. Increased or high surgical risk was considered

Table 1. Study population

Ballon aortic valvuloplasty (BAV) Bremen 6/88
Total number of patients n = 78, 33 men, 45 women
Mean age 73,5 ± 10 years (25–88)

Age distribution			
	< 70	n = 16	(20%)
	70–79	n = 40	(52%)
	≥ 80	n = 22	(28%)

Table 2. Estimation of surgical risk of valve replacement

Valve replacement estimated risk				
age	contraind.	high	increased	good candidate
≥ 80 (22)	6	9	7	–
75–79 (20)	1	8	11	–
< 75 (36)	4	8	11	13

in 65 of the patients due to age over 75 and/or concomitant non-cardiac diseases as well as severely depressed left ventricular function (Table 2). The diagnosis of aortic stenosis was assessed in all patients by clinical and two-dimensional echo/Doppler examination, in a few cases, a previous diagnostic heart catheterization was available.

In most cases, the BAV was performed in combination with the diagnostic procedure. Except for a single brachial approach, all other dilatations were performed via the retrograde femoral artery route. The technical details were previously described (16). In our early experience we used cylindrical single balloons of 15, 18, 19, and 20 mm (Mansfield or Schneider) or the triangular 3×12 mm Trefoil balloon (Schneider); later we tried to use the 23 mm balloon (Mansfield) as the final size. When available, we used balloons with proximal pressure measurement and pigtail end as well as a double-size shape, which allowed a complete dilatation procedure with one balloon, simultaneous gradient measurement and final aortography with no need for a second arterial puncture. Cardiac output was routinely measured by thermodilution three or four times before and after dilatation, and in a few cases by the Fick method. Aortic valve area was estimated during the procedure by the Kakki-formula (10) and later corrected by the accepted Gorlin equation (9). Coronary angiography was performed in those patients who had predominantly angina pectoris symptoms.

Repeat catheterization was offered to nearly all patients except the very frail, initially after an interval of three months and since July 1987, at six months. Restenosis was defined as loss of more than 50% of the initial valve area improvement. Follow-up two-dimensional echo/Doppler evaluations were also performed and a questionaire was sent to the entire group regarding evolution in symptoms.

Results

Seventy-nine procedures were successfully completed; 69 were a first dilatation and 10 a second. Ten attempts had to be prematurely terminated because of either complications, patient's intolerance, or technical difficulties in carrying out the procedure (Table 3). During first BAV, peak aortic gradient decreased from 79.6 ± 29 to

Table 3. First, second and incomplete ballon valvuloplasty procedures

Balloon aortic valvuloplasty (BAV)	
Total number of procedures	n = 89
First valvuloplasty	n = 69
second valvuloplasty	n = 10
incompleted BAV	n = 10

Causes of interruption:	
3	complication
2	iliac tortuosities
1	failure to cross the valve
2	patient tolerance
2	failure to place the balloon

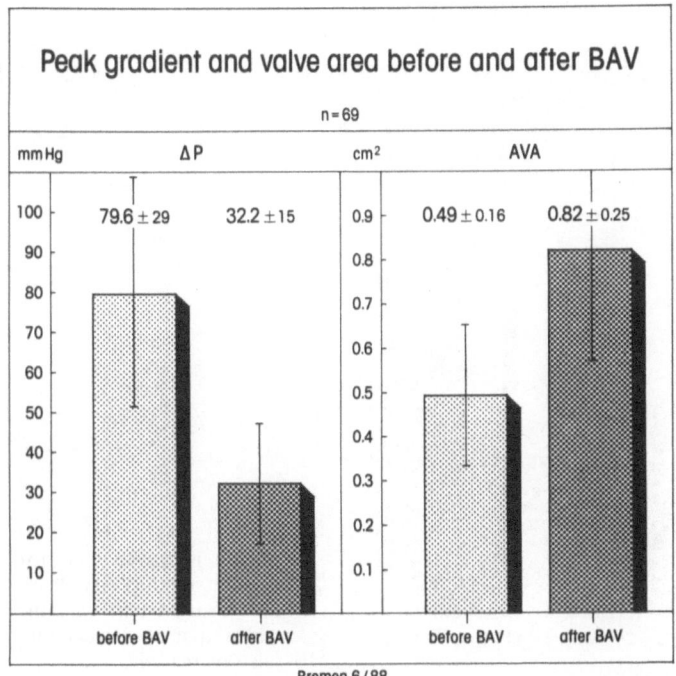

Fig. 1. Peak gradient and valve area before and after BAV

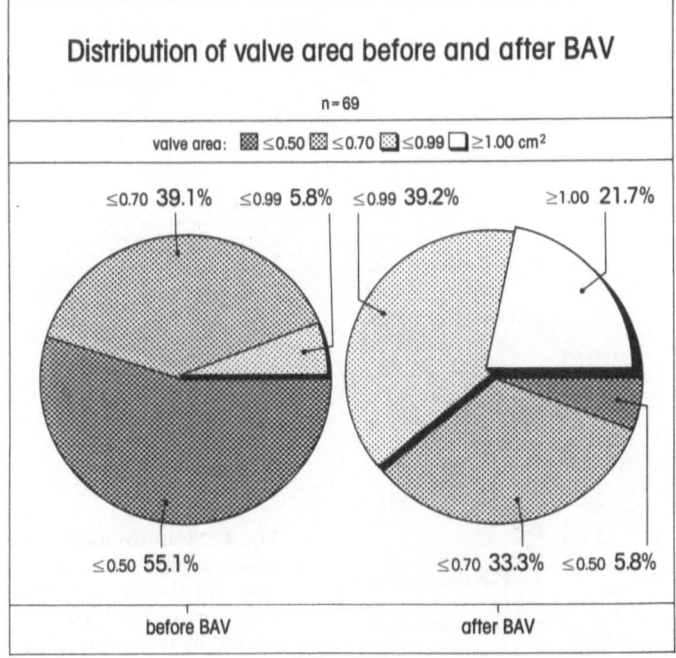

Fig. 2. The distribution of valve area before and after valvuloplasty

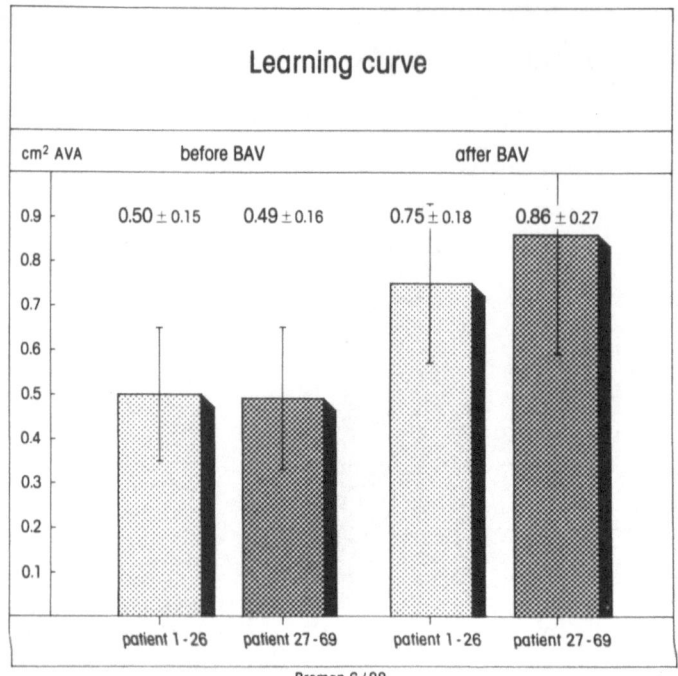

Fig. 3. Learning curve for aortic valvuloplasty. With increasing experience, the valve area post procedure also increased

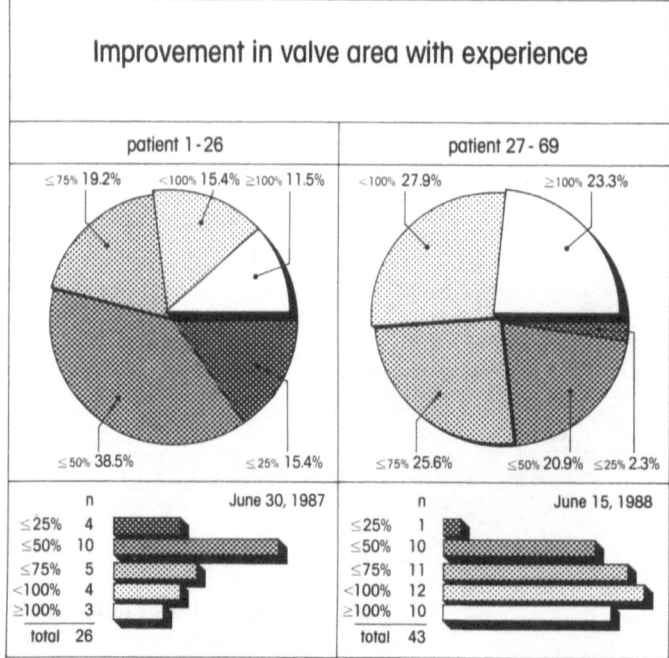

Fig. 4. Improvement in valve area with experience; for the last year, the valve area could be improved by more than 75% in one-half of the cases

82

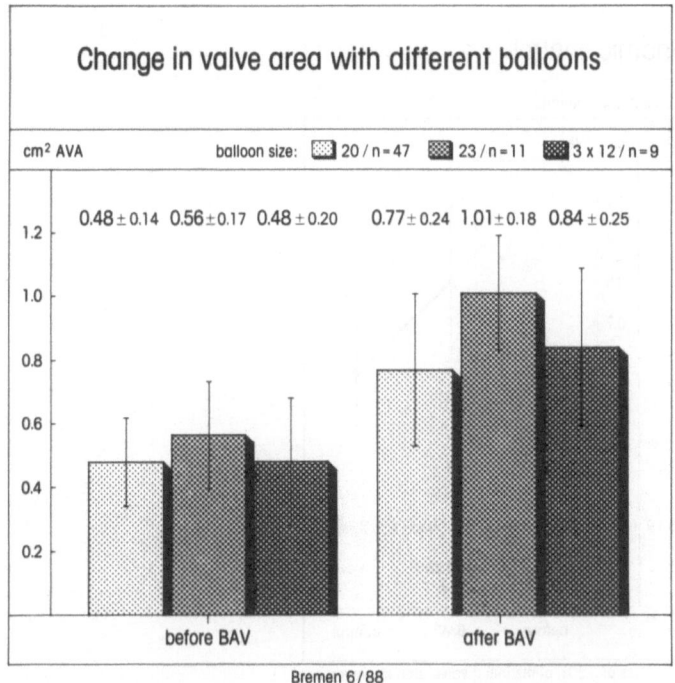

Fig. 5. Change in valve area as related to balloon size used

Table 4. In-hospital mortality after BAV

	Early mortality n = 4 (5,1 %)					
	age	sex	funct. cl.	concom. disease	cause of death	delay
Procedure-related	71	w	IV	marasmus, malignoma	sepsis with DIC	72 h
	76	w	IV	renal/pancreas failure	low output	BAV
non-related	68	m	IV	pneumonia (aspiration)	persistent low output	9 d
	84	m	IV	renal/liver failure	persistent low output	5 d
Bremen 6/88						

32.2 $\pm$ 15 mm Hg, AVA increased from 0.49 $\pm$ 0.16 to 0.82 $\pm$ 0.25 cm^2 (Fig. 1). The distribution of valve area before and after valvuloplasty is depicted in Fig. 2. With increasing experience, valve area improvement tended to become better. For the last year the average dilatation result has been 0.86 cm^2 and in one half of the cases the initial valve area could be improved by more than 75% (Figs. 3, 4). The final valve area depended largely on the balloon size used. A post-dilatation valve area of mean 1.0 cm^2 was obtained with the use of the cylindrical 23 mm balloon as the final size, the balloon related differences are shown in Fig. 5.

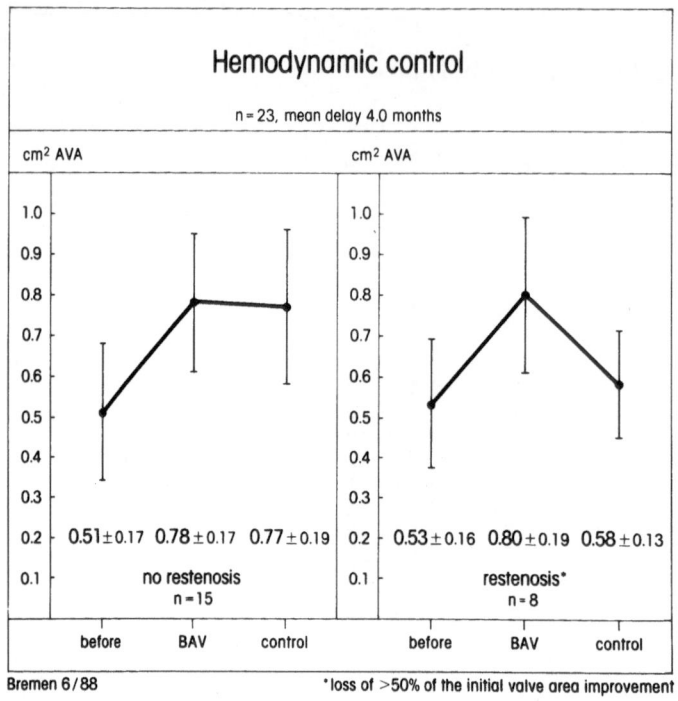

Fig. 6. Invasive follow-up in 23 patients at a mean of 4 months show eight cases (35%) of restenosis

Table 5. Clinical follow up after 6 and 12 months

Clinical follow up n = 78		
Free of symptoms or markedly improved	6 months 26/50 (52%)	12 months 7/31 (22%)
Valve replacement (total)	20/78 (26%)	
Death (total)	13/78 (17%)	

Clinically, 66 patients were in the NYHA class I or II after BAV, eight patients remained in class III and four patients in class IV. The complications of the 89 BAV attempts include two cases of death, five vascular lesions requiring surgical repair, one reversible stroke, two severe regurgitations, and one dissection of the aortic root. Two additional in-hospital deaths occurred, which were not related to the the dilatation procedure (Table 4).

The follow-up data obtained by invasive measurement of 23 patients show eight cases (35%) of restenosis after four months (Fig. 6). Clinically 14 (60%) of these patients were in functional class I or II at that time. Six months after dilatation, 52% of the patients were markedly improved, one year after BAV 22% remained in a stable condition with no or only mild symptoms (Table 5). There were nine late deaths among the discharged patients between one to 11 (mean 6.6) months after BAV, listed in Table 6. Two of them died after aortic valve replacement.

Table 6. Late mortality. COLD denotes chronic obstructive lung disease, CHD coronary heart disease, AVR aortic valve replacement

Late mortality n = 9 (11,5%)

Age	sex	estimated surgical risk high	increased	good	valve area after BAV (cm²)	cause of death	delay (months)
84	m	+			0,49	pneumonia	11
59	w	+ COLD, tumor			0,54	sudden death	4
82	w	+ poor state			0,61	sudden death	2
70	w			+ hypertens./diabetes	0,89	stroke	7
75	m	+ severe CHD, EF 38%			1,33	sudden death	1
73	w	+ poor state, CI 1,6 l/minxm²			0,53	stroke	5
80	m	+			0,67	?	10
67	w			+ COLD	0,61	pneumonia/emergent AVR	10
88	m	+			1,16	pneumonia/AVR (early restenosis)	4

| Total number of patients n = 78 | | | | | | | Bremen 6/88 |

Discussion

Very soon after the first reports of successful aortic valvuloplasty, a controversial discussion – still continuing – developed regarding its value (14). The subject of this debate mainly concerns the possible immediate result, the restenosis rate, as well as early and late mortality compared with the available surgical data (2, 6). First of all it should be emphasized that three years ago, the majority of our patients would never have been recommended for heart catheterization due to the assumed risk of any intervention. Therefore, to date truly comparable surgical series do not exist.

Although recent reports indicate a considerable decrease in mortality of valve replacement in the elderly, the risk remains strongly dependent on patient selection (8). Octogenarians are considered to have a surgical mortality of 30% (8), patients with low ejection fraction, low output, class IV symptoms, cachexia or need of emergency operation are also at high risk (4,8). On the other hand, the prognosis in the spontaneous course of the disease is very poor with a one- and two-year respective mortality of 43% and 73% (12, 17). Summarizing our data, significant clinical improvement after BAV was observed in 84% of the patients. Hemodynamically, the postdilatation valve area remained below 0.70 cm² in 40% of the cases, indicating a persistent severe aortic stenosis, whereas 1.0 cm² or more could be achieved in 20% of the patients. The hemodynamic results vary considerably between the different groups (1, 13, 15). Recent large series demonstrate that an average valve area of 0.90–1.1 cm² is possible (6, 15).

Our results show that often balloons of more than 20 mm diameter are needed, which confirms the experience of others (6, 13). However, two serious regurgitations occurred with obviously oversized balloons, requiring valve replacement. Therefore a careful and gradual increase of the balloon diameter is advised. The early mortality of four patients was clearly correlated to very ill patients in a very advanced state. None of them was a surgical candidate. The restenosis rate in our series was 35%

after four months, as found on repeat invasive measurement in a group overrepresented by symptomatic patients. After six months, the clinical restenosis rate was 48% and a majority of the others may have hemodynamic restenosis as well. Similar to the immediate results, the data of the available reports are quite different concerning time and rate of restenosis (1, 6, 7, 15). In series with minor improvement of valve area the dilatation effect may only last some weeks (1, 6). Safian et al. demonstrated that 50% of the patients can clinically improve for more than one year (15). Therefore similar to Cribier, we suggest that better immediate results may lead to later restenosis, even if in a given patient the outcome is not predictable (6). This question needs further long-term evaluation. Nevertheless, even a one- to two-year improvement qualifies BAV as a palliative treatment for special subgroups of patients with aortic stenosis. For good surgical candidates it is no alternative to surgery, except perhaps in children and young adults with congenital aortic stenosis and less degenerated valves, whose long-term follow-up seems to be much better (18). There is considerable late mortality after BAV. In part, this reflects the general poor prognosis of the very elderly and frail patients with multiorgan impairment (15). In some cases, BAV has been used as a bridge to surgery (3). If patients refuse surgery or have a continued high surgical risk, BAV may be repeated.

In conclusion, BAV should not be seen in competition with surgery. If the assumed surgical risk is high, BAV should be offered. In situations requiring a delay of surgery either due to urgent noncardiac surgical interventions or severely decompensated left ventricular function, BAV can bridge the time until valve replacement will be safer. Despite its limitations, therefore, aortic valvuloplasty is a useful new complementary tool, but it is far from solving all problems in the treatment of aortic stenosis in the elderly or surgical high risk patient.

References

1. Bernard Y, Bassand JP, Anguenot et al. (1988) Early and late evaluation of percutaneous aortic valvuloplasty. A combined hemodynamic and doppler-echocardiographic study. J Am Coll Cardiol 14A
2. Berland J, Cribier A, Savin T et al. (1988) Postvalvuloplasty follow-up of elderly patients with severe aortic stenosis and low ejection fraction. J Am Coll Cardiol 11:15A
3. Block PC (1988) Aortic valvuloplasty – a valid alternative? N Engl J Med 319:169
4. Carabello BA, Green LK, Grossman W et al. (1980) Hemodynamic determinants of prognosis of aortic valve replacement in critical aortic stenosis and advanced congestive heart failure. Circulation 62:42
5. Cribier A, Savin T, Saoudi N et al. (1986) Percutaneous transluminal valvuloplasty of acquired aortic stenosis in elderly patients. An alternative to valve replacement? Lancet I, 63
6. Cribier A, Letac B (1988) Two year experience of percutaneous balloon valvuloplasty in aortic stenosis. Herz 13:110
7. Desnoyers MR, Isner JM, Salem DN et al. (1987) Clinical and non-invasive hemodynamic follow-up of patients treated with balloon valvuloplasty for calcific aortic stenosis. Circulation 76, Suppl IV, 303
8. Edmunds LH, Stephenson LW, Edie RN et al. (1988) Open heart surgery in octogenarians. N Engl J Med 319:131
9. Gorlin R, Gorlin SG (1951) Hydraulic formula for calculation of the area of the stenotic mitral valve, other cardiac valves and central circulatory shunts. Am Heart J 41:1
10. Hakki AH, Iskandrian AS, Bemis CE et al. (1981) A simplified valve formula for the calculation of stenotic cardiac valve areas. Circulation 63:1050

11. McKay RG, Safian RD, Lock JE et al. (1986) Balloon dilatation of calcific aortic stenosis in elderly patients. Post mortem, intraoperative and percutaneous valvuloplasty studies. Circulation 74:119
12. O'Keefe JK, Vlietstra RE, Bailey KR et al. (1987) Natural history of candidates for balloon aortic valvuloplasty. Mayo Clin Proc 62:986
13. Pop TR, Erbel R, Henrichs KJ et al. (1988) Perkutane Angioplastie der stenosierten Aortenklappe: Ergebnisse, haemodynamische Auswirkungen, Komplikationen. Z. Kardiol 77:337
14. Robicsek FN and Harbold NB (1987) Limited value of balloon dilatation in calcified aortic stenosis in adults:direct observations during open heart surgery. Am J Cardiol 60:337
15. Safian RD, Berman AD, Diver DJ et al. (1988) Balloon aortic valvuloplasty in 170 consecutive patients. N Engl J Med 319:125
16. Scherer HE, Hörmann E, Engel HJ (1987) Ballondilatation verkalkter Aortenstenosen. Dtsch med Wschr 112:1694
17. Turina J, Hess O, Sepulcri F et al. (1987) Spontaneous course of aortic valve disease. Eur Heart J 8:471
18. Vogt A, Rupprath G, Tebbe U (1988) Verlaufsbeobachtungen nach Ballondilatation angeborener und erworbener Aortenstenosen. Z Kardiol 77 Suppl 1:86

Experience with mitral valvuloplasty

U. Babic, P. Pejcic, M. Vucinic, Z. Djurisic, S. Grujicic

Cardiovascular Center Dragisa Misovic, Beograd, Yugoslavia

A meaningful experience in non-surgical mitral valvuloplasty has been accumulated over the past five years. The pioneer of this non-surgical, interventional cardiologic procedure was Inoue (1). After Inoue's report, Lock (3), Al Zaibag (4), Vahanian (8) and many other authors reported their modifications of the transvenous mitral balloon valvuloplasty (9–14). The reported results are very encouraging. At our institution the first mitral balloon valvuloplasty was performed in February 1985, using the percutaneous transarterial approach (2).

Since balloon mitral valvuloplasty is absolutely analagous to surgical closed commissurotomy, the indications, contraindications, complications, and expected results should be similar. However, it must not be forgotten that surgeons have over 40 years experience in this field, during which time much has been learned about patient selection, risk factors, and clinical outcome. A good relationship between the interventional cardiologist and the well-experienced surgeon is thus useful for both the cardiologist and the patient.

Indications for transarterial mitral valvuloplasty at our instituion are: symptomatic mitral stenosis (MS) without left atrial thrombi or heavy calcifications of the mitral apparatus; the absence of ilio-femoral arterial disease; asymptomatic mitral stenosis in women who desire a pregnancy in the near future.

Indications for transvenous mitral valvuloplasty at our institution are: symptomatic MS in a patient with ilio-femoral arterial disease or in a patient with an implanted biological prosthesis in the mitral position.

Contraindications to mitral balloon valvuloplasty at our institution are: left atrial thrombus echocardiographic visualized; heavily calcified MS; recent embolic event; no informed consent.

Technique

Our transarterial technique has been described (2, 5, 6). One or two long guidewires (3.5 meter) are introduced from the right femoral vein trans-septally through the left atrium, left ventricle, and into the aortic root where they are caught and exteriorized through the femoral arteries. Over these guidewires, the dilatation balloon catheter is introduced transarterially across the mitral valve and inflated. In the majority of our patients the double balloon technique is used.

Patient population

Of the 183 patients treated, the majority were females aged 30–40 years with long-standing atrial fibrillation. All except five were symptomatic. These were planning pregnancies, and therefore were accepted for dilation although they were not symptomatic.

Results

At the beginning of our experience the procedure took almost 2 h, while in the last 100 patients, the average time needed for accomplishment of the double balloon

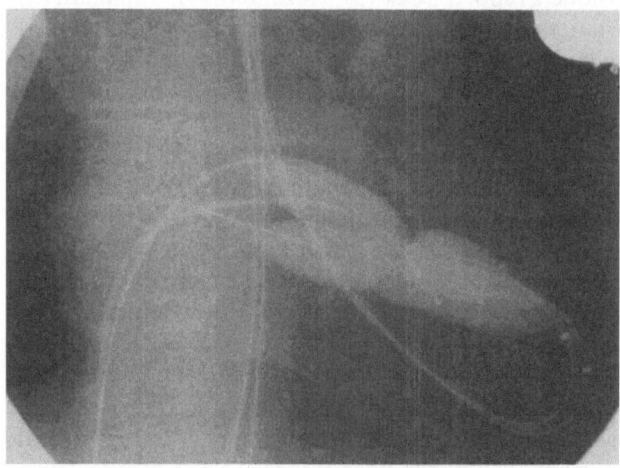

a

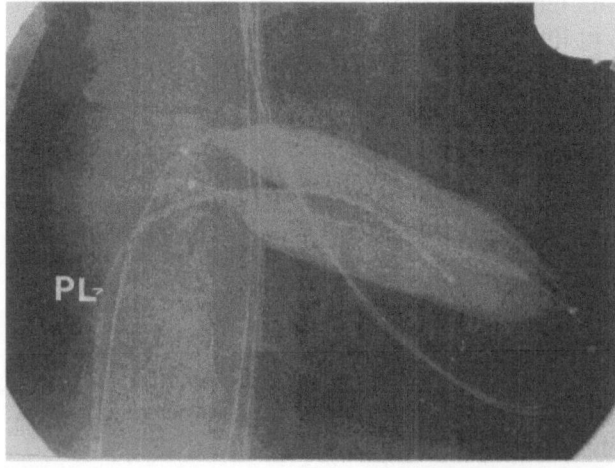

b

Fig. 1. (a, b) Two balloons of 5.5 cm in length (18 and 20 mm) placed transarterially across the mitral valve and semi-inflated with "waisting" (a) and fully inflated (b). PL = pacemaker lead

Table 1. Complications of mitral balloon valvuloplasty in 183 patients

Stroke	4 (1 death*)	2.1%
Coronary embolism	1 (1 death*)	0.5%
Mitral regurgitation	5 (2-IV°, 2-III°, 1-I°)	2.7%
Vascular	5	2.7%
Death**	2	1.1%

mitral valvuloplasty is 40–45 min. The single balloon procedure requires 10–15 min less. The 5.5 cm balloons can be more easily stabilized during inflation than the 3 cm balloons. Each dilation that showed an indentation ("waisting") of the balloon proved to be successful (Figs. 1a and 1b). In some younger patients with very pliable mitral valves, the "waisting" could not be visualized by flouroscopy, but only by cineangiography.

The mitral valve area could be enlarged on the average by 100%. The enlargement was more prominent in patients with a pliable mitral valve. The mitral pressure gradient could be improved significantly but not abolished (19 to 8 mm Hg). Clinical improvement was best registered during the follow-up period but many patients noticed a clinical relief as soon as one day after the procedure. For follow-up, cardiothoracic ratio, echocardiography (two-dimensional mitral valve area and left atrial diameter) and Swan-Ganz right heart catheterization on an out-patient basis were employed. These parameters showed long-term persistence of the hemodynamic improvement. The restenosis rate was relatively low (about 4%) over more than three years. Surprisingly, patients with residual stenosis did not show a higher restenosis rate in the follow-up period.

Complications

The complications are summarized in Table 1. The most serious is stroke. Although two-dimensional echo can easily visualize a large, well organized thrombus of the left atrium, it is not sensitive enough to exclude all thrombi, especially those located in the auricula. The transesophageal echocardiographic technique is certainly more sensitive, but is poorly tolerated by many patients. In some high-risk patients, we used an emboli protection device. This is a selfopening six-wire construction that is introduced transarterially through an 8-French long sheath into the aortic root where it is opened. The heparinized nylon net assumes an umbrella-like position and provides a barrier to the possible embolic particles (Fig. 2 a, b, c). The device can be used only during the transvenous procedure. We used it in patients with Ionescou-Shiley mitral bioprostheses and in patients with a history of recent embolic events.

Mitral regurgitation occurred in 2.7% of patients and required elective surgery. A trace of mitral insufficiency was present in about 25% of dilated patients. Two patients died due to embolic events. Local arterial problems could be managed promptly without any residual morbidity.

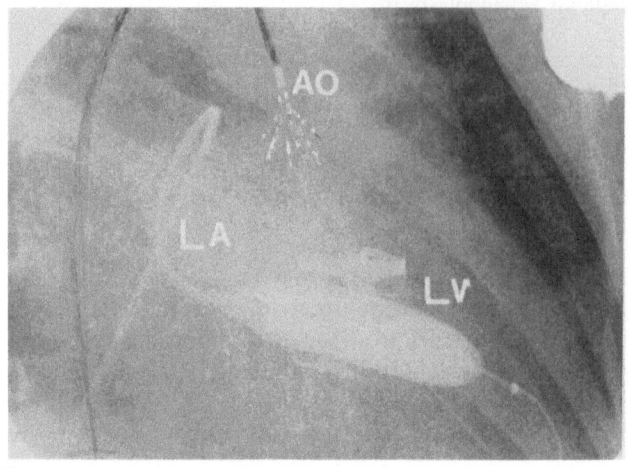

a

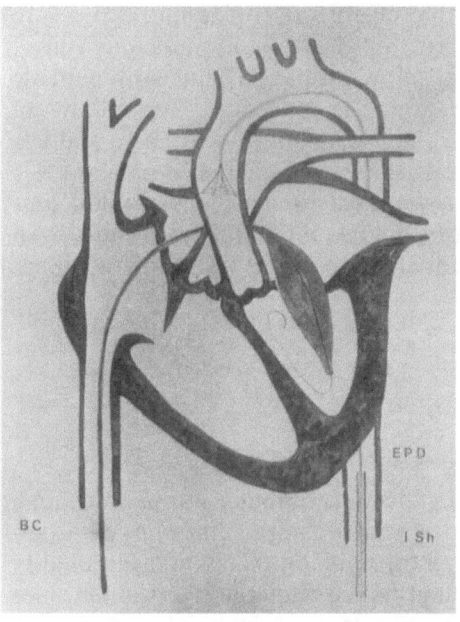

b

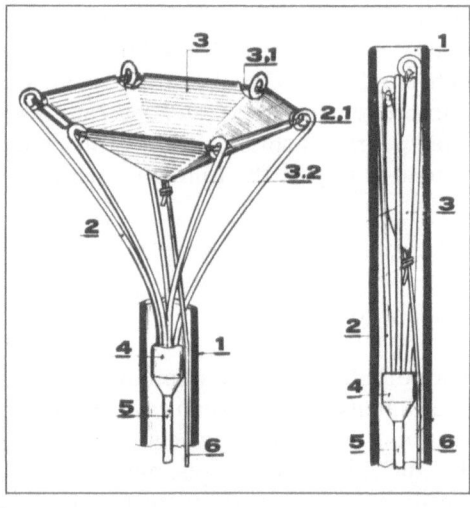

c

Fig. 2. (a, b, c) Transvenously placed balloon across the bioprosthetic (Ionescou-Shiley) stenotic mitral valve while the emboli-protector-device (EPD) is placed into the aortic root. AO = aorta; BC = balloon catheter; ISh = introducer long sheath; LA = left atrium; LV = left ventricle. (a) cineangiographic (b) schematic image (c) drawing of the emboli-protecting device. 1 = introducer sheath; 2 = self-opening wires; 3 = nylon net; 4 and 5 = body of the device

Discussion

There is an unamity of reports that the mitral valve can effectively be dilated with balloons (1–14). The two main approaches to the mitral valve are transvenous and

92

Table 2. Frequency of ASD creation during the transvenous mitral balloon valvuloplasty

Autor	ASD/Pts	%	QP/QS
Diver DJ. (7)	5/14	36	
Vahanian A (8)	3/62	5	1.5
Cunningham MJ (9)	10/43	23	1.4
Ruiz EC (10)	4/41	10	
Alzaibag MA (11)	3/30	10	
Cunninghamm MJ (12)	14/60	23	1.5
Vahanian A (13)	10/81	12	
Come PC (14)	12/37	32	1.6
TOTAL	61/368	16	1.5

ASD = atrial septal defect; QP/QS = pulmonary to systemic flow ratio; PTs = patients

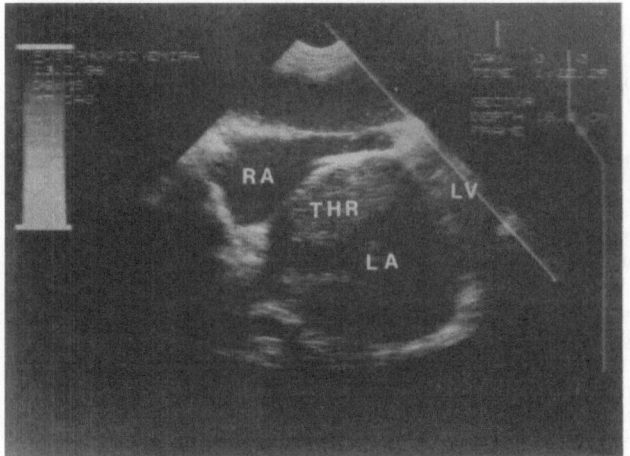

Fig. 3. A large thrombus (THR) is seen inside the left atrium (LA). LV = left ventricle; RA = right atrium. Note the bulging of the septum towards the RA

transarterial. The transvenous route has three or four modifications, all claimed to be superior and advantageous. The crucial question is, can the interatrial septum be perforated with two large balloons without creation of a hole that could be hemodynamically significant and thus affect results?

This question has not yet been answered. Individual reports based on intraoperative observations in patients previously dilated do not provide convincing proof to disprove the presence of an atrial septal defect. The incidence of this complication after transvenous mitral valvuloplasty is 16% (Table 2). According to our own studies on cadaver hearts, each transvenous mitral valvuloplasty that uses two balloons through the same septal hole produces a hemodynamically significant defect (6). The interatrial septum in patients with mitral stenosis bulges towards the right atrium, sometimes like an aneurysm (Fig. 3) and each "slit" in it could have high flow capacity. The transarterial technique is free of this complication. The creation of mitral regurgitation should be equal in incidence in both the transvenous and transarterial technique. The best prevention of thromboembolism is good patient selection. However, bearing the surgical experience in mind, which itself is not free of embolic complications, it is not realistic to expect that balloon mitral valvotomy will not have embolic complications. The mortality rate can probably be expected to be lower than after closed surgical commissurotomy, but it will not be possible to totally eliminate it.

References

1. Inoue K, Owaki T, Nakamura T et al. (1984) Clinical application of transvenous mitral commissurotomy by a new balloon catheter. J Thorac Cardiovasc Surg 87:394
2. Babic UU (1985) Percutaneous transarterial balloon valvuloplasty for mitral valve stenosis: a new technique. In: Vucinic M. (ed): Yugoslav-French Int. Seminar on Cardiac Surgery. Belgrade, Studio Plus, p. 17–25
3. Lock JE, Khalilullah M, Shrivasta et al. (1985) Percutaneous catheter commissurotomy in rheumatic mitral stenosis. N Engl J Med 313:1515
4. Al Zaibag M, Kasab SA, Ribeiro PA et al. (1986) Percutaneous double balloon mitral valvotomy for rheumatic mitral stenosis. Lancet 1:757–761
5. Babic UU, Pejcic P, Djurisic M et al. (1986) Percutaneous transarterial balloon valvuloplasty for mitral valve stenosis. Am J Cardiol 57:1101
6. Babic UU, Pejcic P, Djurisic et al. (1988) Percutaneous transarterial balloon mitral valvuloplasty: 30 months experience. Herz 13:91
7. Diver DJ, Berman AD, Lock JE et al. (1987) Percutaneous balloon mitral valvuloplasty: Acute results and long-term follow-up. JACC 9:14
8. Vahanian A, Michel PL, Cormier B et al. (1988) Perkutane transluminale Valvuloplastie der Mitralklappe. Herz 13, 84.
9. Cunningham MJ, Diver DJ, Berman AD et al. (1987) Balloon mitral valvuloplasty: hemodynamic results and long-term follow-up. Circulation 76:1972
10. Ruiz EC, Lau FYK (1987) Percutaneous double balloon valvuloplasty (PDBV) in 41 adults with mitral stenosis. Circulation 76:304
11. Alzaibag MA, Ribeiro P, Alkasab S (1988) One year follow-up results after percutaneous double balloon mitral valvotomy. JACC 11:15
12. Cunningham MJ, Diver DJ, Berman AD et al. (1988) Acute hemodynamic results and clinical follow-up in patients undergoing balloon mitral valvuloplasty JACC 11:15
13. Acar J, Vahanian A, Michel PL et al. (1988) Percutaneous mitral commissurotomy: a report of 90 cases. JACC 11:220
14. Come PC, Riley MF, Diver DJ et al. (1988) Noninvasive assessment of mitral stenosis before and after percutaneous balloon mitral valvuloplasty. Am J Cardiol 61:817

Assessment of left ventricular function during aortic balloon valvuloplasty by transesophageal echocardiography

K. J. Henrichs [1], R. Erbel [1], A. Cribier [2], T. Pop [1], S. Sack [1], B. Letac [2], J. Meyer [1]

[1] II. Medical Clinic, University of Mainz, FRG
[2] Department of Cardiology, University of Rouen, France

Introduction

Several reports have documented the feasability and utility of balloon aortic valvuloplasty as a palliative treatment for high-surgical-risk patients with critical aortic valve stenosis (1–3).

Evaluation of left ventricular function after the procedure demonstrated either improvement or no change of left ventricular functional variables in the majority of cases. However, in a minority of cases, worsening of left ventricular function was observed after the procedure in comparison with the pre-valvuloplasty condition. Some patients developed left ventricular pump failure, indicating that the procedure may be harmful in some patients (4).

Accordingly, the purpose of the present study was to assess the acute effects of balloon dilatation of the aortic valve on left ventricular performance by the use of transesophageal echocardiography in a group of adult patients with critical aortic stenosis.

Methods

Study population

The study group was comprised of 20 patients (seven males, 13 females) with a mean age of 74 years (range: 55–92 years). All patients were symptomatic with a history of syncope, angina, or dyspnea on exertion, or congestive heart failure. All patients had previously undergone echocardiography and hemodynamic examination where critical aortic stenosis could be documented. None of the patients had significant coronary artery disease at coronary angiography prior to the valvuloplasty procedure. Eight patients were offered valve replacement but refused such a procedure. Seven patients who were offered a choice of either valvuloplasty or surgical valve replacement preferred the valvuloplasty procedure. All patients gave informed consent for balloon aortic valvuloplasty after being informed of the risks and potential complications of the procedure.

Aortic valvuloplasty procedure

All patients underwent left heart catheterization from a percutaneous femoral approach. Right heart catheterization was performed from either the left or right femoral vein with a Swan-Ganz-balloon-tipped catheter. The left ventricular cavity was approached by either a pigtail catheter (USCI) or Sones catheter with a straight-tipped guidewire to cross the aortic valve. In 10 patients an additional left ventricular cavity catheter was placed via a transseptal approach.

Hemodynamic calculation of aortic valve area was performed according to the Gorlin formula (5). Echocardiographic evaluation of aortic valve area was performed by using the continuity equation (6).

In those patients with an aortic regurgitation greater than II+ at preceding evaluation, valvuloplasty was not attempted. The valvuloplasty procedure was begun by exchanging the left chamber catheter with a 300-cm guidewire, where an additional curve had been placed at the distal tip to minimize the chance of subsequent left ventricular perforation.

Balloon dilatation was performed by advancing a 15-mm valvuloplasty balloon catheter (Mansfield, BSIC, Hilden, FRG) over the guidewire and positioning the balloon into the plane of the aortic valve. Ballon inflations were performed by hand injection of a saline-contrast medium mixture. The duration of balloon inflation varied between 10 and 30 s. Repeated inflations were performed using larger balloon catheters (up to 23 mm) depending on repeated evaluations of the aortic valve area.

Finally, a pigtail catheter was exchanged over the guidewire into the left ventricle and left ventricular angiography, then hemodynamic evaluation and aortic root angiography were performed.

Transesophageal echocardiography

Transesophageal echocardiographic studies were performed using a Toshiba SSH-65 A phased array sector scanner and a fiber-echoscope (ESB-37 SR, Toshiba, Delft, Netherlands) with a 3.75 MHz transducer.

Each patient's history was evaluated to exclude any esophageal disease which was considered a contraindication for the procedure. Before insertion of the probe local anesthetic spray (Lidocain, Astra Chemicals) was applied to the pharyngeal region and 0.3 mg buprenorphine (Temgesic, Boehringer Mannheim) were administered intravenously. The echoscope was advanced blindly. For the esophageal studies, additionally, informed consent of the patients was obtained. After advancing the scope at a length of 35–40 cm from patient's incisors into the stomach and at anteflexion of the distal portion of the scope, cross-sectional images of the left ventricle (short axis views) at the midpapillary muscle level were obtained; care was taken that the ventricular cavity appeared in a circular rather than an elliptical shape. After drawing back the scope with the tip at a distance of 25 to 30 cm from patient's incisors the left ventricle could be imaged in the long-axis view and the transducer was focused on the mitral valve. Doppler flow patterns across the mitral valve were obtained. During each balloon inflation the echoscope was kept in either position for continous monitoring. Periods of interest (preinflation, inflation period, postinflation) were recorded on videotape for later detailed analysis.

ECG and left ventricular pressure, as well as aortic pressure were continuously recorded during the procedure.

Quantitative assessment of left ventricular function

Epicardial and endocardial borders were traced, and by the aid of a graphics tablet and a semiautomatic computer system (Kontron 200, Munich, FRG) enddiastolic and endsystolic areas of the short-axis view of the left ventricle were calculated. Enddiastole was defined at the peak of the R wave in the electrocardiogram which was recorded simultaneously. Endsystole was defined as the smallest ventricular silhouette. From these variables left ventricular area ejection fraction and endocardial circumferential shortening could be calculated. Short-axis views of the left ventricle at the midpapillary muscle level were considered representative of left ventricular volume, because previous papers confirm that minor axis shortening is closely correlated to stroke volume (7, 8).

Additionally, in those patients where left ventricular pressure was continuously monitored, left ventricular meridional wall stress as a quantitative index of myocardial afterload could be calculated (9).

Turbulent regurgitant jets across the mitral valve were traced and the regurgitant jet area was used as a semiquantitative measure of mitral regurgitation.

Left ventricular short-axis dimensions and mitral regurgitation were evaluated throughout the cardiac cycle before, during, and after balloon insufflation.

Documentation

Enddiastolic and endsystolic left ventricular area, as well as area-ejection-fraction are shown as obtained before and during balloon inflation and 90–120 s after deflation of the valvuloplasty balloon. Individual values and means ± standard error are presented.

Results

As shown in Table 1, the mean peak-to-peak pressure gradient across the aortic valve was found at 86 ± 6 mmHg and mean aortic valve area was 0.59 ± 0.03 cm² in our patient group. After the procedure, aortic valve area was found at 1.02 ± 0.09 cm² with a mean peak-to-peak gradient of 44 ± 5 mmHg. Enddiastolic left ventricular cavity area considerably increased during balloon inflation but returned to nearly preinflation levels within 2 min after balloon deflation, as shown in Fig. 1; accordingly, left ventricular area-ejection-fraction decreased during the balloon inflation period, but left ventricular function returned to nearly pre-inflation levels after balloon deflation (Fig. 2).

Recovery of left ventricular function was not impaired with each subsequent balloon inflation.

Table 1. Aortic valve gradient and area before and after valvuloplasty

	Before valvuloplasty	After valvuloplasty
Gradient mm Hg (SEM)	86 (6)	44 (5)
Valve Area (cm²)	0.59 (0.03)	1.02 (0.09)

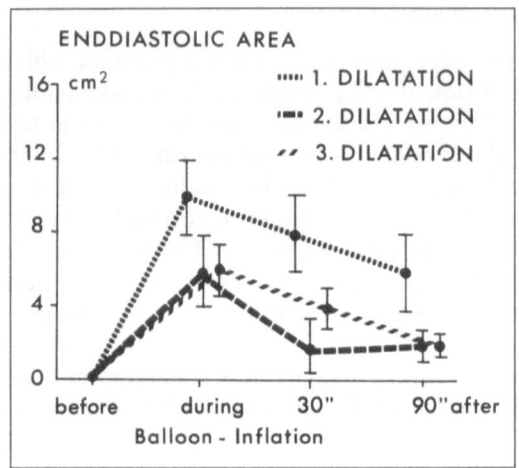

Fig. 1. Enddiastolic left ventricular cavity area as obtained in the short-axis view shows an increase during balloon inflation at the valvuloplasty of the aortic valve; after balloon deflation left ventricular enddiastolic cavity area gradually returned to near baseline levels

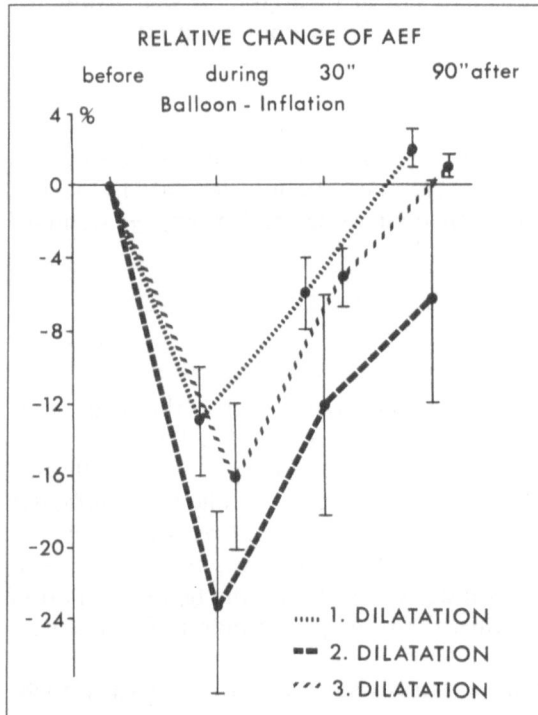

Fig. 2. Left ventricular area-ejection-fraction decreased as a result of increased afterload and returned to preinflation levels within 2 min after balloon deflation during aortic valvuloplasty

Evaluation of color Doppler flow across the mitral valve showed an increase of mitral regurgitation during balloon inflation in the majority of cases with return to preinflation levels within 2 min after balloon deflation (Fig. 3). In one patient, considerable decrease of mitral regurgitation was found after valvuloplasty when compared with prevalvuloplasty values.

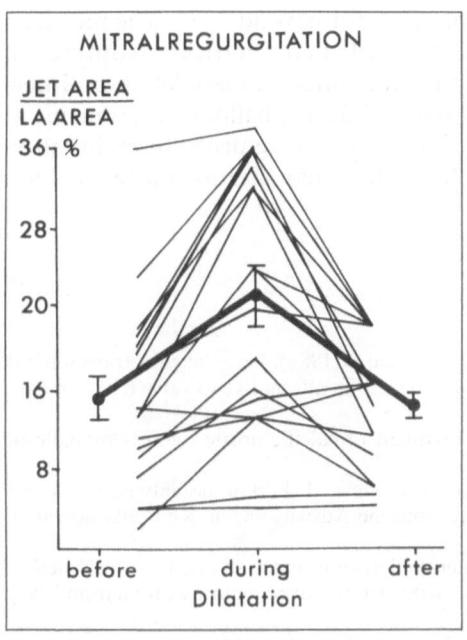

Fig. 3. Mitral regurgitation, as assessed by color Doppler imaging, increased during aortic valvuloplasty as a result of increased afterload, but returned to baseline levels after balloon deflation

Conclusion

Percutaneous aortic valvuloplasty appears as a feasible, but yet palliative treatment in a selected group of patients with critical aortic stenosis because of limited immediate and long-term efficacy (10), but in addition, because a variety of procedure-related complications, such as pump failure have been observed (1–4).

Pump failure could be related to ischemic events because of compromised coronary perfusion due to reduced perfusion pressure during prolonged balloon inflation; but also left ventricular perforation has been observed during aortic valvuloplasty.

Transesophageal echocardiography has proven to be a valuable method for continuous and on-line observation of regional and global left ventricular function during cardiological interventions. Complications such as ventricular perforation with subsequent pericardial effusion or tamponade can be readily detected by this approach. Furthermore, transesophageal echocardiography allows direct visualization of the valvuloplasty balloon which can be used for the optimal transvalvular balloon placement (11); imaging of aortic valve leaflets and planimetry of the aortic valve area appears to be useful for immediate evaluation of the valvuloplasty effect obviating the need for repetitive angiography.

Our data show that in all cases balloon inflation results in abrupt and considerable increase of left ventricular afterload with increase of enddiastolic and endsystolic left ventricular volumes. Reduction of contraction was marked during the balloon inflation period. Increase in left ventricular afterload implements an increase of left ventricular wall stress, this – together with a reduction in coronary perfusion pressure – could result in ischemic alterations during prolonged periods of balloon inflation. In our series with balloon inflation time not beyond 30 s, ischemic alteration of left ventricular pumping was not observed. Left ventricular contraction variables returned to preinflation levels within 2 min after balloon deflation. Interestingly, with an increase of left ventricular afterload during balloon inflation mitral regurgitation was shown to be considerably increased, but returned to preinflation levels in most cases with the reduction of left ventricular afterload after balloon deflation.

References

1. Cribier A, Saouch N, Berland J, Savin T, Rocha P, Letac B (1986). Percutaneous transluminal valvuloplasty of aquired aortic stenosis in elderly patients: an alternative to valve replacement? Lancet 1:63–7
2. Isner JM, Salem DN, Desmayers MR, et al. Treatment of calcific aortic stenosis by balloon valvuloplasty. Am J Cardiol 1987; 59:313–7
3. Pop T, Erbel R, Henrichs KJ, Todt M, Bednarczyk I, Meyer J. Perkutane Valvuloplastie der stenosierten Aortenklappe: Ergebnisse, haemodynamische Auswirkungen, Komplikationen. Z Kardiol 1988; 77:337–45
4. Mc Kay RG, Safian RD, Lock JE, et al. Assessment of left ventricular and aortic valve function after aortic balloon valvuloplasty in adult patients with critical aortic stenosis. Circulation 1987; 75:192–203
5. Braunwald E (ed). Heart Disease. Philadelphia, London, Toronto, 1988
6. Zoghbi WA, Farmer KL, Soto L, et al. Accurate noninvasive quantification of stenotic aortic valve area by Doppler echocardiography. Circulation 1986; 73:452–5
7. Rankin JS, McHale PA, Arentzen CE, et al. Three dimensional dynamic geometry of the left ventricle in the conscious dog. Circ Res 1976; 39:304–13
8. De Bruijn NP, Clements FM. Transesophageal Echocardiography. Boston, Dordrecht, Lancaster, 1987
9. Quirmones MA, Mukotoff DM, Nouri S, et al. Noninvasive quantification of left ventricular wall stress: validation of method and application to assessment of chronic pressure overload. Am J Cardiol 1980; 45:782–90
10. Serruys PW, Kijten HE, Beatt KJ, et al. Percutaneous balloon valvuloplasty for calcific aortic stenosis. A treatment "sinecure"? Eur Heart J 1988; 9:782–94
11. Cyran SE, Kimball TR, Schwartz DC, et al. Evaluation of balloon aortic valvuloplasty with transesophageal echocardiography. Am Heart J 1988; 115:460–2

3. New techniques for revascularization

Percutaneous transluminal atherectomy of the peripheral and coronary arteries

J. B. Simpson

Department of Cardiology, Sequoia Hospital, Redwood City, California, USA

Introduction

Since the first coronary angioplasty was performed in 1977 by Gruentzig, angioplasty has gained wide acceptance as a treatment for coronary artery disease. Angioplasty is a less invasive and less costly alternative to bypass surgery and has a lower morbidity. Over the last decade improvements in the equipment have allowed for expanded indications for angioplasty, thereby increasing the number of patients able to be treated with this procedure. Angioplasty, however, has been plagued with a recurrence rate of approximately 30%, as well as acute occlusions resulting from dissections. In addition, eccentric lesions do not respond well to angioplasty and hard, fibrous or calcified lesions often fail to dilate. Atherectomy is one of several new techniques currently being developed to address these shortcomings.

Catheter design

The atherectomy catheter is designed to remove atheromatous obstructions from peripheral as well as coronary arteries. The distal end of the catheter is composed of a hollow metal cylinder (housing), with a longitudinal opening (window) on one side and a balloon on the other side. Distal to the housing is a flexible collection chamber. A fixed spring tip, which helps negotiate the catheter through the vessel, is attached to the distal end of the catheter. Inside the housing is a cylindrical cutting blade which is attached to a cable. The cable runs through one of the two lumens of the catheter and is attached to a handheld battery-operated motor at the proximal end of the catheter.

Technique

Following angiography to confirm the location of the lesion, the atherectomy catheter is introduced percutaneously and the distal end of the catheter placed across the stenosis (Fig. 1). Once positioned across the lesion, the balloon is inflated to 20–40 psi, which is enough pressure to hold the housing firmly against the atheroma, but is not high enough to create much angioplasty effect, thus minimizing the creation of dissections. The motor is then turned on and the cutter, spinning at approximately 2 000 rpm, is slowly advanced forward, shaving off any obstructing atheroma hanging into the window opening. The strip of shaved atheroma is pushed

101

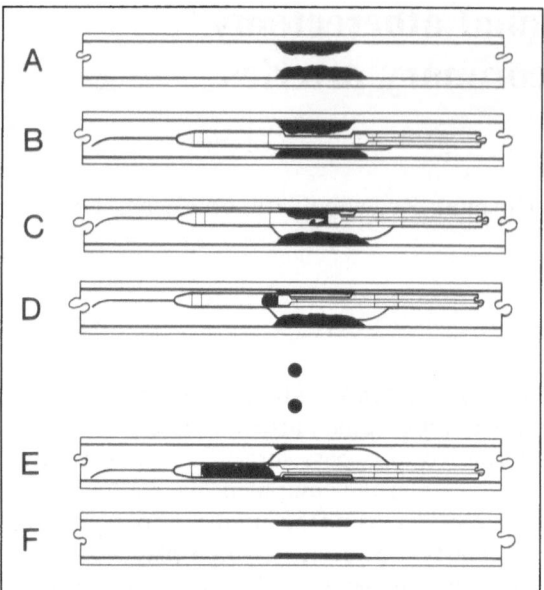

Fig. 1. Diagram of the atherectomy procedure A) the lesion before atherectomy B) the atherectomy catheter across the stenosis C) the atherectomy catheter during the first cutter advancement D) completion of the first cutter advancement with the atheroma shaving pushed into the collection chamber E) the collection chamber full after multiple cutter advancements F) the artery after atherectomy

forward into the distal collection chamber, the balloon is deflated and the cutter torqued so the window is facing another area of atheroma. This sequence is repeated until the lesion is reduced to less than 30%. Upon removal of the catheter from the artery, the specimens are retrieved from the collection chamber, fixed in 10% buffered formalin and sent to our pathologist for histopathologic examination.

Peripheral atherectomy

Since August 1985, we have performed 160 peripheral atherectomy procedures on over 200 lesions, retrieving at least 1 600 specimens. The majority of the stenoses (82%) were in the superficial femoral artery. Fig. 2 shows the pre- and post- angiograms of an atherectomy of an SFA lesion, as well as the specimens removed from the stenosis. The remaining lesions treated were in the iliac, popliteal, anterior tibial or posterior tibial artery. The primary success rate was 92%. The mean degree of stenosis pre atherectomy was 79% and was reduced to 24% postatherectomy . For those lesions treated with a complete atherectomy, defined as a reduction of the lesion to a less than 30% residual stenosis, the restenosis rate was 16%. Of the 160 procedures performed, three complications occurred. There was one probable distal embolization resulting in calf pain that resolved spontaneously within 48 h. One localized thrombus occurred which resolved following intra-arterial infusion of

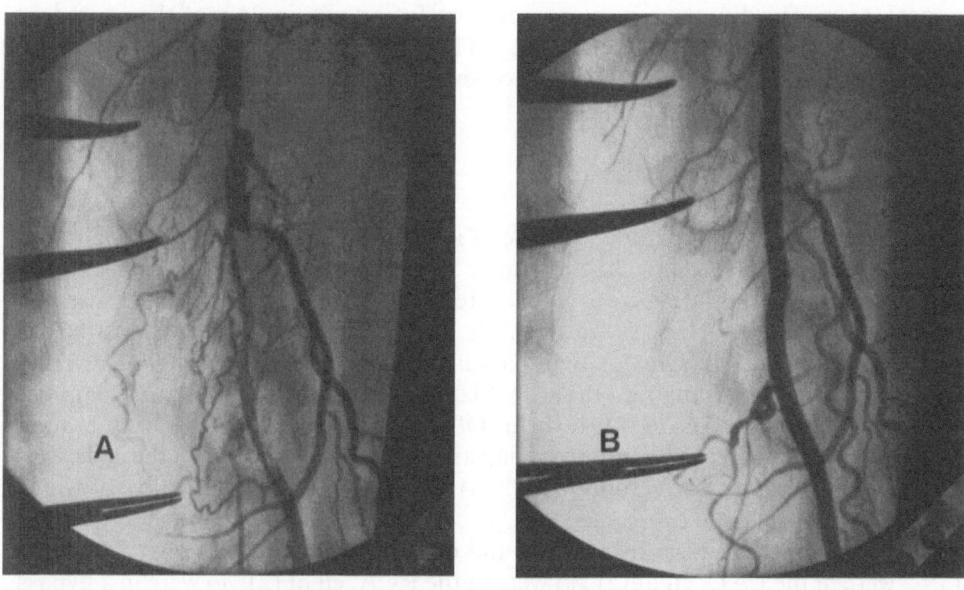

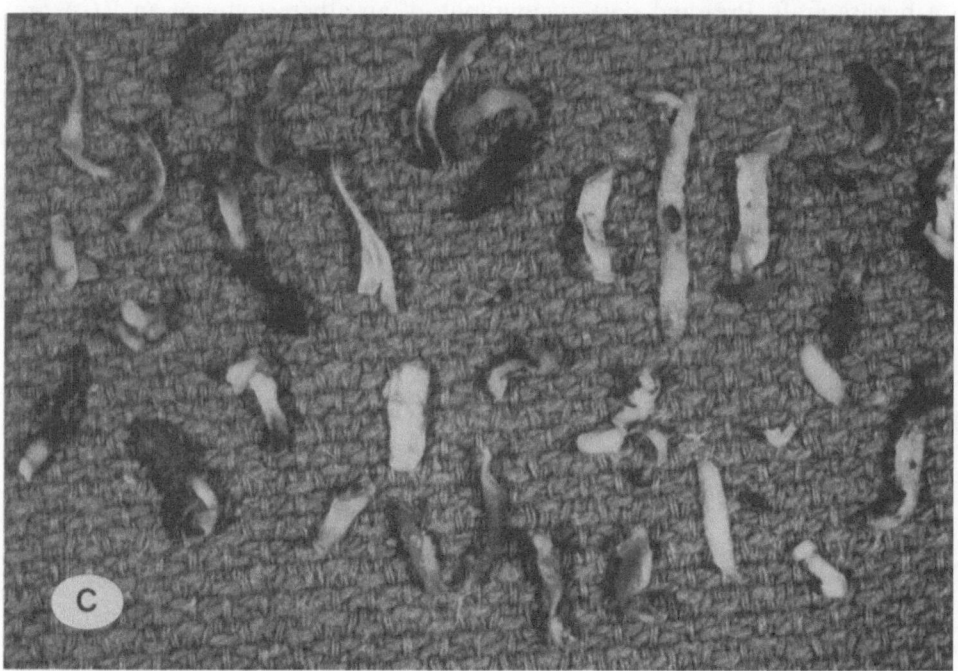

Fig. 2. A) pre-atherectomy angiogram of an SFA B) post-atherectomy angiogram of the same artery C) multiple specimens obtained from the same artery

streptokinase. Thirdly, there was one acute occlusion within 24 h of the procedure and the patient was sent to bypass surgery. There were four dissections noted angiographically, but none were occlusive. No perforations occurred.

Coronary atherectomy

More recently, we have expanded the use of atherectomy into the coronary circulation. Coronary atherectomy catheters range in size from 4.7F through 8F and are used over a movable 0.014- inch guide wire. An 11F guiding catheter is used to introduce the catheter (Fig. 3). To date, we have performed 64 coronary atherectomies on 58 patients. The majority of patients (91 %) were male and 39 (67 %) had Class II or III NYHA angina (Table 1). Sixty-seven lesions have been attempted, retrieving tissue from 51 (76 %) of them. Of those 51 lesions, (75 %) were treated definitively with atherectomy, not requiring any additional therapy. Of the 38 lesions treated with definitive atherectomy, 31 (82 %) were restenosis lesions from a previous PTCA.

Table 2 shows the vessel location of the definitively treated lesions. Seventeen (45 %) were in the LAD, eight (21 %) were in the RCA, eight (21 %) were in a bypass graft, two (5 %) were left main stenoses, and one was a lesion at the site of a stent in a bypass graft. Pre- and post-angiography of an atherectomy of an RCA are shown in Fig. 4. Below the angiograms are the specimens removed.

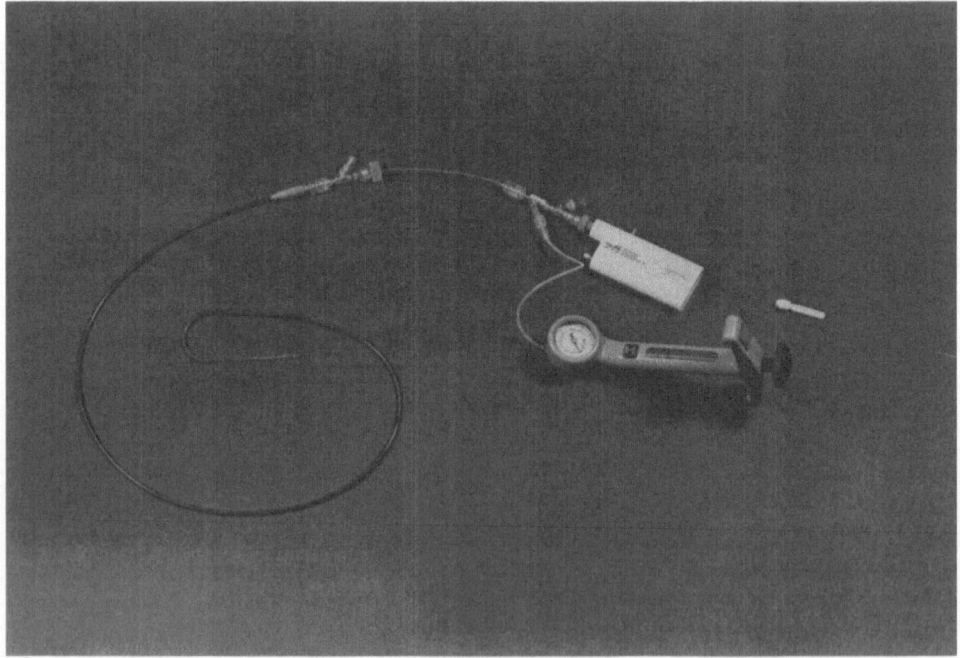

Fig. 3. The coronary atherectomy system including an inflation/deflation device, a 0.014 guide wird an a 7F coronary atherectomy device advanced through an 11F guiding catheter

Table 1. Characteristics and clinical classification of 58 patients treated with the coronary atherectomy catheter

	No.	%
Total Patients	58	100
Age (years)		
Mean Age	58	
Range	18–71	
Sex		
Male	53	91
Female	5	9
NYHA Angina Classification		
Class I	8	14
Class II	23	40
Class III	16	27
Class IV	11	19

Table 2. Lesion distribution of 38 coronary lesions treated definitively by atherectomy

Vessel	No.	%
LAD	17	45
RCA	8	21
Bypass Graft	8	21
LCX	2	5
Left Main	2	5
Stent in Bypass Graft	1	3
Total lesions	38	100

Table 3. Comparison of early and recent results with coronary atherectomy

Procedure	No. of Patients	Patients with Tissue Retrieved	Definitive Atherectomy
1–32	32	20 (63%)	11 (55%)
33–64	32	28 (88%)	24 (86%)

During the early stages of the investigation, while the equipment and technique were both evolving, the success rate was considerably lower than the more recent atherectomies. This is shown in Table 3 by comparison of the first 32 procedures with the last 32 procedures. The percentage of patients from which tissue was retrieved went from 63% in the early group to 88% in the more recent group. Definitive treatment increased from 55% in the early group to 86% in the later group.

Of the 64 procedures, we have had four complications, including one worsened run-off followed successfully with PTCA, one thrombotic occlusion treated success-

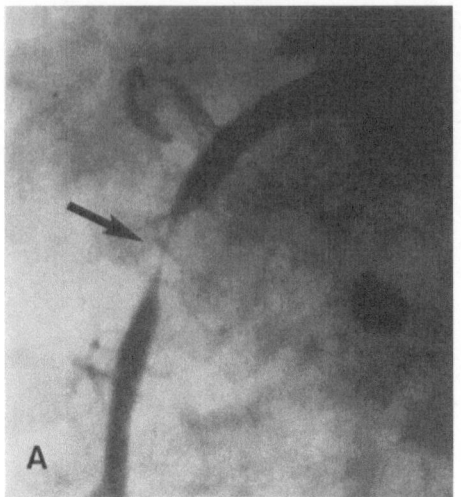
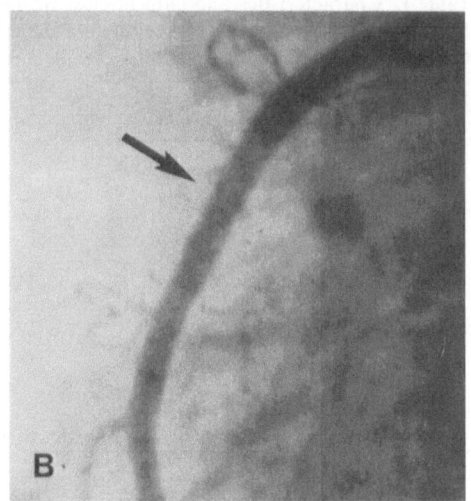
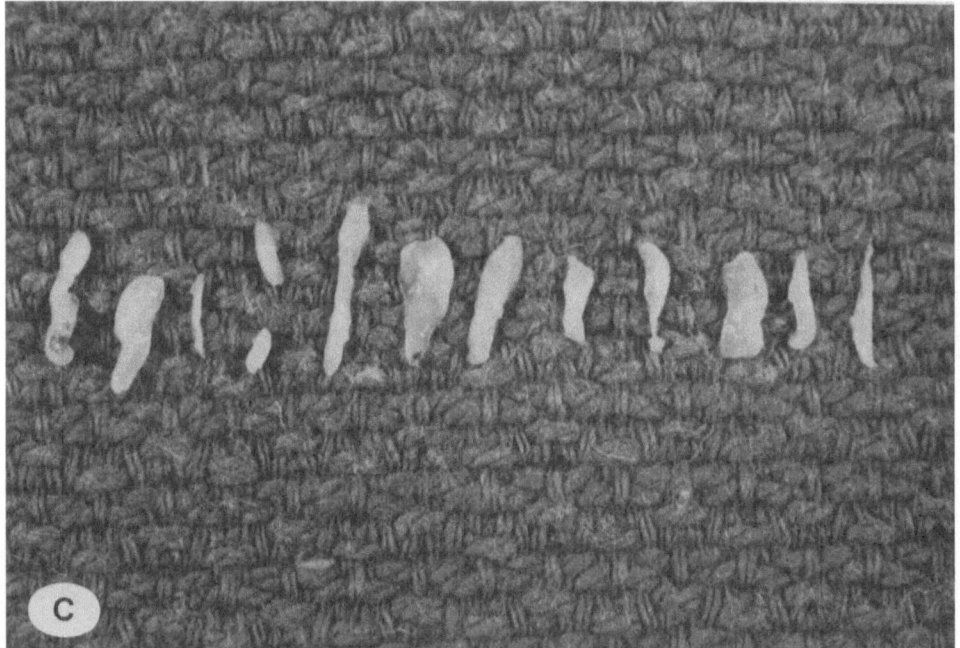

Fig. 4. A) pre-atherectomy angiogram of a proximal RCA stenosis B) angiogram of the RCA post-atherectomy C) specimens removed from the RCA lesion

fully with PTCA, one air embolization which resolved on its own without sequelae, and one dissection which occluded within 12 h and the patient was sent to bypass surgery. There have been no perforations, myocardial infarctions, or deaths.

Histopathology was performed on all tissue specimens removed from both the peripheral as well as coronary arteries. After the specimens were fixed in formalin, they were embedded in paraffin blocks, cut into 4-micron thick sections and stained with various solutions. Overall, tissue from original lesions which had not been previously treated with any prior intervention, were composed of typical atheromatous plaque, consisting primarily of densely collagenous and often lipid-laden tissue. Some had surface thrombus or microcalcification. Specimens removed from restenosis lesions however, often consisted of two separate and distinct layers. One layer was the original atheroma, while the other more recent layer consisted of smooth muscle cell proliferation. Often the restenosis tissue had cracks in the atheroma caused from the angioplasty, with hemorhage filling in the splits.

In conclusion, atherectomy is a safe and predictable method for treating patients with peripheral or coronary artery disease. The luminal borders are smoother and more well-defined than with angioplasty, and the fewer number of dissections created should lower the thrombogenicity and acute occlusion rate. In addition, atheroma is removed rather than just displaced, which may reduce the recurrence rate. Although it is too early to predict what the restenosis rate in the coronary arteries will be, the restenosis rate in the peripheral arteries appears to be about onethird that of angioplasty. Because the tissue is actually removed, it provides us with a unique opportunity to study the atheromatous deposits which will hopefully aid in our understanding of atherosclerosis in general, and restenosis specifically.

Histological findings from "atherectomy" specimens

D. Backa[1], A. v. Pölnitz[1], A. Nerlich[2], B. Höfling[1]

Department of Medicine I[1], Klinikum Großhadern and Institute of Pathology[2], Ludwig Maximilians-University, Munich, FRG

Introduction

The Simpson atherectomy catheter (10) allows the excision of obstructive material from peripheral vessels (4). For the first time this method enables the histological evaluation of percutaneously removed plaques and perhaps the study of primary lesions and their restenoses will give further insight into this rapidly progressing atherosclerotic model.

Methods

We examined the excised specimens from 52 primary stenoses (iliac n = 5, superficial femoral artery n = 44, popliteal n = 3) of 24 patients (mean age 64.4 $\pm$ 8.8 years, 21 male, 3 female). Angiographically the lesions were reduced from 84.4 $\pm$ 14.4% to 16.5 $\pm$ 12.5%. In addition, 7 restenoses from 5 patients (all taking salicylates) occurring at a mean of 5.4 $\pm$ 2.5 months were reatherec tomized and histologically evaluated.

Histological preparation and fixation process

The atherectomy specimens were initially fixed in 6% formaldehyde followed by dehydration in solutions of increasing alcohol concentrations, and then by imbeddment in paraffin. Four to seven micron thick layers could thus be sliced via microtome. After removal from paraffin and rehydration, the preparations were treated with Haemotoxylin-Eosin (HE) and Elastic-van Gieson stains (EvG). With HE staining, basophilic cytoplasm, nucleii and calcifications appear blue while eosinophilic cytoplasm collagenous connective tissue and elastic fibers stain red. Elastic membranes stain light pink. EvG stain nucleii and elastic fibers black, collagenous connective tissue red, and cytoplasm, muscular fibres and fibrin yellow.

Results

Macroscopic appearance

A mean of 5.9 $\pm$ 4.5 desobliterates (max. 20 min. 1) were "atherectomized" from the stenoses. Altogether a total of 305 specimens with a mean length of 4.9 $\pm$ 2.4 mm (max. 13 mm) and width of 1.3 ± 0.5 mm (max. 2 mm) were examined. Macroscopically they appeared to be mainly soft, white, and glistening tissue specimens, sometimes with yellow streaks. In addition, several were of a more calcified nature and significantly, apparent thrombi were often present.

Histological findings in primary stenoses

A total of 305 specimens from 52 stenoses (= 100%) were examined. Intima was present in all stenoses, the internal elastic lamina in 42.3% whereas media could be found in 55.8% of lesions. In addition, 75% of stenoses showed overlying thrombi (Fig. 1). It is striking that endothelium was found in only 3.8%; this could be attributed to disruption of the cell wall due to the atherectomy itself or to the histological preparation process. It is important to note that neither the external

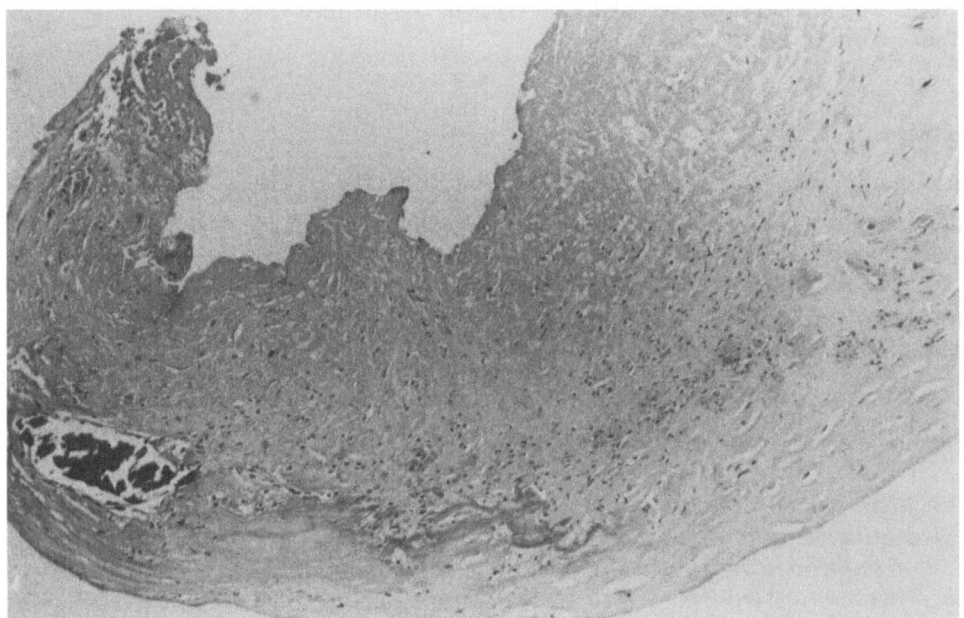

Fig. 1. Thrombotic material with beginning organization overlying a fibrous thickened intima. On the left calcified mass is to be seen (HE, 10 ×)

Table 1. Pathologic changes in 52 primary stenoses

Thickened fibrotic intima	100.0%	(52 stenoses)
Foam cells, inflammartory infiltrates, cholesterol clefts	34.6%	(18 stenoses)
Calcification	15.4%	(8 stenoses)
Thrombi	75.0%	(39 stenoses)
fresh (only fibrin)		(18 stenoses)
organized		(21 stenoses)

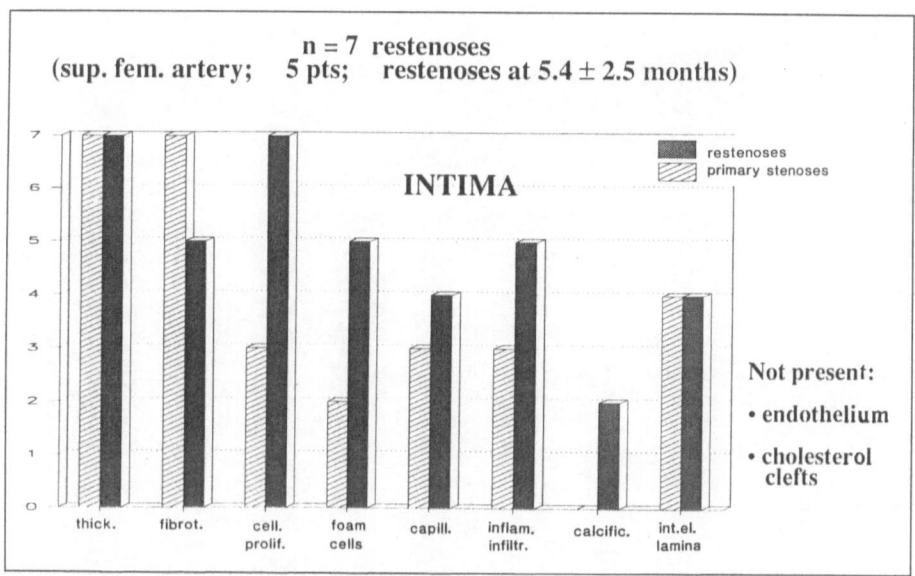

Fig. 2. Histological findings in restenoses compared with their primary lesions

elastic lamina nor the adventitia could be detected in any specimen. The pathological changes found in the primary lesions are described in Table 1. All intimal sections showed irregular fibrosis and thickening, and atherosclerotic plaque material such as foam cells, severe sclerosis, neocapillarization or calcification were found in up to 34.6% of stenoses. Fresh or organized thrombi with cellular infiltration were found overlying 75% of lesions and the classical atheromatous bed with cholesterol clefts could be detected in 5.8%.

Histological findings in restenoses

The histology of the pathological findings within the intima of the restenoses as compared to their primary lesions is shown in Fig. 2. The restenoses (Fig. 3) showed more cellular proliferation, foam cells, and inflammatory infiltration. In addition, the media was reached in all restenotic lesions, and 6 of the 7 had overlying organized thrombi.

Discussion

In the transverse sections of an atherosclerotically altered arterial wall (5, 6, 12) the intima shows initial edema and thickening, then fatty infiltration with smooth muscle cell invasion and foam cell development, followed by fibrosis with neo- capillarization and rupture of the internal elastic lamina. An atheromatous bed with cholesterol clefts and reactive inflammatory infiltrates is also classically described (7, 8) and lies deep within the fibrous thickened intima. Ulceration of this atheroma

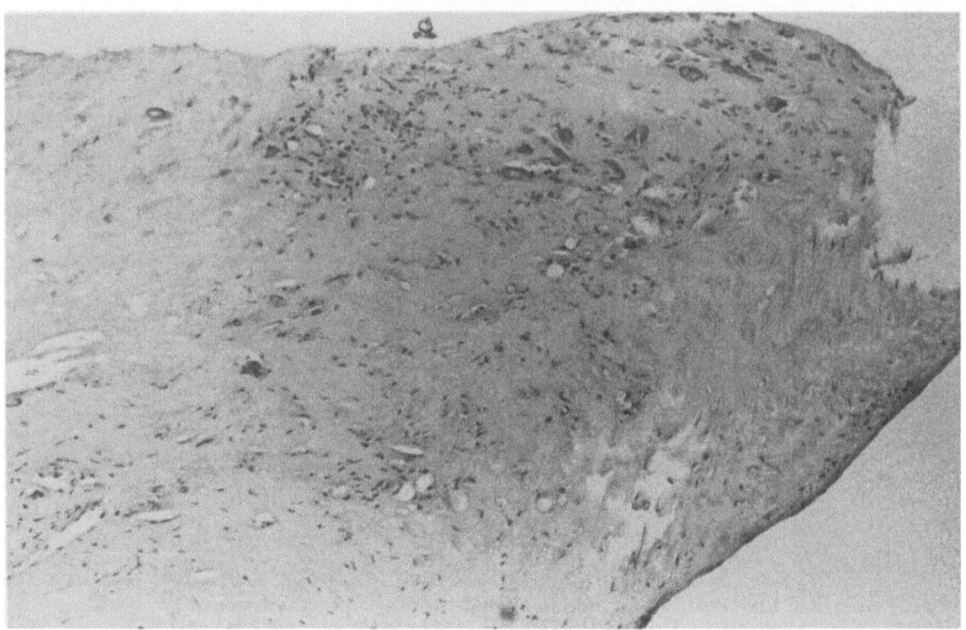

Fig. 3. Specimen of restenosis with irregular cell proliferation, spotty calcification and capillarization (HE, 10 ×)

to the luminal surface induces a thrombotic reaction and probable progression of the stenosis.

Our histological evaluation of removed atherectomy specimens showed a predominance of fibrous intimal thickening, although atherosclerotic plaque material was also obtained, and the classic atheromatous bed was only rarely present. A possible interpretation could be that it is the thickened, fibrotic intima and thrombus overlying the actual plaque which accounts for the hemodynamically relevant stenosis and it is this material which is mainly removed by atherectomy. Alternatively, it might be due to the excision of abundant fibrotic material adjacent to, or from the wall opposite to, the true plaque. Plaque ulceration is difficult to detect on atherectomy specimens due to the disruption of the material secondary to the procedure itself thus making it often not possible to define the luminal surface.

Importantly the media was reached in 55.8 % of stenoses, while the external elastic lamina and the adventitia were never found. This verifies the safety of the atherectomy procedure itself. Evaluation of 7 restenoses compared with their primary lesions showed a slight shift in their morphologic components with more frequently detectable foam cells as well as cellular proliferation and inflammatory infiltrates typical of granulation tissue. In addition, organized thrombus was found in the majority (6/7) of restenoses.

At the present time salicylates and calcium antagonists are most often used post-intervention. The histological findings after atherectomy may help to further guide the prophylaxis of restenosis.

112

References

1. Buss H (1984) Arteriosklerose/Atherosklerose. In: Remmele, W. (ed) Pathologie I. Springer Verlag Berlin, Heidelberg, New York, Tokyo, pp 198–209
2. Feigl W (1987) Morphogenese der Arteriosklerose:Progression und Regression. VASA Suppl 20:41–44
3. Höfling B, Backa D, von Arnim Th, Jauch KW, Simpson JB (1987) Methode, angiographische und klinische Ergebnisse bei perkutaner Atherektomie. VASA Suppl 20:337–342
4. Höfling B, von Pölnitz A, Backa D, von Arnim Th, Lauterjung L, Jauch KW, Simpson JB (1988) Percutaneous atherectomy: a new technique for non-operative removal of obstructive plaques in peripheral vascular disease. Lancet Feb. 20:384–386
5. Hort W (1986) Kreislauforgane/Arterien. In: Eder M, Gedik P (eds) Lehrbuch der Allgemeinen Pathologie und der Pathologischen Anatomie. 32. Aufl., Springer Verlag Berlin, Heidelberg, New York, Tokyo, pp 353–36
6. Llombart-Bosch A (1986) Gefäßsystem/Arterienerkrankungen. In: Grundmann E (ed) Spezielle Pathologie, 7. Aufl, Verlag Urban und Schwarzenberg, München, Wien, Baltimore, pp 35–40
7. Robbins SL, Cotran RS, Kumar V (1984) Blood vessels. In: Pathologic Basis of Disease, 3rd edition. W.B. Saunders Company, Philadelphia, London, Toronto, Mexico City, Rio de Janeiro, Sydney, Tokyo, pp 502–519
8. Ross R, Wight Th N, Strandness E, Thiele B (1984) Human atherosclerosis: I. cell constitution and characteristics of advanced lesions of the superficial femoral artery. Am J Pathol 114:79–93
9. Simpson JB Atherectomy device and method. European patent application Nr. 0 163 502, 4.12.1985
10. Simpson JB, Johnson DE, Thapliyal HV, Marks DS, Braden LJ (1985) Transluminal atherectomy: a new approach to the treatment of atherosclerotic vascular disease. Circulation 72:Suppl 2, III–146
11. Thomas C (1986) Histopathologie. Lehrbuch und Atlas für die Kurse der allgemeinen und speziellen Pathologie. 10. Aufl., Schattauer Verlag Stuttgart New York, pp 2–4
12. Titus JL, Kim HS (1985) Blood vessels and lymphatics. In: Kissane M.J. (ed) Anderson's Pathology, 8th edition, The C.V. Mosby Company, St. Louis, Toronto, Princeton, pp 684–697

Cell culture of human atheromatous plaque material

P. C. Dartsch[1], G. Bauriedel[2], B. Höfling[2], E. Betz[1]

[1] Institute of Physiology I, University of Tübingen, and [2] Department of Medicine I, University of Munich, FRG

Atherosclerosis is an arterial disease that is known to be the main cause of death in Western Europe and in the United States. Consequently, different animal models and experimental designs have been developed to study the progress of this disease. Migration and proliferation of arterial smooth muscle cells from the media into the subendothelial space in response to injury or exposure to potential pathogenic factors are characteristic features in the pathogenesis of atherosclerosis (1–5). Morphology, function and metabolic alteration of endothelial and smooth muscle cells from atherosclerotic arteries of man and of animals have been widely investigated (6, 7). Atheromas contain cells with increased amounts of rough endoplasmatic reticulum and mitochondria, polynuclear and hypertrophied cells (8–12). This investigation describes the isolation of cells from human atheromatous plaque material, their growth in cell culture and characteristic features of these cells.

Materials and methods

In patients with severe arterial occlusive disease, atherosclerotic plaque material was obtained from iliac, femoral, and popliteal arteries with a Simpson atherectomy device (13). The selective capture of material from stenosing tissue of femoral and popliteal arteries was guided by angioscopy (14). Ninety-nine protruding atherectomy specimens from 12 patients were cultivated in an explant technique (15, 16) or cut into small pieces and disaggregated fractionally as follows: for isolation of endothelial cells, specimens were incubated for 20–40 min at 37 °C in dispase grade II (2.4 U/ml, Boehringer Mannheim) containing 1 mg/ml collagenase Worthington CLS III (229 U/mg, Biochrom). The free floating cells were centrifuged after addition of 20% human serum and seeded into cell culture dishes. For isolation of smooth muscle cells, samples were again incubated for another 180 min at 37 °C in the following enzyme mixture: 10 ml of HEPES-buffered culture medium (Ham F 12) containing 18 mg collagenase Worthington, 2 mg elastase from porcine pancreas (Boehringer Mannheim) and 10 mg of trypsin inhibitor from soybean (Serva), pH 7.2. After addition of human serum, isolated cells were centrifuged and plated. Since trypsin damages cells and prevents attachment, its activity had to be blocked.

Cultures were incubated in a moist atmosphere of 37 °C gassed with 7% CO_2. For cell culturing, a mixture of Waymouth's MB 752/1 medium and Ham F 12 (1:1, v/v) supplemented with 10%–15% pooled and heat-inactivated human serum of healthy donors and standard amounts of penicillin and streptomycin (Gibco BRL) were

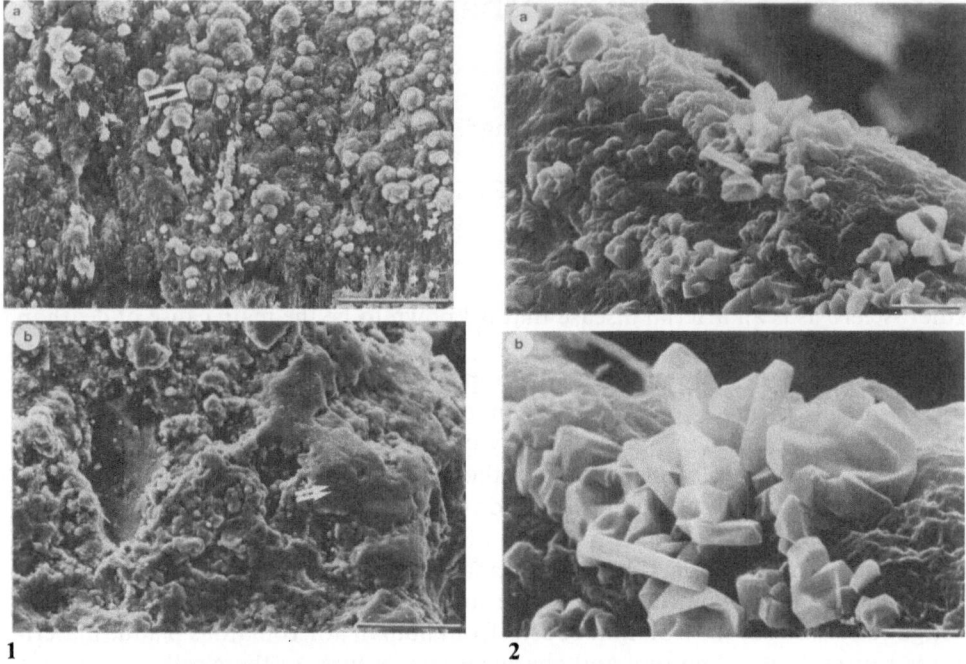

Fig. 1. Scanning electron micrographs of crystalline structures in human atheromatous plaque material selectively removed by the Simpson atherectomy catheter. Note spherical (arrow) and amorphous (double arrow) deposits of calcium phosphate (hydroxyl and carbonate apatite). Scale bars – 10 μm.

Fig. 2. Sodium chloride crystals in different modifications as sometimes observed at edges of atherectomy specimen. Scale bar – 1 μm (a) and 0.5 μm (b).

used. All culture dishes were coated with collagen type I from lathyritic rat skin (Boehringer Mannheim).

For immunological identification and characterization of the cytoskeleton, cells were grown on round glass coverslips. Attached and completely spread cells were fixed in methanol (6 min at −20 °C). Indirect immunofluorescence microscopy with specific antibodies against factor VIII-related antigen (von Willebrand factor; Ortho Diagnostic Systems), smooth muscle α-actin (Biomakor), α- and β-tubulin (Amersham Buchler), vimentin (monoclonal antibodies were a gift of Dr. M. Osborn, Göttingen) and desmin (Biomakor) was carried out as previously described (17). FITC- or TRITCconjugated goat anti-mouse IgG and goat anti-rabbit IgG (secondary antibodies) were purchased from Dianova and Miles Scientific. Fluorescent staining of nuclei and DNA, respectively, was performed with Hoechst stain 33 258 (Farbwerke Hoechst) or with DAPI (4′, 6-Diaminidino-2-phenylindole · 2 HCL; Serva).

Cells were examined and photographed with an inverted microscope Nikon Diaphot TMD (phase contrast) or with a Nikon Optiphot microscope equipped for epifluorescence with appropriate filters sets for green, blue and UV illumination using a Nikon Planapo 40/1.0 or a Nikon Planapo 60/1.4 oil lens. Phase micrographs

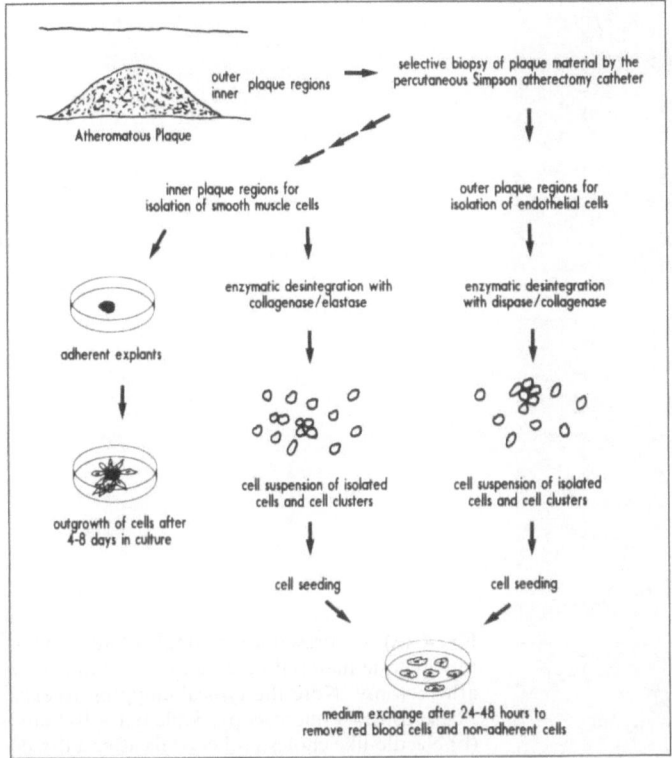

Fig. 3. Schematic presentation of techniques used for isolation of cells from human atheromatous plaque material

were recorded on Kodak Technical Pan 2415 film at 100 ASA rating and epifluorescence micrographs on Kodak Tri-X Pan film at 1 600 ASA rating. Cell proliferation and cell size was measured with a cell counter CASY 1 (Schärfe Systems, Kirchentellinsfurt, FRG).

For scanning electron microscopic examination, atheromatous plaque material was fixed for 3 h in 3.5% formaldehyde, washed with distilled water and air dried. Samples were sputtered with gold palladium (thickness: 20 nm) and crystalline structures were examined by use of a Stereoscan 250 scanning electron microscope (Cambridge Instruments). Element analysis was carried out with an EDAX 9100 X-ray analysis system.

Results and discussion

Within 4–8 days after adhesion, the first cells grew out of the explants. After 10 days, a compact cell layer around the explants had developed. The vast majority of cells exhibited numerous vacuoles around the nuclei and granules on cell surface. At the level of light microscopy, cells exhibited a very pronounced actin filament network, i.e., abundant stress fibers within the cytoplasm. Enzymatically obtained cells were

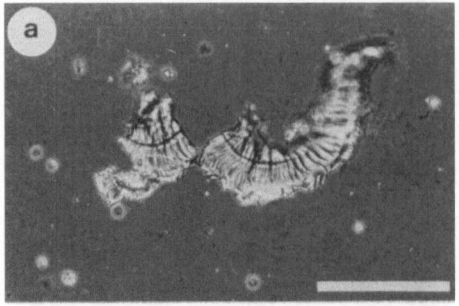

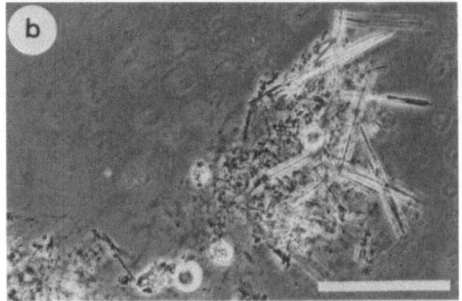

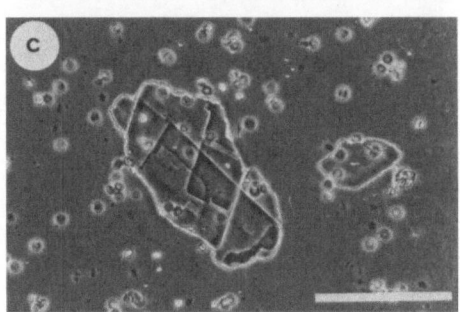

Fig. 4. (a) A representative sample of atheromatous plaque material obtained by percutaneous atherectomy. Note the typical chipping tracks. Phase contrast microscopy. Scale bar – 100 µm. (b) Needle-like cholesterol crystals after a three-hour-enzymatic disintegration of plaque material with collagenase/elastase. Phase contrast microscopy. Scale bar – 100 µm. (c) Rhomboid crystals as sometimes observed in primary cultures after enzymatic disintegration of plaque material. Phase contrast microscopy. Scale bar – 100 µm

attached and spread within 48 h after isolation and seeding, at which time culture medium was exchanged to remove red blood cells. Cell clusters did not attach to culture dishes. Sometimes, insoluble rhomboid crystals were present. Isolated and cultured cells from human atheromatous plaques were not infected with mycoplasmas as checked by a cytochemical technique for DNA demonstration (18).

Most cells (mono- or polynucleated) were elongated and resembled fibroblasts, but polygonally shaped cells, probably endothelial cells, were also detectable. This observation of two morphologically different cell types in culture is confirmed by the results of Haust (10) who examined fatty dots and streaks from the aorta of 12 patients post mortem. He observed two types of binuclear cells and described them as elongated slender cells and as ovoid, probably mesenchymal cells.

In indirect immunofluorescence microscopy, however, the vast majority of isolated and cultured cells of atheromatous plaques exhibited an intense positive reaction with antibodies against smooth muscle α-actin which was shown to be specific for smooth muscle cells only (19, 20). This observation is confirmed by previous elec-

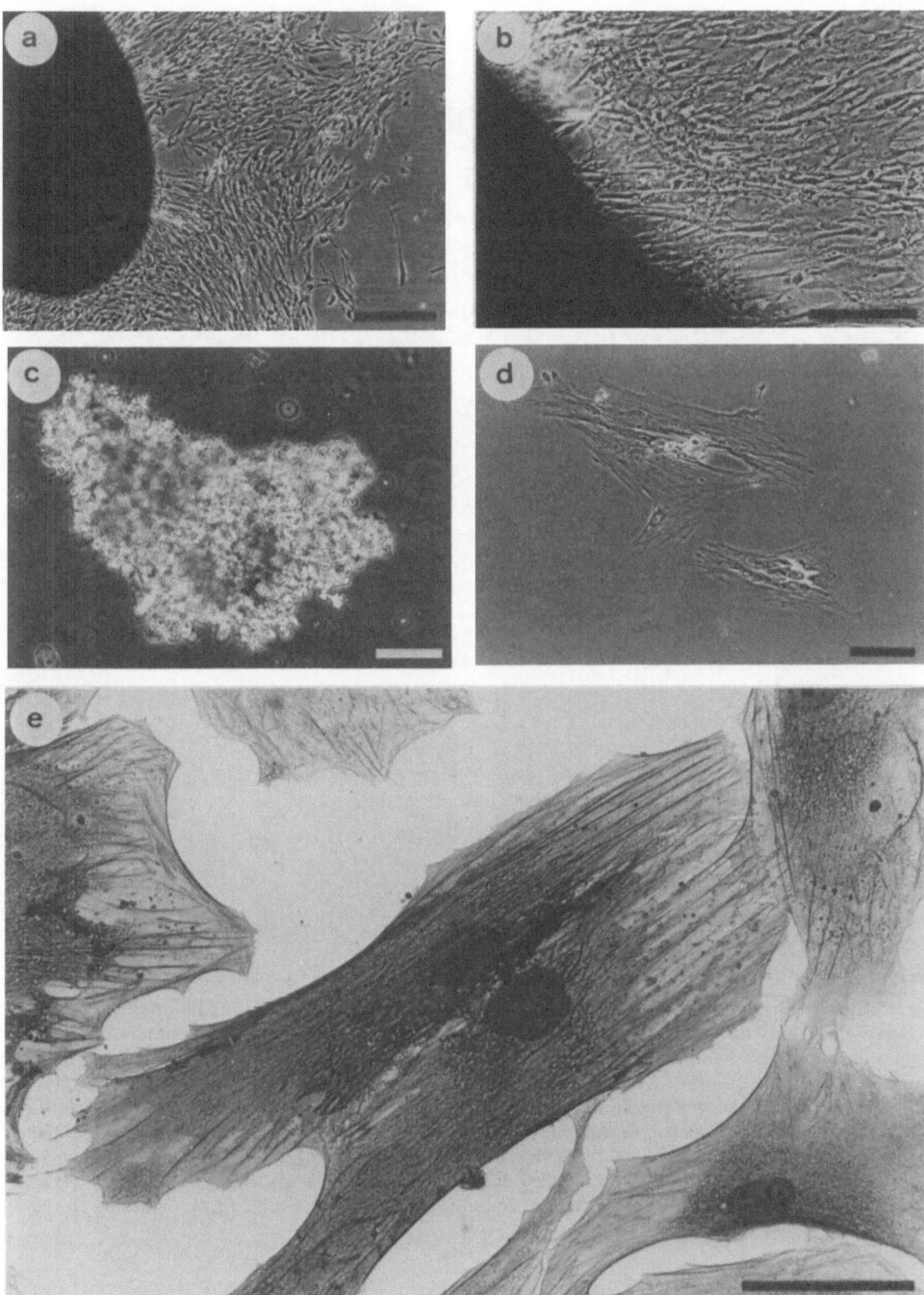

Fig. 5. Cells from atheromatous plaque material in primary cultures and subcultures. (a) and (b) Outgrowth of cells from adherent explants after 14 days in culture. Phase contrast microscopy. Scale bar – 500 µm (a) and 300 µm (b). (c) Undigested cell cluster after enzymatic desintegration with collagenase/elastase. Cell clusters did not attach to petri dish. Phase contrast microscopy. Scale bar – 100 µm. (d) Completely spread cells 48 hours after enzymatic digestion and seeding exhibiting abundant "stress fibers" within the cytoplasm. Phase contrast microscopy. Scale bar – 100 µm. (e) Elongated cell from atheromatous plaque in first subculture. Staining with 0.02% coomassie and 5% giemsa solution. Bright field microscopy. Scale bar – 50 µm.

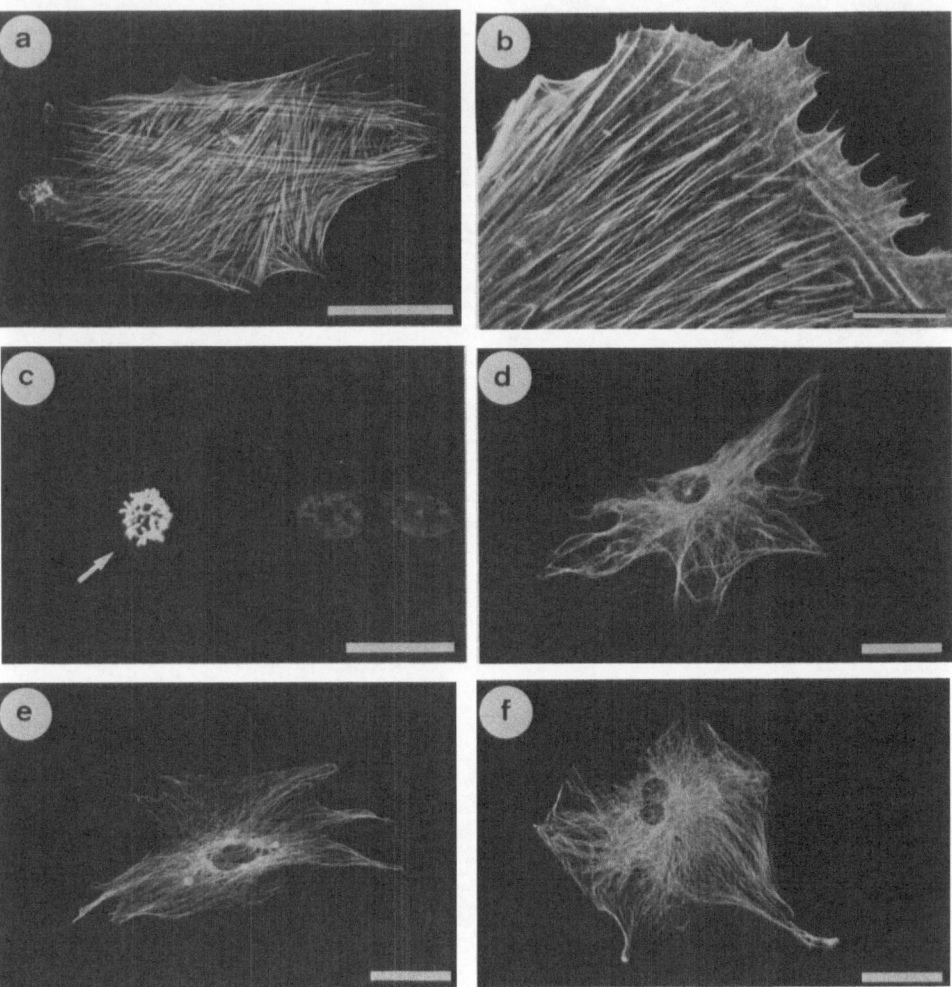

Fig. 6. Indirect immunofluorescence microscopy of cells from atheromatous plaques. (a) and (b) Positive reaction with antibodies against smooth muscle α-actin. Note the three-dimensional network in (a) and the ruffling membrane with microspikes in (b). Epifluorescence microscopy. Scale bar – 50 μm (a) and 10 μm (b). (c) Double fluorescence with antibodies against factor VIII-related antigen and DAPI for counterstaining of cell nuclei. Cells do not react with antibodies against von Willebrand protein, but nuclei are stained intensely. A dividing cell in prophase (arrow) exhibits the elongated chromosomes. Epifluorescence microscopy. Scale bar – 20 μm. (d) Vimentin filaments of a fibroblast-like plaque smooth muscle cell. Epifluorescence microscopy. Scale bar – 50 μm. (e) and (f) Three-dimensional microtubule network of plaque smooth muscle cells. Epifluorescence microscopy. Scale bars – 50 μm

trophoretic results of Gabbiani et al. on human atheromatous plaques (21). Additionally, Gabbiani could also demonstrate a predominance of the β-actin isoform. A positive reaction with antibodies against factor VIII-related antigen, a typical marker for endothelial cells (22–26) was not observed. These data from cell culture indicated that the main portion of isolated and cultivated cells of plaques were

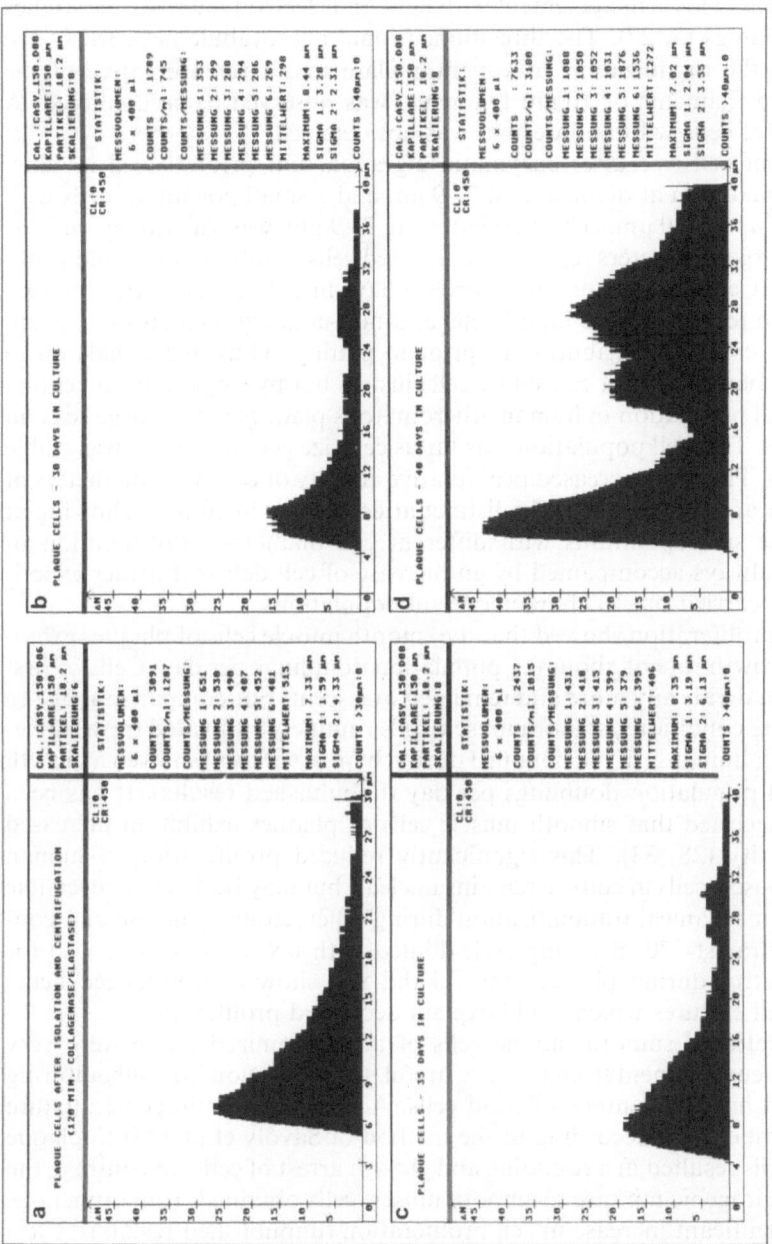

Fig. 7. Cell size blots of smooth muscle cells from atheromatous plaques. (a) Cell size distribution directly after enzymatic disintegration with collagenase/elastase and centrifugation showing a large debris peak at 7–9 μm and a portion of cells with diameters up to 30 μm. (b) Cell size blot after 30 days in culture exhibiting the debris peak at 7–9 μm and an appearing cell population at about 28 μm. (c) Cell size distribution after 35 days in culture. The cell population with a diameter of 26–30 μm becomes more pronounced. (d) Cell size blot after 40 days in culture. The cell population appearing after 30 to 35 days in culture is much more pronounced and can be divided in at least two subpopulations with different diameters of about 20 μm and 28 μm

121

smooth muscle cells. This is in agreement with light and electron microscopic studies on intimal thickenings (3, 27). The three-dimensional microtubule network of the plaque cells and the organization of vimentin filaments, a representative of the intermediate sized filaments or 10 nm filaments, was observed to be unaltered. A positive reaction of cells with anti-desmin was not detected.

Measurement of cell size after enzymatic digestion, but prior to cell seeding, showed a clear maximum at diameters of 7–9 µm and a small portion of cells with larger diameters up to 30 µm. The maximum at 7–9 µm was caused by cellular debris, whereas larger diameters represented isolated cells of different size and probably cell clusters. Cell size measurements after 5 days in culture, i.e., after the first medium exchange to remove red blood cells and non-adherent cell clusters, again showed the same cell size distribution as prior to plating. Thus, the signals up to 30 µm in cell size blots were not caused by cell clusters but by single cells indicating a homogenous cell population in human atheromatous plaques with a large scale in cellular diameters. This cell population – as far as cell size is concerned – was stable for about 30 days. Then, an increased proliferative activity of cells with diameters of about 28 µm appeared and was clearly distinct after 40 days in culture, showing at least two definite subpopulations with different cell diameters. Proliferation of plaque cells was always accompanied by an increase of cell debris. Further experiments have to be carried out to characterize subpopulations.

Studies of cell proliferation showed that the smooth muscle cells of plaques exhibited a very low growth rate of about 0.1 population doublings per day. Cells of first subculture did not divide any more and remained quiescent. For comparison, by use of the same culture conditions, smooth muscle cells routinely cultivated from saphenous veins of adult humans (tissue obtained during bypass surgery) showed a growth rate of 0.3 to 0.4 population doublings per day (unpublished results). It has been shown and/or suggested that smooth muscle cells of plaques exhibit an increased proliferative activity (28–33). This significantly reduced proliferation of human plaque smooth muscle cells in culture remains unclear, but may be due to irreversible injury caused by mechanical traumatization during atherectomy. The use of a contrast reagent (Ultravist-370, Schering AG, diluted with 0.9% saline 1:1, v/v) for angiographic control during plaque removal did not show a pronounced acute cytotoxicity in cell cultures which could explain decreased proliferation.

Isolated and cultured smooth muscle cells of atherectomized tissue were very sensitive against environmental changes. Careful trypsinization for subculturing cells resulted in a high percentage of dead cells. Addition of a mitogenic mixture isolated from bovine brain according to the method of Savoly et al. (34) to plaque smooth muscle cells resulted in a rounding and growth arrest of cells. In contrast, the addition of this mitogenic mixture to smooth muscle cells obtained from saphenous veins caused a significant increase in cell proliferation (unpublished results). A few recent studies of the growth characteristics of cells from human lesions have shown similar results, i.e., cells from human lesions exhibited a low proliferation rate and failed to respond to mitogens (35) or became quiescent in second passage (36). Ross et al. (35) have suggested that decreased proliferative activity of lesion smooth muscle cells is a manifestation of the cells having undergone a greater number of cell doublings in vivo than smooth muscle cells from the media and thus have become senescent (37).

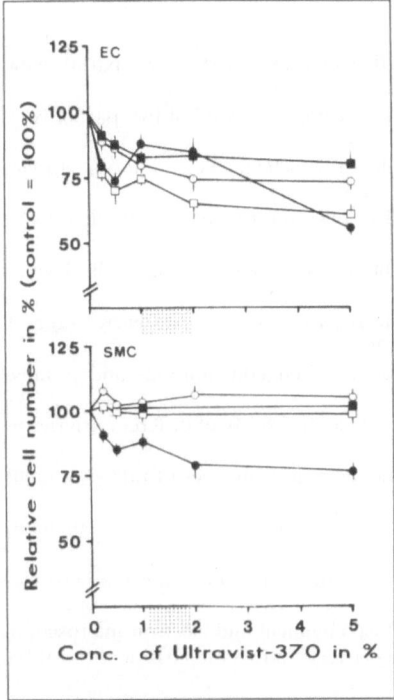

Fig. 8. Cytotoxic effect of the contrast reagent (Ultravist-370) as used for angiographic control during plaque removement. An acute cytotoxic effect after an eight-hour-incubation at 37 °C was not observed. To determine a late cytotoxic effect appearing after further incubation, Ultravist-370 was removed after eight hours and replaced by culture medium. After two days of incubation in culture medium, cell numbers were measured. Under these conditions, endothelial cells were more sensitive than smooth muscle cells. The absolute Ultravist-370 concentrations occuring under in-vivo-conditions of angiography is pointed out. □−□ Ultrasvist undiluted; ○−○ Ultravist/0.9% saline (1:1); ■−■ Ultravist/0.9% saline (1:1) + 2 IU/ml heparin; ●−● cell number after a continuous incubation with Ultravist/0.9% saline (1:1) for 2 days at 37 °C

Scanning electron microscopic studies demonstrated that a minority of atheromatous plaque material removed by the Simpson atherectomy catheter showed areas of amorphous and spherical calcium phosphate deposits (hydroxyl and carbonate apatite). Sometimes, at edges of the specimens sodium chloride crystals in different modificatons were detectable, those possibly being artifacts caused by the one-to two-day delay for transportation of plaque material using HEPES-buffered culture medium with antibiotics.

The results presented here show that isolation and cultivation of cells from selectively removed atheromatous plaque material by the Simpson atherectomy catheter is possible. Cultivation of the cells may represent a suitable in vitro model to investigate growth characteristics and cytoskeletal and metabolic alterations of smooth muscle cells in human atherosclerotic plaques.

Acknowledgements

This work was partially supported by Ministerium für Wissenschaft und Kunst, Baden-Württemberg, Forschungsprojekt No. 26. The authors are indebted to A. Lüttge and Prof. P. Metz, Mineralogisch-Petrographisches Institut der Universität Tübingen, for help and suggestions with the analysis and SEM examination of atheromatous plaque material, and Prof. C. Hemleben and H. Hüttemann, Geologisch-Paläontologisches Institut der Universität Tübingen, for providing SEM facilities. The authors thank H. Kratzer for photographic assistance.

References

1. Ross R and Glomset JA (1976) The pathogenesis of atherosclerosis (first of two parts). New Engl J Med 295:369–377
2. Ross R and Glomset JA (1976) The pathogenesis of atherosclerosis (second of two parts). New Engl J Med 295:420–425
3. Haust M (1983) Atherosclerosis and smooth muscle cells. In: Biochemistry of Smooth Muscle, Vol. II, NL Stephens (ed), pp. 189–250 (Boca Raton, CRC Press)
4. Schwartz SM, Campbell GR and Campbell JH (1986) Replication of smooth muscle cells in vascular disease. Circ Res 58:427–444
5. Ross R and Glomset JA (1973) Atherosclerosis and the arterial smooth muscle cell. Science 180:1332–1339
6. Velican C and Velican D (1986): Coronary intimal necrosis occurring at an early stage of atherosclerotic involvement. Atherosclerosis 39:479–496
7. Vesselinovitch, D (1979) Animal models in atherosclerosis, their contributions and pitfalls. Artery 5:193–206
8. Greditzer HG and Fischer VW (1978) A sequential ultrastructural study of different arteries in the hypertensive rat. Exp Mol Path 29:12–28
9. Aikawa M and Koletzky S (1970) Arteriosclerosis of the mesenteric arteries of rats with renal hypertension. Am J Path 61:293–304
10. Haust M (1980): The nature of bi- and trinuclear cells in atherosclerotic lesions in man. Atherosclerosis 36:365–377
11. Haust MD (1974) Reaction patterns of intimal mesenchyme to injury and repair in atherosclerosis. Adv Exp Med Biol 43:35–57
12. Parker F and Odland GF (1966) A light microscopic histochemical and electron microscopic study of experimental atherosclerosis in rabbit coronary artery and a comparison with rabbit aorta atherosclerosis. Am J Path 48:451–481
13. Höfling B, v. Pölnitz A, Backa D, v. Arnim Th, Lauterjung L, Jauch KW and Simpson JB (1988) Percutaneous removal of atheromatous plaques in peripheral arteries. Lancet I:384–386
14. Bauriedel G, Backa D, Stäblein A and Höfling B (1987) Angioskopie bei Patienten vor und nach perkutaner Atherektomie. VASA 16 Suppl 20:334–336
15. Chamley-Campbell JH, Campbell GR and Ross R (1979) The smooth muscle cell in culture. Phys Rev 59:1–61
16. Kocan RM, Moss NS and Benditt EP (1980) Human arterial wall cells and tissues in culture. Meth Cell Biol 21 A:153–165
17. Dartsch PC (1987) Das Zellskelett von kultivierten Gefäßwandzellen. Mikrokosmos 76:33–39
18. Russel WC, Newman C and Williamson DH (1975) A simple cytochemical technique for demonstration of DNA in cells infected with mycoplasmas and viruses. Nature 253:461–462
19. Owens GK, Loeb A, Gordon D and Thompson MM (1986) Expression of smooth muscle-specific α-isoactin in cultured vascular smooth muscle cells: Relationship between growth and cytodifferentiation. J Cell Biol 102:343–352
20. Skalli O, Ropraz P, Trzeciak A, Benzonana G, Gillessen D and Gabbiani G (1986) A monoclonal antibody against α-smooth muscle actin: A new probe for smooth muscle differentiation. J Cell Biol 103:2787–2796
21. Gabbiani G, Kocher O, Bloom WS, Vandekerckhove J and Weber K (1984) Actin expression in smooth muscle cells in rat aortic intimal thickening, human atheromatous plaque and cultured rat aortic media. J Clin Invest 73:148–152
22. Hoyer LW, de los Santos RP and Hoyer JR (1973) Antihemophilic factor antigen. Localization in endothelial cells by immunofluorescent microscopy. J Clin Invest 52:2737–2744
23. Jaffe EA (1984) Culture and identification of large vessel endothelial cells. In: Biology of Endothelial Cells, Jaffe EA (ed), Martinus Nijhoff Publishers, Boston, The Hague, Dordrecht, Lancaster, pp. 1–13
24. Jaffe EA, Nachman RL, Becker CG and Minick CR (1973) Culture of human endothelial cells derived from umbilical veins. Identification by morphologic and immunologic criteria. J Clin Invest 52:2745–2756

25. Jaffe EA, Hoyer LW and Nachman RL (1973) Synthesis of antihemophilic factor antigen by cultured human endothelial cells. J Clin Invest 52:2757–2764
26. Wagner DD, Olmsted JB and Marder VJ (1982) Immunolocalization of von Willebrand protein in Weibel-Palade bodies of human endothelial cells. J Cell Biol 95:355–360
27. Mosse PRL, Campbell GR, Wang ZI and Campbell JH (1985) Smooth muscle phenotypic expression in human carotid arteries. Comparison of cells from diffuse intimal thickenings adjacent to atheromatous plaques with those of the media. Lab Invest 53:556–562
28. Schmitt H, Knoche H, Junge-Hülsing G, Koch R and Hauss WH (1970) Über die Reduplikation von Aortenwandzellen bei arterieller Hypertonie. Z Kreislaufforsch 59:481–487
29. Ross R, Glomset JA and Harker L (1977) Response to injury and atherogenesis. Am J Path 86:675–684
30. Hassler O (1970) The origin of the cells constituting arterial intima thickening. An experimental autoradiographic study with the use of H^3-thymidine. Lab Invest 22:286–293
31. Burns ER, Spaet TH and Stemerman MB (1978) Response of the arterial wall to endothelial removal: An autoradiographic study. Proc Soc Exp Biol Med 159:473–477
32. Goldberg ID, Stemerman MB, Ransil BJ and Fuhro RL (1980) In vivo aortic muscle cell growth kinetics. Differencies between thoracic and abdominal segments after intimal injury in the rabbit. Circ Res 47:182–189
33. Orekhov AN, Kosykh VA, Repin VS and Smirnov VN (1983) Cell proliferation in normal and atherosclerotic human aorta. Flow cytofluorometric determination of cellular deoxyribonucleic acid content. Lab Invest 48:395–398
34. Savoly SB, Halle W, Heder G and Loose R (1987) Zur Wirkung eines proliferationsfördernden Rinderhirnpräparates auf Endothelzellkulturen aus Kälberaorten. Biomed Biochem Acta 46:285-291
35. Ross R., Wight TM, Strandness E and Thiele B (1980) Human atherosclerosis. Cell constitution and characteristics of advanced lesions of the superficial femoral artery. Am J Path 114:79–93
36. Melnick JL, Petrie BL, Dreesman GR, Burek J, McCollum CH and DeBakey ME (1983) Cytomegalovirus antigen within human arterial smooth muscle cells. Lancet:644–647
37. Ross R. and Kariya B (1980) Morphogenesis of vascular smooth muscle in atherosclerosis and cell culture. In: Handbook of Physiology: Vascular Smooth Muscle, Bohr D (ed), Am Physiol Soc, Washington DC, pp. 69–91

Low-speed rotational angioplasty – clinical results in 53 patients with chronic occlusions

C. Vallbracht[1], I. Prignitz[4], W. Beinhorn[4], D. Liermann[2], H. Landgraf[3], W. Bamberg[1], F. J. Roth[4], J. Kollath[2], W. Schoop[5], M. Kaltenbach[1]

Departments of Cardiology[1], Radiology[2], Angiology[3], University Hospital Frankfurt; Departments of Radiology[4] and Angiology[5], Aggertalklinik Engelskirchen, FRG

Today the limits of non-operative dilatation of atherosclerotic arteries (4) are very tight stenoses, which cannot be passed with a guide wire or balloon catheter, and importantly, total occlusions. Occlusions of peripheral vessels of more than 10 cm in length (16) and subacute coronary occlusions (8, 9, 11) can be reopened successfully only in about 50% – 60% of cases. The chance of recanalization decreases with the duration of occlusion and the amount of calcification. The new technique called low speed rotational angioplasty (6, 14, 15) uses a very flexible, blunt, rotating catheter.

Experimental investigations in postmortem human arteries (14) could demonstrate that even old and calcified occlusions in which conventional techniques had failed, could be reopened with a speed of only 200 rpm. No perforations occurred and histologic and angioscopic examinations showed a relatively smooth surface of the created channel, which could be dilated further with conventional balloon catheters or special rotating elastic elements.

Because of these encouraging results we started our clinical investigations in December 1986 (15), and the results in our first 53 patients will be described.

Patients

Between December 1986, and June 1988, 53 patients (41 men and 12 woman, ages 35 to 84 years; mean age 68.6 years) were treated with the new technique. In 41 patients, the superficial femoral artery, in 11 patients the popliteal artery, and in one patient the iliac artery was completely occluded. Twenty-one patients were treated in the University Hospital, Frankfurt and 32 patients in the Aggertalklinik in Engelskirchen. Patients were divided into three groups:

Group 1: 11 patients with rotational angioplasty as the primary intervention and a length of occlusion of less than 10 cm (mean 5.3 cm);
Group 2: 24 patients with rotational angioplasty as the primary intervention and a length of occlusion of more than 10 cm (mean 14.5 cm, longest occlusion 30 cm);
Group 3: 18 patients after failure of conventional techniques.

Functional and angiographic findings

Forty-eight patients were in Fontaine stage II with a walking distance before claudication between 30 m and 300 m with a mean of 110 m. Five patients were in Fontaine

127

stage IV with pain at rest and local gangrene; four were considered inoperable by the vascular surgeons and amputation was impending.

The Doppler-pressure index (12, 13) was between 0 and 0.86 (mean 0.51). Duration of occlusion was estimated from patients' histories and ranged from five to 48 months (mean 18.2 months). In seven patients, durations of six to 36 months had been documented by previous angiographic examinations. The length of occlusion measured four to 30 cm (mean 10.9 cm). In 30 of 53 patients, the occluded arteries showed marked calcification.

Technique, documentation and medication

After puncture of the femoral artery and injection of 5 000 units of heparin an 8-F sheath was introduced and angiography was performed. With a second injection a digital subtraction angiogram followed (road mapping). The rotating catheter (outer diameter 2.2 mm) consisting of four 0.2mm V2A-steel coiled wires with an inner lumen and a suitable rounded tip covered with a highly flexible polyolefin or teflon shrinking tube (Fig. 1) was introduced through the hemostatic valve of the sheath (Fig. 2), which was perfused with a combination of 2 000 units of heparin and 100 000 units of urokinase per h throughout the intervention. The speed range of the small motor unit (Fig. 3) was infinitely variable with the help of a foot switch. Rotational angioplasty was performed at low speed up to 200 rpm with only slight axial thrust.

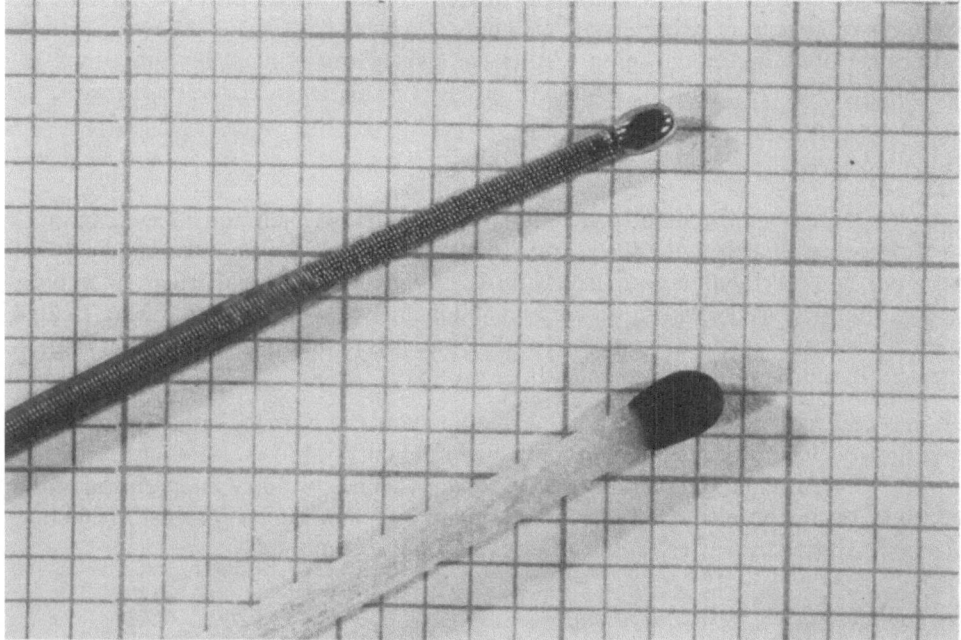

Fig. 1. Rotating catheter (4 × 0.2 mm V$_2$A-steel coiled wires) with teflon shrinking tube and blunt tip

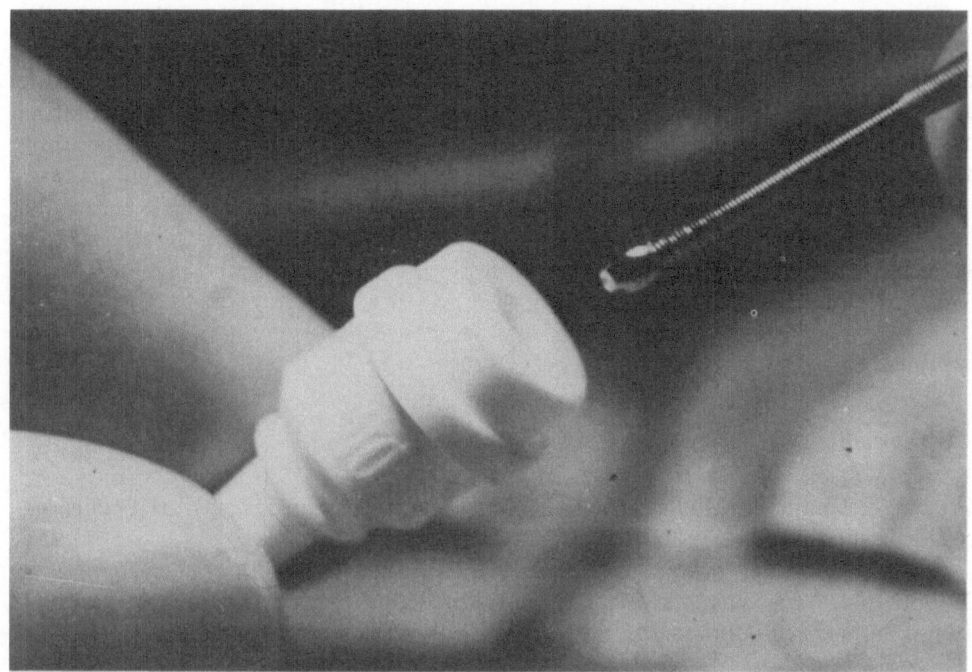

Fig. 2. The rotating catheter gets introduced through the 8-French-sheath

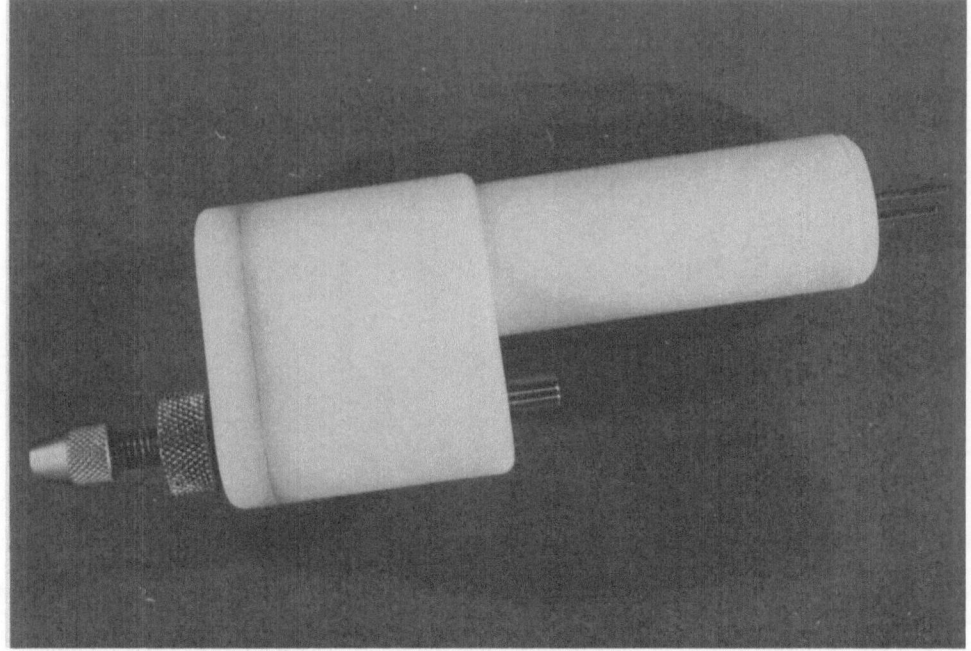

Fig. 3. Motor unit with infinitely variable speed (0–300 rpm)

The passage through the occlusion was documented on video film followed by the injection of contrast medium through the rotating catheter to document the intraluminal localization. Thereafter, an 0.35″-exchange wire was introduced through the rotating catheter and placed distal to the occlusion. After retraction of the rotating catheter, the new channel was documented by angiography and further dilated using a conventional balloon catheter.

All patients received aspirin 500–1 500 mg/day (1) at least one week before the intervention; 1 000–1 200 units of heparin were given intravenously for at least 24 h starting immediately after the intervention.

Results

Angiographic

Group 1 (11 patients with occlusion < 10 cm in length; mean 5.3 cm): All occlusions could be successfully recanalized (Fig. 4).

Group 2 (24 patients with occlusion > 10 cm in length; mean 14.5 cm): In 19 of 24 patients, the occlusions of up to 30 cm in length and of up to a 36 months' angiographically documented duration could be successfully reopened (Figs. 5 and

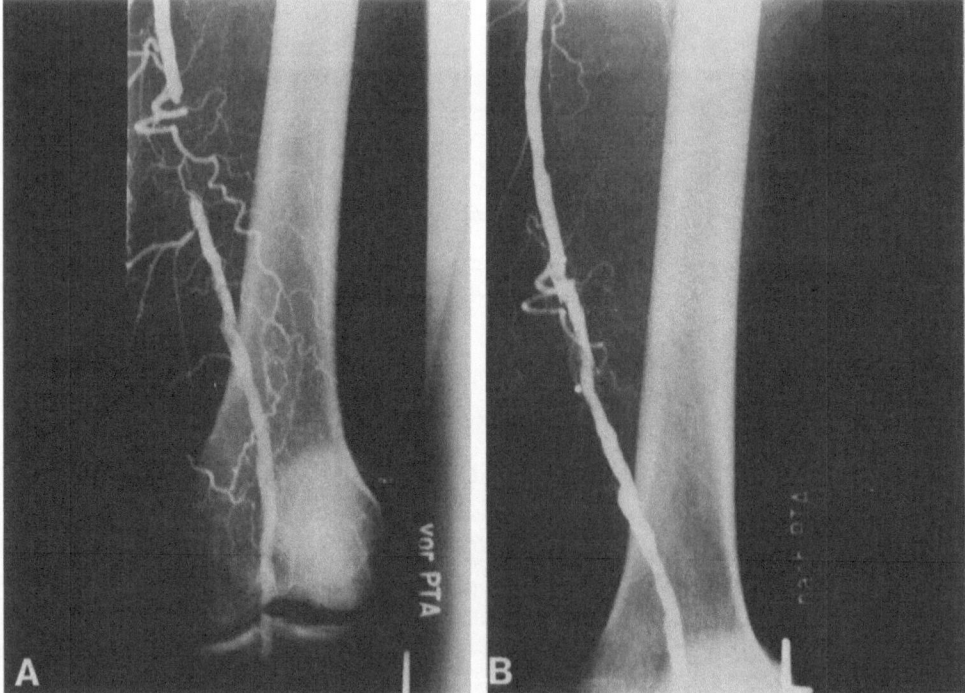

Fig. 4. Short occlusion (4 cm) of the superficial femoral artery. (A) Before (B) After rotational angioplasty and balloon dilatation

130

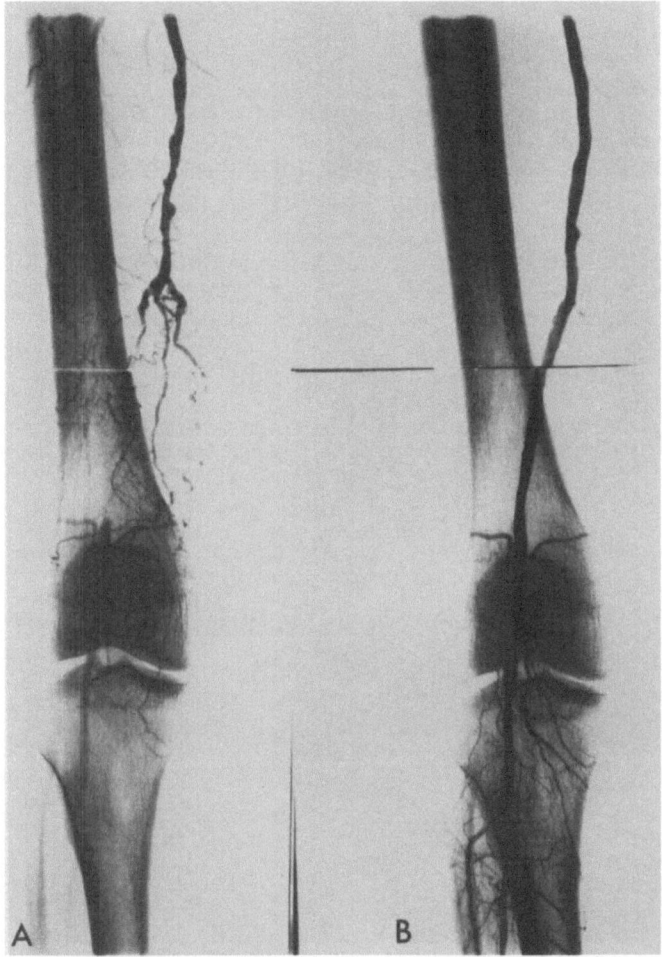

Fig. 5. Superficial femoral artery with narrowings up to 60% in the proximal and total occlusion of 10.4 cm in the distal part. (A) before (B) after rotational angioplasty and balloon dilatation

6). In four patients, the severely calcified occlusions could not be crossed and in one patient the intervention had to be stopped after 50 min because of increasing restlessness of the patient.

Group 3 (18 patients after failure of conventional techniques): 14 of 18 patients were treated with rotational angioplasty more than four weeks after the conventional attempt; in nine out of these 14 patients the occlusions could be successfully reopened (in one patient there had been two unsuccessful attempts with conventional techniques before and in one patient the unsuccessful attempt dated back to 1985 (Fig. 7). In one patient with a short occlusion of the superficial femoral artery, a large collateral vessel exited proximal to the occlusion and the rotating catheter entered the collateral, as had been the case with the conventional technique before. There was no damage of the collateral branch.

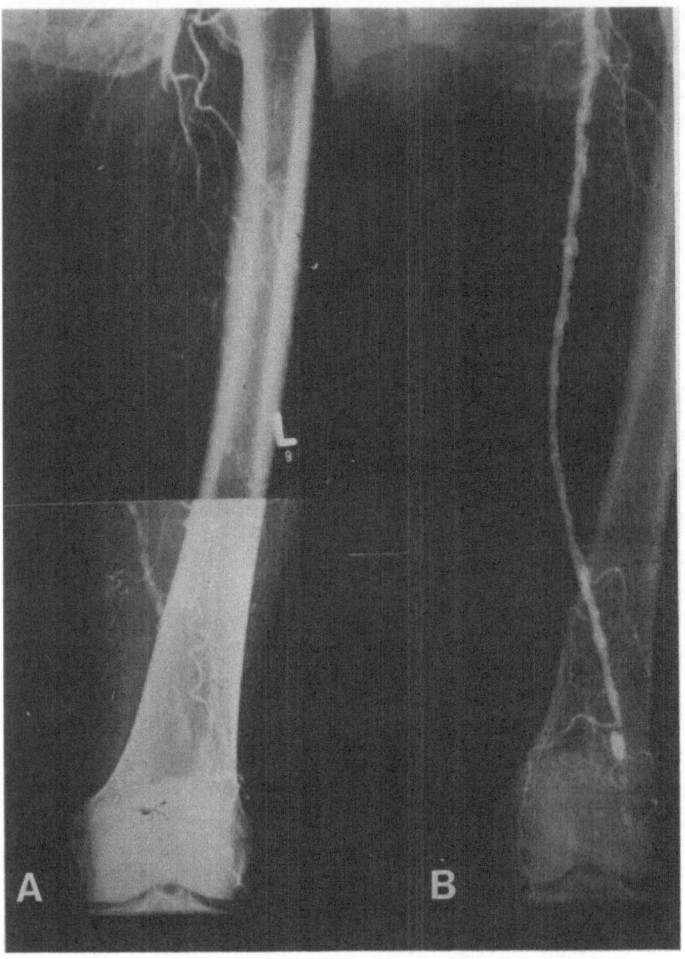

Fig. 6. Total occlusion of the left superficial femoral artery in a 78 year old female diabetic patient (25 cm). (A) before (B) after rotational angioplasty and balloon dilatation

Functional

Twenty-four of 39 successfully treated patients could walk without claudication after the procedure. In three of four inoperable patients the reopening of the vessel prevented amputation. In one 78-year old female diabetic with gangrene of the foot and pain at rest, the reopening of the entire superficial femoral artery resulted in warming of the lower leg and a marked decrease in pain. Although the occlusion of the popliteal artery was unchanged she could walk approx. 300 m and the gangrene healed (Fig. 6).

The ankle-brachial-index of Doppler pressure measurements increased from a mean of 0.51 to 0.89.

132

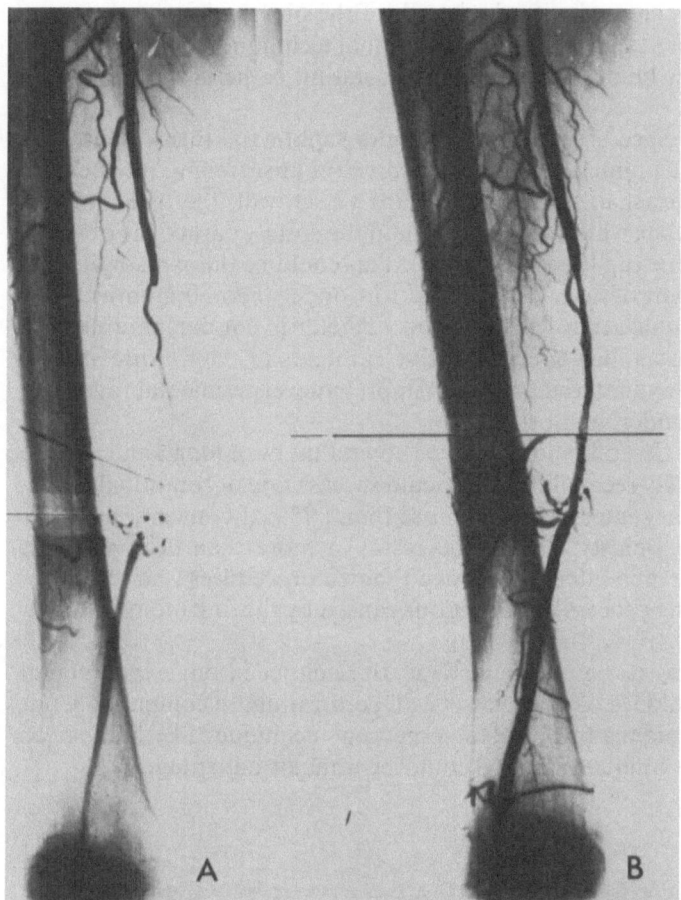

Fig. 7. Total occlusion (11 cm) of the right superficial femoral artery in which the conventional technique had failed several weeks before. (A) before (B) after rotational angioplasty and balloon dilatation

Complications

In none of our 53 patients did a perforation or other severe complication occur. In three patients, minor dissections and in one patient a small peripheral embolism was observed but caused no sequelae. In three patients there was bleeding at the puncture site; in one of them a transfusion was necessary.

Discussion

In non-operative recanalization of chronic atherosclerotic obstructions, the danger of dissection or perforation is increased because of the underlying ulceration of the plaque which originally led to the occlusion of the vessel. This possibility of exiting

133

the true lumen is further increased with the length of the obstruction. Therefore, a relatively thin strainght wire as used in the conventional technique seems to be more dangerous than our large, blunt, flexible, slowly rotating catheter with an outer diameter of 2.2 mm (15).

Our concept is that low-speed rotation while under slight axial thrust allows the catheter to discover the true lumen of the occluded vessel in searching for the path of least resistance. In contrast to the sick and hard vessel wall, the true lumen is usually occluded by thrombus which seems to remain the softest part of the obstruction for a long period of time (up to several years). This could be the explanation for our successful recanalization of arteries occluded for longer than 30 months.

The mechanism of recanalization with our new catheter is not comparable with other new techniques such as high-speed abrasive catheters (7, 10). Expression of fluid without removal of any material as shown in previous experimental investigations (5) seems to be the underlying principle.

The acute results in our first 53 patients have shown that even long and calcified occlusions can be successfully recanalized; the acute success rate of rotational angioplasty, if used as the primary intervention is more than 80 %. If conventional techniques fail, rotational angioplasty can be successful in more than 60 % of these patients, provided that the time interval between the two procedures is at least four weeks because of the healing process of dissections caused by the first (conventional) attempt.

The new technique seems to be particularly gentle; neither in our experimental nor in our clinical cases could we observe vessel wall perforation. In comparison, not only to conventional techniques but also to some new techniques like high-speed rotation (7, 10) or laser techniques (2), this could be a major advantage.

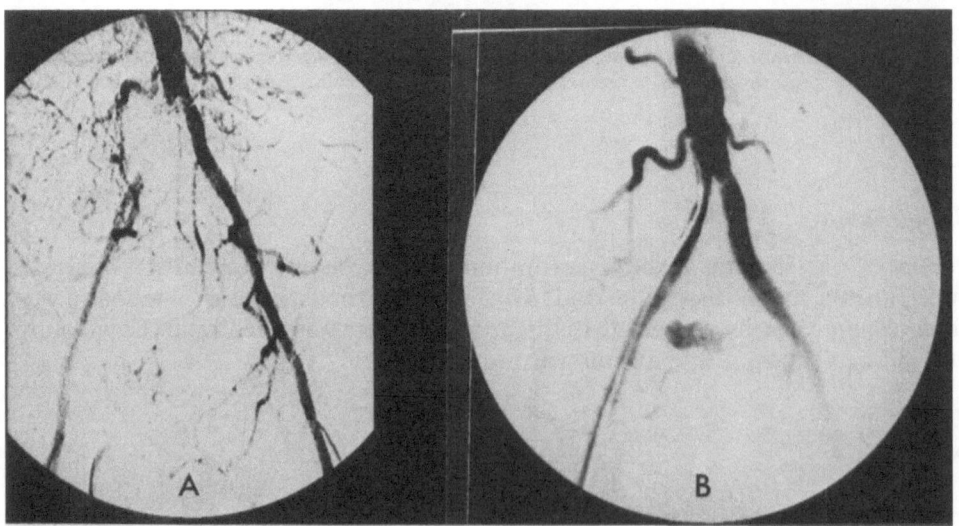

Fig. 8. Occlusion of the right iliac artery (6 cm). (A) before (B) after rotational angioplasty and balloon dilatation (DSA; the exchange-wire is still in place)

In previous studies, long-term results after reopening of long occlusions have been disappointing (3). Whether the capability of our catheter to apparently find the true lumen may improve even the long-term outcome remains to be seen.

Because of these encouraging results in chronic femoral and popliteal occlusions, an extension of indications could be expected. A first step in this direction was made with the first successful reopening of a totally occluded iliac artery (Fig. 8).

References

1. Breddin HK (1982) Treatment with platelet function inhibitors in: Kaltenbach, Grüntzig, Rentrop, Bussman (eds) Transluminal coronary angioplasty and intracoronary thrombolysis. Springer Verlag, Heidelberg-New York, p 41–43
2. Fourrier JL, Marache P, Brunetaud et al. (1987) Human percutaneous laser angioplasty with sapphire tips: results and follow-up. Circulation 76 Suppl IV:919
3. Gallino A, Mahler F, Probst P, Nachbur B: Percutaneous transluminal angioplasty of the arteries of the lower limbs: a five-year follow-up. Circulation 70:4:619
4. Grüntzig A, Hopff H. (1974) Perkutane Rekanalisation chronischer arterieller Verschlüsse mit einem neuen Dilatationskatheter. Modifikation der Dottertechnik. Dtsch Med Wschr 99:2502
5. Kaltenbach M, Beyer J, Klepzig H et al. (1982) Effect of 5 kg/cm² pressure on atherosclerotic vessel wall segments in Kaltenbach, Grüntzig, Rentrop, Bussman (eds) Transluminal coronary angioplasty and intracoronary thrombolysis. Springer Verlag, Heidelberg-New York
6. Kaltenbach M, Vallbracht C (1987) Rotationsangioplastik-ein neues Katheterverfahrn. Fortschr Med 105:21:412
7. Kensey K, Nash J, Abrahams C et al. (1986) Recanalization of obstructed arteries using a flexible rotating tip catheter. Circulation 74 Suppl II:1821
8. Kober G, Vallbracht C, Lang H et al. (1985) Transluminale koronare Angioplastik 1977–1985. Erfahrungen bei 1000 Eingriffen. Radiologe 25:346
9. Meier B, Grüntzig A (1984). Resultate der transluminalen Koronardilatation. Dtsch Med Wschr 109:675
10. Ritchie JL, Hansen DD, Vracko H, Auth D (1986) In vivo rotational thrombectomy-evaluation by angioscopy. Circulation 74 Suppl II:1822
11. Savage R, Hollman J, Grüntzig AR et al. (1982) Can percutaneous transluminal coronary angioplasty be performed in patients with total occlusions? Circulation 66:Suppl II:330
12. Schoop W (1976) Die Ultraschall-Doppler-Methode in der Diagnostik der arteriellen und venösen Störungen in den Exdtremitäten. Internist 17:580
13. Thulesius O, Gjörjes JE. (1971) Use of Doppler shift detection for determining peripheral arterial blood pressure. Angiology 22:594
14. Vallbracht C, Kress J, Schweitzer M et al. (1987) Rotationsangioplastik – ein neues Verfahren zur Gefäßwiedereröffnung und -erweiterung. Z Kardiol 76:608
15. Vallbracht C, Schweitzer M, Kress J et al. (1987) Low speed rotational angioplasty-preliminary clinical results. Circulation 76 Suppl IV:111
16. Zeitler E (1985) Die perkutane transluminale Rekanalisation chronischer Stenosen und Verschlüsse peripherer Arterien. Wien Med Wschr 135:384

Laser angioplasty: 1988

T. A. Sanborn

Department of Medicine, Division of Cardiology, Mount Sinai Medical Center, New York City, USA

While laser angioplasty has the potential to serve as an adjunct to alternative conventional angioplasty by recanalizing chronic total occlusions (1) and reducing restenosis (2, 3), a great deal of work is still required to solve the two main problems with the cardiovascular use of laser, namely, vessel perforation and small recanalized channels which have poor long-term patency.

Currently, there is a tremendous variety of cardiovascular lasers available, with different systems and in various stages of experimental and clinical investigation

Table 1. Characteristics of current clinical cardiovascular lasers

	Lasers			
	Excimer	Argon	Nd:YAG	CO_2
Laser characteristics				
Spectral Region	Ultraviolet	Visible	Near Infrared	Infrared
Wavelength (nm)	308	488,514	1,060	10,600
Temperal Mode	Pulsed (P)	Continuous Wave (CW)	P, CW	CW
Delivery Systems	Fiberoptic	Fiberoptic, metal cap combined metal cap – sapphire tip, lensed tip	Fiberoptic, metal cap, sapphire tip, laser-balloon	Rigid Instrument
Pathophysiological mechanisms				
Vaporization	+	+	+	+
Thermal Compression	–	+	+	–
Sealing	–	–	+	–

Table 2. Early trials with bare argon fiberoptics on femoro-popliteal stenoses and occlusions

	Improved lumen	Perforations
Ginsberg et al. (4)	8/17 (47%)	3/17 (18%)
Cumberland et al. (5)	10/15 (67%)	2/15 (13%)
Total	18/32 (56%)	5/32 (16%)

Table 3. Current laser angioplasty approaches

1. *Modified Fiberoptic Tip*
   - Laser Probe
   - Sapphire Tip
   - Combined Metal Cap-Sapphire Tip
   - Lensed Tip
   - Laser-Balloon Catheter
2. *Short Pulse Laser Delivery*
   - Excimer
   - Q-switched Nd:YAG
3. *Improved Plaque Recognition*
   - Angioscopy
   - Spectroscopy
   - Ultrasound
4. *Selective Plaque Ablation*
   - Endogenous chromophores (cartenoids)
   - Exogenous chromophores (HPD, Tetracycline)
5. *Other Engery Source*
   - Electrical
   - Chemical

(Table 1). These clinical cardiovascular laser systems are often separated by their laser wavelength (excimer, argon, Nd:YAG, and CO_2) however, the specifics of the delivery system may ultimately determine which system is most successful.

Historically, clinical trials in peripheral arteries began with established bare fiberoptic laser systems such as the argon (4, 5) and Nd:YAG (6); however, these early series only achieved clinical success in one-half to two-thirds of the patients and were complicated by perforation in 15% – 20% of the cases (Table 2). Thus, a variety of different approaches are now being investigated in order to improve on these results and to decrease the incidence of laser perforation (Table 3).

Modified fiberoptics

Modification of the fiberoptic tips was the first approach to improve upon these results with bare fiberoptics. The first, but certainly not the last modified laser delivery system to demonstrate a high incidence of successful laser recanalization with a low incidence of vessel perforation is an argon laser heated metallic-capped fiberoptic device (Laserprobe-PLR, Trimidyne Inc, Santa Ana, California).

The laserprobe is a fiberoptic delivery system (7) which allows transmission of argon laser energy from the laser generator to the desired target and conversion of this light energy into controlled thermal energy at the distal end of the probe. In the first 2 s of argon laser energy delivery, the temperature on the surface of the probe rises sooner and higher at the probe tip and decreases towards the neck of the probe, but by 5 s the temperature distribution of the probe is nearly uniform (8). When brought in contact with atherosclerotic tissue, the laser probe conducts this heat to the tissue and vaporization of the tissue occurs. As expected, increased laser energy resulted in greater depth of ablation. Interestingly, in this study increasing the force

138

applied by the laser-heated device also resulted in more efficient ablation of tissue (8). While this greater tissue ablation may simply be because of less thermal resistance from improved contact of the probe with the tissue, another possibility is that vacuolated tissue is compressed by the rounded probe. In a comparative study in this same report, irradiation of aortic tissue with bare argon optical fibers was found to result in a split, fragmented appearance on the surface of the aortic tissue and extensive dissection of the subintima while the injury resulting from the laser probe was more controlled without evidence of vessel dissection. In this study, the laser-heated probe was also more effective in ablating fibrofatty plaque than non-atherosclerotic aorta. It can be speculated that this difference in thermal properties could explain the clinical observation that the laser probe preferentially vaporizes obstructive atheroma and thrombus during laser recanalization rather than the vessel wall and that this explains why the incidence of vessel perforation is reduced.

Experimental in vivo results. Three in vivo experimental studies have now been published which demonstrate not only improved safety and efficacy of this laser-heated probe compared to bare fiberoptics (9, 10) but also less restenosis than conventional balloon angioplasty (2). First, in a series of atherosclerotic rabbit iliac artery stenoses (9), angiography revealed greater widening of luminal stenoses in animals treated with the laser probe device as compared to the standard fiberoptic system. More importantly, while perforation of the vessel wall occurred frequently with the fiberoptic fiber, only 1 mechanical perforation occurred in 12 animals treated with the laser probe.

Acute histology revealed striking differences with these two fiberoptic systems. With direct laser radiation from the bare fiberoptic, a deep localized laser crater was noted along one side of the vessel wall with charring and considerable thrombus formation (Fig. 1, top). On histologic cross-sections of eccentric lesions, the major portion of the atherosclerotic lesion was often missed by the narrow laser beam. In contrast, those vessels treated with the laser-heated metallic probe showed histologic evidence of thermal injury distributed evenly around the entire luminal circumference with minimal charring and thinner, flatter thrombus formation (Fig. 1, bottom). These histologic data suggest that circumferential rather than localized distribution of energy is a factor in these improved results.

These results were confirmed in a series of postmortem human coronary artery zenographs transplanted into canine femoral arteries (10). Angiography demonstrated recanalization in all five arteries treated with a laser-heated probe compared to three of five arteries treated with a bare fiberoptic. There was also less vessel perforation with the metallic-capped fiber, compared to the bare fiberoptic.

Recent follow-up angiographic and histologic studies in the rabbit model demonstrated good long term patency with laser thermal angioplasty in comparison to conventional balloon angioplasty (2). While the immediate enlargement of the angiographic luminal diameter was similar for both procedures, the vessels treated with 1.5–2.0 mm laser probe devices had less angiographic restenosis and a significantly larger mean luminal diameter than those treated with balloon angioplasty. On histology, four weeks after the laser procedure, there was a larger lumen, minimal thrombosis or smooth muscle cell proliferation, and a thin neointimal covered with a fibrous cap (Fig. 2, top). In contrast, those vessels treated with balloon angioplasty

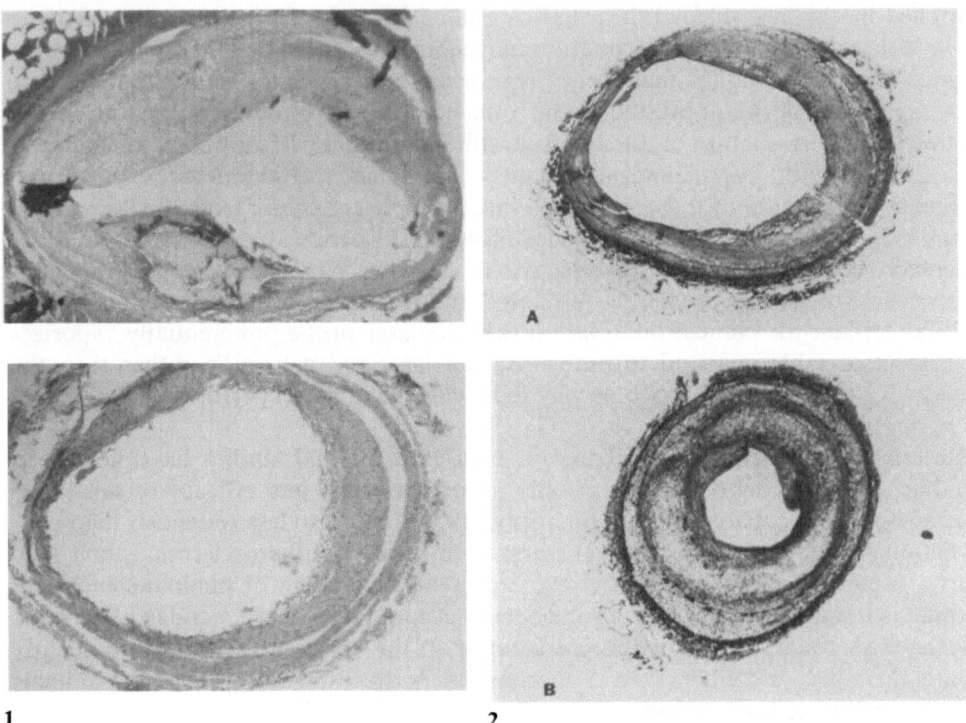

1   2

Fig. 1. (Top) Histological specimens of iliac artery. Example of direct argon laser radiation resulting in a localized laser defect along one side of the vessel wall which extends through the neointima into the media. A gradient of thermal injury characterized by cell swelling and tissue edema is also noted. In addition, considerable thrombus is present which fills the newly formed laser defect. (Bottom) Example of laserprobe thermal injury distributed evenly around the entire luminal circumference. Hematoxylin-eosin stain, magnification × 80. Reproduced with the permission of Sanborn TA et al. and the American College of Cardiology (J Am Coll Cardiol 5:934–938, 1985)

Fig. 2. A, cross-section of the patent rabbit iliac vessel four weeks after laser thermal angioplasty, demonstrating minimal fibrocellular proliferative response and a thin, condensed fibrous cap. B, histologic section four weeks after balloon angioplasty, revealing moderate fibrocellular proliferation caused by the dilatation which, partially filled the lumen and obliterate the prior dissection planes between the neointimal and the media (Verhoff-van Gieson elastin stains; original magnification × 26). Reproduced with the permission of Sanborn TA and the American Heart Association (Circulation 75:1281, 1987)

demonstrate evidence of prior fracture and dissection of the vessel wall (11) with more of a fibrocellular proliferative response and ongoing thrombus formation (Fig. 2, bottom). Morphometric analysis of these histologic cross-sections confirmed a significantly larger luminal area after laser thermal angioplasty compared with balloon angioplasty. Thus, laser thermal angioplasty was associated with less restenosis and produced a significantly larger mean luminal diameter and mean luminal area than conventional balloon angioplasty. The differences in the pathophysiology of these techniques is probably responsible for these observations. That is, with laser recanalization of these high-grade stenotic lesions there is (a) partial laser vaporization or removal of atherosclerotic material, and (b) perhaps more importantly, a smoother, less thrombogenic surface is left behind compared with balloon angioplasty. Whether there is an additional thermal effect on the arterial wall which inhibits platelet accumulation and/or smooth muscle cell proliferation is another intriguing concept.

Clinical laser recanalization with the argon laser-heated probe in peripheral vessels. After demonstrating the safety and efficacy of this device in experimental animals, a clinical trial was initiated to investigate its role in performing percutaneous laser thermal angioplasty as an adjunct to balloon angioplasty in patients with severe peripheral vascular disease (1, 12). The initial aims were two-fold: first, to demonstrate the safety of this laser device, and second, to determine whether this procedure could add to conventional balloon angioplasty by (a) increasing the initial success rate in peripheral artery total occlusions, and (b) recanalizing occlusions in which balloon and guidewire techniques had failed. In an initial report laser recanalization was achieved in 50 of 56 (89%) femoropopliteal and iliac artery occlusions (1). From a previous assessment of the angiogram and/or gentle probing of the proximal origin of the occlusion with a guide wire, the lesions were subjectively classified as easy (n = 17) or difficult (N = 21) to cross by conventional angioplasty methods. Eighteen occlusions were classified as impossible either because previous angioplasty attempts had failed (n = 11), or because they were considered unsuitable for conventional angioplasty (n = 7). All 17 easy, 19 of 21 difficult and 14 of 18 impossible occlusions were successfully recanalized. Since there were 2 acute reocclusions in the first 24 hours, the overall initial clinical success rate was 86%. These results compare favorably to recent clinical success rates of 72% – 78% for conventional balloon angioplasty (13, 14).

In this initial series, the perforation rate was less than 2% and the one perforation was attributed to excess mechanical pressure within a hard calcified occlusion rather

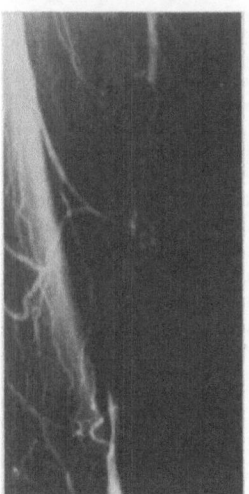 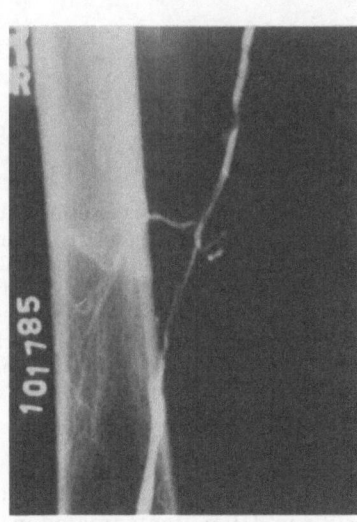 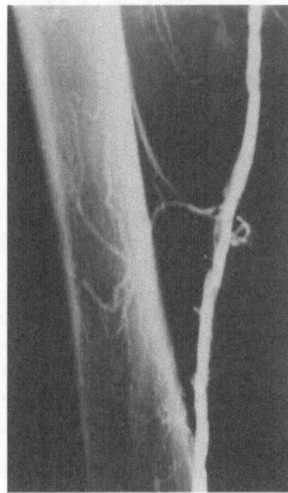

Fig. 3. Angiogram of a 6 cm high grade stenosis of the superficial femoral artery (left panel) in which the luminal diameter was enlarged with the laser probe (middle panel). This allowed conventional balloon angioplasty to be performed more easily (right panel). Reproduced with permission of Sanborn TA et al. (J Vascular Surgery 5:83, l987)

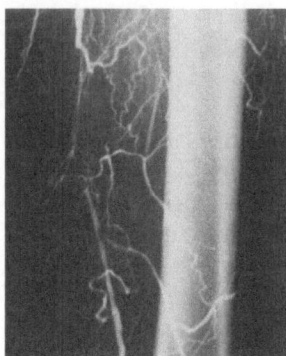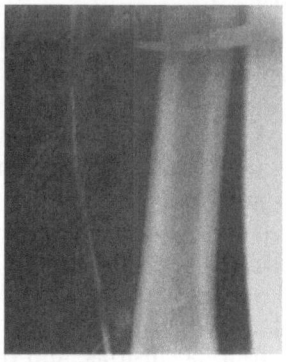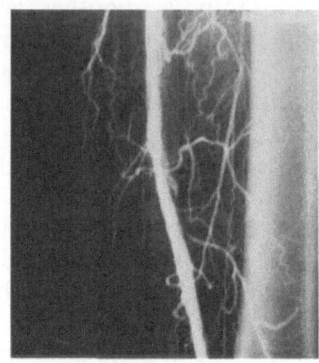

Fig. 4. Angiograms of a 4 cm total occlusion of the superficial femoral artery (left panel) which was recanalized with three pulses of 12 watts of argon laser energy delivered by the laserprobe for ten seconds duration each (middle panel). This was followed by balloon angioplasty to yield a good angiographic result (right panel). Reproduced with permission of Sanborn TA et al. (J Vascular Surgery 5:83, 1987)

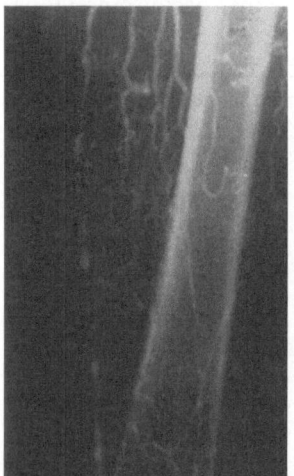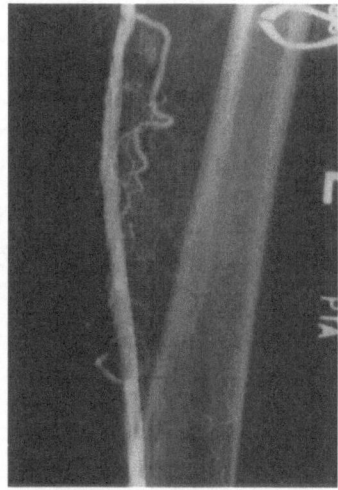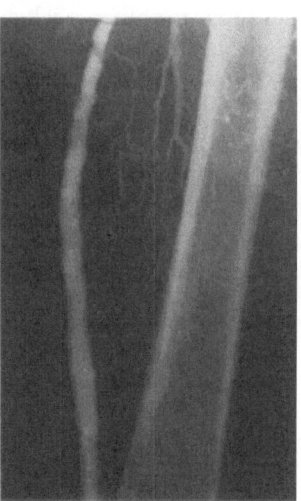

Fig. 5. Angiography of a 4 cm superficial femoral artery occlusion with a tortuous 8 cm stenosis proximal to the occlusion. (A) Image obtained before angioplasty (B) Image obtained immediately after laser-assisted balloon angioplasty. Traversing the tortuous proximal stenosis required shaping a curve in the 0.014-inch guide wire attached to the laser probe. With the curved guide wire, it was possible to torque the laser probe through the stenosis. After the occlusion had been crossed with the laser-heated probe, the probe was slowly withdrawn through the occlusion and the stenosis with continuous laser-pulse delivery to further enlarge the entire lumen before balloon angioplasty. (C) Image obtained at repeat angiography two months later, at the time of angioplasty of the opposite leg. Reproduced with permission from Radiology 168:121, 1988

than a thermal perforation. There was no clinical sequelae as a result of this perforation. Based on additional results in 219 patients treated in 10 medical centers, this laser probe device was approved for clinical use in February 1987, for peripheral artery lesions considered difficult or impossible to treat by conventional means. Angiographic examples of laser-assisted balloon angioplasty are shown in Figs. 3–5.

142

Clinical follow-up results with the laser probe in peripheral arteries. While recanalization with laser devices may be a useful adjunct to improve the initial chance of a successful angioplasty in peripheral artery total occlusions, the real challenge will be to determine whether laser angioplasty by whatever pathophysiological mechanism (vaporization, thermal compression, sealing, Table 1) can actually improve long-term clinical patency and reduce recurrence. At present, the laser probe is the only laser catheter with adequate clinical experience for assessment of long-term results; one year cummulative results were recently reported and compared to results of recently published series for conventional balloon angioplasty (3).

When examining long-term results of peripheral angioplasty, recurrence rates varied considerably depending on the type of lesion (stenosis vs occlusion), lesion length, and the definition of recurrence. With subgroup analysis of this initial series, a potential benefit of combined laser recanalization and balloon angioplasty was suggested in femoropopliteal arteries (Table 4). For example, the one year cumulative recurrence rates for stenoses and short occlusion (1–3 cm in length) were only 5% and 7%, respectively (3). These results were considerably better than recent balloon angioplasty series in which one year recurrence rates of 20% to 30% or more were reported for stenoses and recurrence rates of 7% to 33% or more were reported for short occlusions (14–16). The definition of clinical patency is important in comparing these results as a 12% to 29% redilation rate was not considered a recurrence in two of these recent series (14, 16). For longer occlusions treated with laser-assisted balloon angioplasty, one-year recurrence rate of 24% for 4–7 cm occlusion and 42% for occlusion > 7 cm are also better than a recurrence rate of 50% for occlusions > 3 cm reported in one series (15).

On one hand, these results are influenced by operator learning experience and the initial development stage of a device; clinical success and patency should improve with more experience and device modifications. On the other hand, these results could be influenced by other patient demographic factors such as case selection, diabetes, smoking, distal vessel run-off, and medications. Obviously, these results have to be confirmed and a multicenter randomized trial should be considered. These initial results do serve as a useful reference for future laser or mechanical devices.

Possible explanation for these lower recurrence rates after laser recanalization and balloon angioplasty are that the technique partially vaporizes or thermally compresses the atherosclerotic lesion and leaves behind a smoother less thrombogenic

Table 4. Comparison of one year cummulative patency rates

Technique	Occlusions			
	Stenoses	< 3 cm	4–7 cm	>7 cm
Laser-assisted balloon angioplasty	95	93	76	58
Balloon angioplasty alone				
Hewes et al. (6)	81*	67*	82*	69*
Murray et al. (7)	72*	86 +		
Krepel et al. (5)	80	93	50 (> 3 cm)	

Note: Values are expressed as percentages
* Redilation rate of 12–20% was not considered recurrence.
+ Value for all occlusions
Reproduced with permission from Radiology 168:121, 1988.

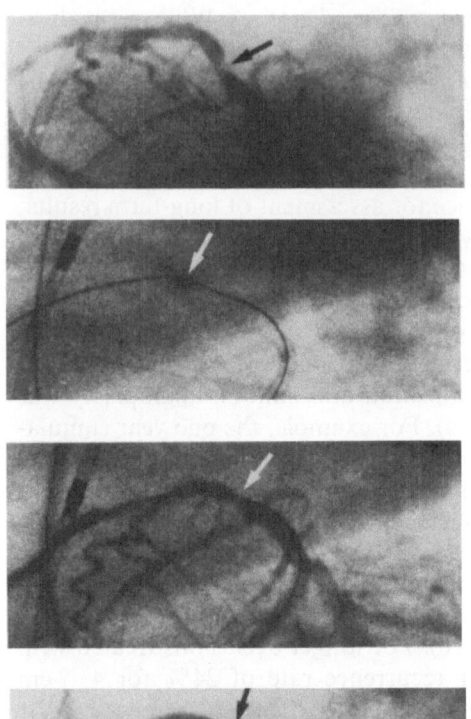

Fig. 6. The 60° left anterior oblique, 10° caudal views of a 90% eccentric left anterior descending artery lesion (arrows) before treatment (top), after laser thermal angioplasty results with the laser probe through the lesion and the angiographic results of laser thermal angioplasty (middle panels) and after balloon angioplasty (bottom). Reproduced with permission of Sanborn TA et al. and the American College of Cardiology (J Am Coll Cardiol 8:1437, 1986)

arterial surface. Obviously, for longer occlusions more atherosclerotic material will have to be removed. Larger probes may be beneficial in removing more material or leaving behind a smoother surface with a larger lumen so that balloon angioplasty may not be required at all. Preliminary clinical experience with larger 2.5 mm devices indicates that this may be possible. The recent study in the smaller (1–2 mm) rabbit iliac arteries discussed earlier suggest that laser recanalization with the laser probe device alone may cause less restenosis than conventional balloon angioplasty (2).

Percutaneous coronary laser feasibility. Based on this experience in peripheral vessels, clinical trials of lasers for percutaneous coronary use were recently initiated using specially designed coronary laser-heated probes (17, 18). These preliminary studies indicated that a coronary laser catheter can be used percutaneously to reduce coronary stenoses angiographically (Fig. 11); however, laser recanalization of the stenoses was limited by the inflexible prototype of the device (17). In addition, a high incidence of myocardial infarction in one study (18) raised concerns about the thrombogenicity or vasospastic nature of these early prototype devices. Currently, laserprobe catheters with improved flexibility, trackability, profile, a central lumen design, and temperature feedback are being investigated and appear promising.

Conclusions

We are definitely entering a new era of interventional techniques. There is already evidence that at least one laser device can supplement the vascular radiologists'complement of balloons and wires to recanalizing lesions which previously could not be treated (1). Perhaps more exciting is the suggestion that long-term results for femoropopliteal angioplasty may be improved with laser techniques (3). We have learned that bare fiberoptics are unsafe and provide inadequate recanalized channels. A second generation of modified fiberoptic tips offer significant improvements in safety and efficacy compared to bare fiberoptics. The improved results are attributed to self-centering rounded tips, circumferential vaporization, thermal compression by the contact devices, and a residual luminal surface that has less fracture, dissection, and restenosis than balloon angioplasty. Experimental research as well as randomized comparative clinical trials are greatly needed to determine which laser devices can improve upon the two major limitations of balloon angioplasty: recanalization of chronic total occlusions and restenosis.

References

1. Cumberland DC, Sanborn TA, Tayler DI et al. (1986) Percutaneous laser thermal angioplasty:initial clinical results with a laserprobe in total peripheral artery occlusions. Lancet I:1457
2. Sanborn TA, Haudenschild CC, Faxon DP et al. (1987) Angiographic and histologic consequences of laser thermal angioplasty: comparison with balloon angioplasty. Circulation 75:281
3. Sanborn TA, Cumberland DC, Greenfield AJ et al. (1988) Percutaneous laser thermal angioplasty: initial results and one-year follow-up in 129 femoropopliteal lesions. Radiology 168:121
4. Ginsberg R, Wexler L, Mitchell RS, Profitt D (1985) Percutaneous transluminal laser angioplasty for treatment of peripheral vascular disease:clinical experience with 16 patients. Radiology 156:619
5. Cumberland DC, Taylor DI, Proctor AE (1986) Laser-assisted percutaneous angioplasty: initial clinical experience in peripheral arteries. Clin Radiol 37:423
6. Geschwind HJ, Boussignac G, Teisseire B et al. (1984) Conditions for effective Nd-YAG laser angioplasty. Br Heart J 52:484
7. Hussein H (1986) A novel fiberoptic laser probe for treatment of occlusive vessel disease. Optical Laser Technol Med 605:59
8. Welch AJ, Bradley AB, Torres JH et al. (1987) Laser probe ablation of normal and atherosclerotic human aorta in vitro: a first thermographic and histologic analysis. Circulation 76:1353
9. Sanborn TA, Faxon DP, Haudenschild C, Ryan TJ (1985) Experimental angioplasty: circumferential distribution of laser thermal energy with a laser probe. J Am Coll Cardiol 5:934
10. Abela GS, Fenech A, Crea F et al. (1985) Hot Tip: another method of laser vascular recanalization. Laser in Surgery and Medicine 5:327
11. Sanborn TA, Faxon DP, Haudenschild CC et al. (1983) The mechanism of transluminal angioplasty: Evidence for formation of aneurysm in experimental atherosclerosis. Circulation 68:1136
12. Sanborn TA, Greenfield AJ, Guben JK et al. (1987) Human percutaneous and intraoperative laser thermal angioplasty: Initial clinical results as an adjunct to balloon angioplasty. J Vasc surg 5:83
13. Zeitler E, Richter EI, Seyferth W (1982) Femoropopliteal arteries. In: Percutaneous Transluminal Angioplasty. Dotter CT, Grüntzig A, Schoop W, Zeitler E (eds) Springer-Verlag Berlin p 105
14. Hewes RC, White RI, Murray RR et al. (1986) Long-term results of superficial femoral artery angioplasty. Am J Radiol 146:1025

15. Krepel VM, van Ardel GJ, van Erp WFM, Breslau PJ (1985) Percutaneous transluminal angioplasty of the femoropopliteal artery: initial and long-term results. Radiology 156:325
16. Murray RR, Hewes RC, White RI et al. (1987) Long segment femoropopliteal stenoses: is angioplasty a boon or a bust. Radiology 162:473
17. Sanborn TA, Faxon DP, Kellett MA, Ryan TJ (1986) Percutaneous coronary laser thermal angioplasty. J Am Coll Cardiol 8:1437
18. Cumberland DC, Starkey IR, Oakley GDG et al. Percutaneous laser-assisted coronary angioplasty. Lancet 2:214

Intraoperative coronary laser angioplasty – first clinical experiences with a new method

R. Moosdorf

Klinik für Herz- und Gefäßchirurgie am Zentrum der Justus-Liebig-Universität Giessen, FRG

With the availability of flexible fiber systems, different laser systems have commanded a growing interest in the field of cardiovascular disease (1, 2).

We started our first experimental investigations on laser angioplasty in 1984, using a continuous wave argon laser system with flexible quartz fibers of different diameters down to 0.4 mm. Our in vitro experiments on human cadaver hearts showed an ablative effect in non-calcified plaques, but the unprotected fiber led to a high rate of perforation due to mechanical or thermal damage (3, 4).

This risk could significantly be decreased by the introduction of specially designed laser-thermalprobes with metal-capped tips, in which laser energy is totally converted into thermal energy and is circumferentially distributed to the affected arterial segment (5, 6). These so called hot tips proved to be safe and effective in experimental settings, so that we started our first clinical trial on intraoperative coronary laser angioplasty with these probes in the beginning of 1987. Besides the totally metal-capped hot tips a newly designed type of a so-called hybrid probe was also used later on. In these hybrid probes, a small sapphire window at the top of the metal cap allows the direct passage of a certain amount of light energy, while the major part of approximately 80% is still converted into heat. Especially suited for total occlusions, the direct laser beam may create a small guiding channel, which then allows passage of the larger metal head.

Based on these two types of probes, differently designed special coronary systems were also used later during our clinical trial, which for example, incorporated special flushing channels for cooling and dye injection, or a small guide wire channel for improved steerability.

In our concept, as with endarterectomy and intraoperative balloon angioplasty, laser angioplasty was considered an adjunct to coronary bypass surgery. To evaluate its intraoperative applicability, safety and efficacy, the indications for a laser angioplasty were limited to proximal tandem lesions, entrapping of one or more non-diseased side branches which were not able to be revascularized, as well as diffuse proximal lesions with impaired run-off to side branches. Longer calcified lesions were still treated by endarterectomy and distal lesions were considered to be an indication for balloon angioplasty (7).

Patients and methods

Within this protocol, between January 1987, and June 1988, 28 patients were additionally treated by an intraoperative argon laser angioplasty during conventional bypass procedures. The patient information is shown in Table 1.

147

Table 1. Clinical characteristics of 28 patients undergoing laser angioplasty. Number of patients 28; male 23; female 5; mean age 58,9 (48–73) years

Preoperative Data:			
NYHA class	II (6)	III (16)	IV (6)
cardiac index	3,95	(3,3–4,4)	
ejection fraction	63,4%	(40%–83%)	
myocardial infarction	13 (1×)	6 (2×)	

According to our protocol the main indication for a laser angioplasty was a tandem lesion of the LAD in 13 patients, of the circumflex system in two patients and of the left main stem and LAD or a diagonal branch in two patients. Finally, 10 patients showed diffuse lesions of the mid-portion of the LAD entrapping major side branches.

The intraoperative procedure was similar to that of conventional bypass surgery. Under cardioplegic cardiac arrest, the target artery was incised distal to the atherosclerotic lesion. Size of the artery, degree of stenosis and distance between incision and the lesion were measured by calibrated probes. Afterwards, the laser probe was introduced and after contact with the target lesion it was activated. In cases of minor lesions, flushing with cardioplegic solution via the aortic root proved to be sufficient during the laser procedure. In cases of subtotal lesions or total occlusion, retrograde flushing was achieved by introducing a small catheter sheath into the coronary artery. The laser probe was then introduced through the central catheter while flushing was performed through a side port, again using cardioplegic solution. Special intraoperative coronary probes with integrated flushing ports allowed a direct fluid irrigation through small side holes in the metal tip of the laser probe. Under continuous fluid irrigation, the activated laser probe was advanced through the lesion under continuous motion; after passage of the lesion it was deactivated and drawn back. The size of the newly created channel was afterwards measured by calibrated probes. In cases of larger caliber coronaries, for which the new lumen seemed too small, a balloon angioplasty was added. Finally, the anastomosis between a segment of the saphenous vein or the internal mammary artery was performed. The result of the entire procedure was then again controlled by perfusion of cardiogreen through the bypass graft.

An intraoperative angiographic control was performed in four cases and proved to be technically difficult and time consuming, so that we no longer use it for routine interventions. In contrast to this, angioscopy in our hands seems to be much more effective and less time consuming. Within the framework of a special study of angioscopy and laser angioplasty, we routinely performed angioscopy prior to and after lasing with a thin 1.00 mm angioscope in our last eight patients. We could visualize the target lesion before laser application, estimate the degree of stenosis, and afterwards could demonstrate the effect of the laser angioplasty including for example dissections or perforations. This control takes approximately five minutes and offers precise images of the intravascular situation. The detailed intraoperative data of our laser procedures are shown in Table 2.

Table 2. Intraoperative date of simultaneous laser procedure

Intraoperative Data:	
Crossclamping time	61 min (38–80 min)
Number of anastomoses	2,8 (2–5)
Additional endarterectomy	2
Mean lasing time	45 sec (15–90 sec)

Within this first protocol which was closely related to the phase one control of the FDA, laser angioplasty proved to be efficient and associated with a low risk of complication. We were unsuccessful in passing the lesion in four patients because of severe calcification and there was only one perforation and one dissection within this first series. We saw no probe-related complication in any of the cases. In the remaining 24 cases, the laser probe could pass the target lesion and create a new channel.

The postoperative complications were also very low. Only one patient showed signs of temporary myocardial ischemia without any sequelae or myocardial infarction. Four patients showed postoperative rhythm disturbances. One patient had previously been under medical therapy for ventricular extrasystoles and a second patient first developed ventricular extrasystoles postoperatively. In both cases drug therapy effectively terminated the arrhythmia. Another two patients developed atrial flutter, a common occurrence after bypass surgery, which could be converted medically.

Conclusion

The first clinical trial of coronary laser angioplasty as an adjunct to conventional bypass surgery could up to now demonstrate the following: The method can effectively be applied in an intraoperative setting. The immediate success rate of 85 % is comparable to other adjunctive methods such as endarterectomy or intraoperative balloon angioplasty. The procedure can be performed with reasonable expenditure and within a reasonable time period. Careful consideration of indications and of laser safety leads to a low risk of complication. The immediate intraoperative control of laser angioplasty can be performed by calibrated probes and direct perfusion with dye solution, moreover angioscopy has proven to be a very efficient control method. Intraoperative fluoroscopy involves extreme technical expenditure and is very time consuming, so that we do not consider it as a routine method. Highly calcified lesions cannot be ablated by this laser system and are still an indication for a conventional endarterectomy, or for yet to be perfected photo-ablative laser systems.

The further evaluation of this method will also depend on its long-term results. Our first clinical protocol did not require routine angiographic control study, however in nine patients, repeat angiographic study between one week and six months after operation, showed improved or partially improved luminal diameter in five patients. One lased segment showed an unchanged status and three segments with formerly longer subtotal lesions were totally occluded. The results of these first angiographic studies must be interpreted carefully, as the patency of the lased segment depends on the retrograde run-off, the length of the treated lesion and also on the anticoagulant therapy. By treating only the second of a tandem lesion, compet-

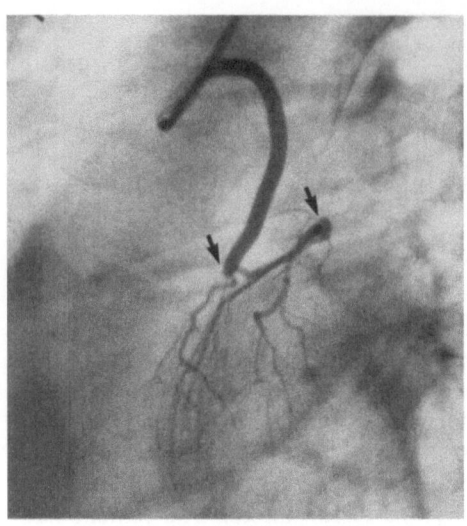

Fig. 1. Lasered distal segment of a tandem lesion (arrows) with retrograde perfusion of formerly entrapped marginal and diagonal branch

itive flow is avoided and patency is mainly influenced by retrograde flow. The segment proximal to entrapped side branches, including the proximal tandem lesion, tends to occlude in the sense of a dead-end street phenomenon (Fig. 1). Among the restenosed or reoccluded vessels, three of four were longer diffuse lesions with only smaller entrapped side branches, in which, in the setting of competitive flow and bad run-off, early reocclusion occurred even after angioscopically demonstrable intraoperative patency.

In addition, the optimal anticoagulant regimen remains open to discussion. In cases of peripheral laser angioplasties, patients are treated with an antiplatelet drug prior to the intervention and remain under therapy during and after angioplasty. This regimen cannot be applied to patients undergoing surgical interventions under extracorporeal circulation. We used heparin at 10 IU/kg/h immediately postoperatively for the first two days. Afterwards, patients received coumadin plus 100 mg of ASA. A follow up study will compare this therapy with an antiplatelet regimen of aspirin/persantine starting on the second postoperative day. Another change in our second protocol is the inclusion of segmental distal lesions which can be treated with specially designed small probes of 1 mm. The first patient with a diffusely affected LAD could be successfully revascularized and showed a patent lased segment on repeat angiography one week postoperatively.

To date, the results of our first clinical protocol on intraoperative coronary laser angioplasty could demonstrate the effectivity and feasibility of the method in an intraoperative setting. A lot of questions concerning technical problems and long-term results remain to be solved before this new technique can be applied as a routine method during operative or even percutaneous procedures.

References

1. Choy DSJ, Stertzer SH, Myler RK, Marco J and Fournial G (1984) Human coronary laser recanalization. Clin Cardiol 7:377–381

2. Ginsburg R, Kim DS, Guthaner D, Toth J and Mitchel RS (1984) Salvage of an ischemic limb by laser angioplasty; Description of a new technique. Clin Cardiol 7:54–58
3. Moosdorf R, Glauber M and Scheld HH (1987) Experimentelle Untersuchungen zur Frage der klinischen Anwendbarkeit des Argon-Lasers in der Herz- und Gefäßchirurgie. Herz-Kreislauf 9:427–431
4. Abela GS, Normann SJ, Cohen DM, Franzini D, Feldman RL, Crea F, Fenech A, Pepine CH, Conti CR (1985) Laser recanalization of occluded atherosclerotic arteries in vivo and in vitro. Circulation 71:403–411
5. Abela GS, Fenech A, Crea F, Conti CR (1985) Hot tip: another method of laser vascular recanalization. Lasers in Surgery and Medicine 5:327–335
6. Sanborn TA, Faxon DP, Haudenschild C, Ryan TJ (1985) Experimental angioplasty: circumferential distribution of laser thermal energy with a laser probe. J Am Coll Cardiol 5:934–938
7. Scheld HH, Görlach G, Kling D, Moosdorf R, Stertmann WA, Hehrlein FW (1987) Technik der koronaren Endarteriektomie. Z f Herz-, Thorax- und Gefäßchirurgie 1:91–96

Laser angioplasty of iliac and femoropopliteal obstructive lesions

M. P. Heintzen, T. Neubaur, M. Klepzig, B. E. Strauer

Medical Clinic and Polyclinic B, University of Düsseldorf, FRG

Introduction

In 1964, Dotter and Judkins (3) published initial results of a percutaneous transluminal approach for the treatment of peripheral arterial occlusive disease. Since then different techniques have been developed to overcome the limitations of their method. The double-lumen balloon catheter was introduced by Grüntzig in 1974, and lead to a widespread application of this technique in peripheral and coronary artery disease (6). In spite of balloon catheter improvement there are still some problems of conventional balloon angioplasty, e.g., long occlusions and calcified lesions are difficult to recanalize and the incidence of restenosis seems to be too high (4, 21, 22). Therefore, new strategies such as laser angioplasty were investigated and introduced into clinical application. Since Ginsburg and coworkers initially performed a percutaneous transluminal laser angioplasty in a high-grade deep femoral artery stenosis of a patient in 1983 (5), laser angioplasty has evolved into an accepted method for the treatment of peripheral arterial occlusive disease.

Different catheter systems (bare-fiberoptics, laser probes, sapphire-tips) were used for the application of laser energy on atherosclerotic tissue. Bare-fiber laser angioplasty offers some advantages over thermal laser angioplasty using laser probes, and accordingly a bare-fiber laser catheter was developed and used in this clinical study (12, 16). A continous-wave Nd:YAG laser (1064 nm) in a chopped mode was coupled to the catheter system to treat 26 patients suffering from stenoses and occlusions of the lower limb (7, 8, 9, 23).

Patients and Procedure

Patients

Twenty-six patients (18 males, eight females) with stenoses (n = 19) and occlusions (n = 7) of the iliac, superficial femoral, and popliteal arteries were treated by laser angioplasty; their age ranged between 42 and 78 years (mean 63 ± 10 years). There were four patients in clinical stage IV (gangrene) according to Fontaine, two patients in stage III (rest pain), 17 in stage II b (severe claudication with a painfree walking distance of less than 200 m) and four patients in stage II a (claudication with a painfree walking distance of more than 200 m).

Method

Laser angioplasty is performed with a novel bare-fiber catheter developed in our institution (12, 16). The catheter consists of a modified 6.3 French polyethylene

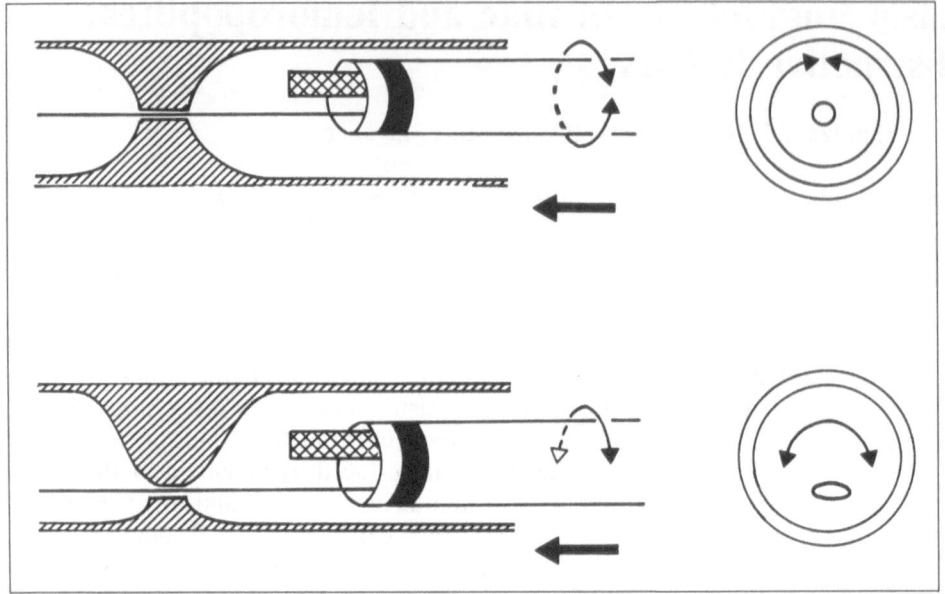

Fig. 1. Laser angioplasty in concentric (above) and eccentric (below) stenoses: In concentric stenoses the laser catheter is rotated around the guidewire within a full circle. In eccentric stenoses the fiber tip is directed under fluoroscopy only to the obstructive material, so a perforation in a region without atherosclerotic tissue can be avoided.

catheter with an oval shaped and x-ray-dense marked tip into which an also marked 0.6 mm-core silica fiber is inserted and fixed in eccentric position. Previous in vitro studies proved laser angioplasty with a melted fiber to be more effective in tissue vaporization (12, 16), so the fiber tip is prepared to melt down during laser irradiation. Furthermore, it is neccessary for controlled tissue vaporization to keep the fiber tip in direct contact to the obstructive tissue. To prevent perforation, the catheter is advanced over an 0.014-inch-guidewire with a flexible, gold-coated wolframite tip. During laser angioplasty the laser catheter is rotated around the guidewire and is slowly advanced forward in order to vaporize an adequate new lumen while the fiber tip is flushed by sodium chloride with an infusion velocity of 15 – 20 ml per min. The laser source is a continous-wave Nd:YAG laser (Medilas 40, MBB, Munich) with a wavelength of 1064 nm used in a chopped mode. Laser energy is applied in series of pulses with a pulselength of 0.2 s at a laser power of 30 watts, resulting in a pulse energy of 6 Joule. The frequency of pulse is 2 per s.

The procedure, including all possible complications, is explained to the patients prior to the treatment and written consent is obtained.

In patients with lesions in the femoropopliteal artery the common femoral artery is punctured by an antegrade stick and an 8-F introducer sheath is placed intraarterially. Patients with iliac artery stenoses have a retrograde common femoral artery puncture on the contralateral side for diagnostic angiography and an ipsilateral retrograde common femoral artery puncture for laser angioplasty. After taking an angiogram the lesion chosen for laser treatment is marked by metal clamps and an x-ray-dense grid and the guidewire for laser angioplasty is passed over the stenosis or occlusion, the laser catheter is advanced under fluoroscopic control over the wire to the obstruction and finally, laser angioplasty is started. The result of the procedure is checked by intermittent injections of diluted contrast material and laser angioplasty is continued until the laser catheter can easily cross the lesion.

As a part of our initial protocol all patients with obstructions in the femoropopliteal arteries were treated by conventional balloon angioplasty following laser angioplasty to reduce residual stenosis and to smooth further irregularities of the vessel wall. As discussed later, an additional balloon dilatation may cause some complications and we therefore decided to treat our patients who had iliac artery stenoses with laser angioplasty alone.

Before and after laser angioplasty all patients received careful clinical investigation, including Doppler measurement; follow-up examinations were performed after three and six months, and then after every six months. The degree of stenosis before and after laser angioplasty was evaluated, Doppler ankle-arm index was calculated, and in patients with iliac artery stenosis direct measurement of the systolic blood pressure gradient across the stenosis was performed. In cases of suspected recurrence digital subtraction angiography was used to visualize the treated region.

The patients wer pretreated with platelet aggregation inhibitors (acetylsalicylic acid 500–1000 mg), mostly in combination with dipyridamole (150–225 mg) for at least one day; the same medication was given during the follow-up period. During the laser angioplasty procedure 5000 to 10000 units of heparine were injected intraarterially; within the following one to two days, 25000 units of heparine were given intravenously. Most patients were discharged within three days after the procedure.

Results

In 25 out of 26 patients (96%) laser angioplasty was initially successful, resulting in recanalization of an obstruction and leaving a residual stenosis of less than 50%. Laser angioplasty failed in one patient with a long, strongly calcified superficial femoral artery occlusion.

In 16 out of 19 patients with lesions treated in the *femoropopliteal region* the clinical Fontaine stage improved; in no case did it deteriorate. The mean degree of stenosis decreased from $91 \pm 12\%$ before laser angioplasty to $31 \pm 19\%$ after laser angioplasty. Additional balloon dilatation further reduced the mean degree of stenosis to $13 \pm 18\%$, but in eight patients dissections of the vessel wall were observed. In three patients Doppler examination was not possible due to sclerosed distal vessels. In the remaining 16 patients the mean Doppler ankler-arm index improved from 0.56 ± 0.25 before treatment to 0.89 ± 0.24 after combined laser and balloon angioplasty. There were no severe acute complications such as vessel wall perforations, acute reocclusions, major bleedings at the puncture site or significant peripheral embolizations. In seven cases microembolizations were detected on the final angiogram after additional balloon dilatation. In none of these cases did any related clinical symptom occur; in two cases spontaneous lysis of these emboli was proven by additional contrast injection. Early digital subtraction angiography three days

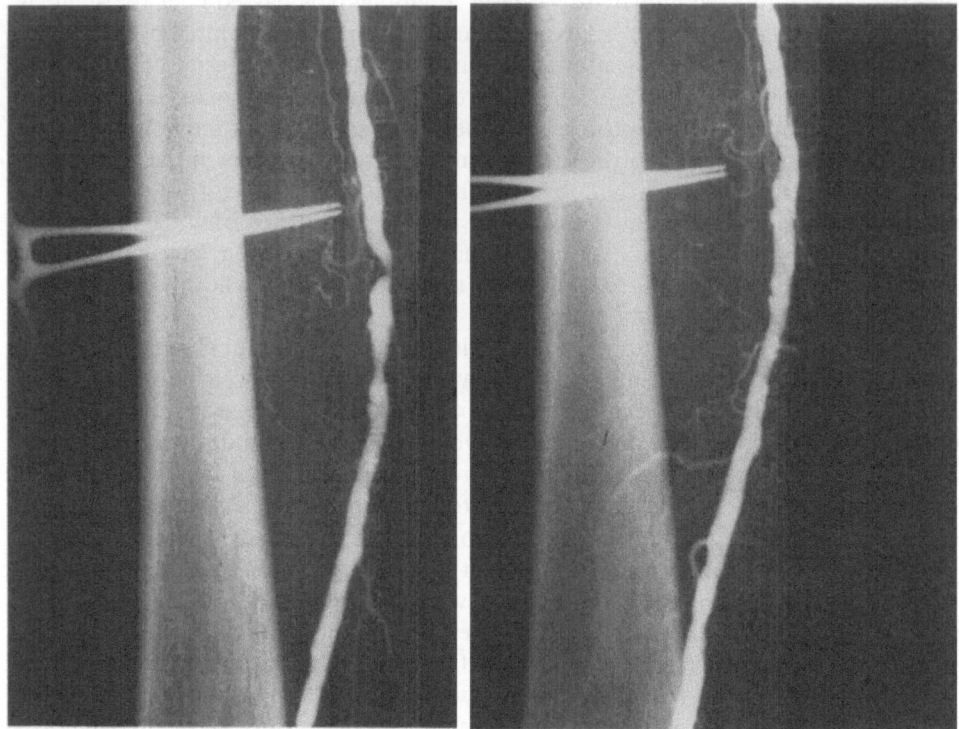

Fig. 2. Angiogram of a 78-year-old male with an eccentric superficial femoral artery stenosis before (left) and after (right) combined laser and balloon angioplasty

after the procedure showed patency of all treated lesions, within the following three months the clinical state remained unchanged, as did the Doppler index (0.82 ± 0.22). Within a total follow-up period of 18–24 months (mean 19.4 months) 17 patients with 19 treated lesions were observed. There were no reocclusions but there were four recurrences with significant stenoses in the formerly treated region resulting in a patency rate (concerning restenosis) of 76%, according to the number of patients, or 79% according to the number of treated lesions. The mean Doppler index was reduced to 0.75 ± 0.32.

All seven patients who had laser angioplasty for *iliac artery stenoses* were treated with primary success (100%) by laser angioplasty alone and the clinical stage improved in each individual. The mean degree of stenosis decreased from 86 ± 10% before laser angioplasty to 22 ± 18% after laser angioplasty. Direct blood pressure measurement showed a reduction of the mean systolic pressure gradient from 65 ± 17 mm Hg to 17 ± 15 mm Hg. Accordingly, the Doppler ankle-arm index improved from 0.61 ± 0.20 to 0.90 ± 0.15. Serious complications requiring surgery did not occur, but in one case extensive hematoma at the puncture site required blood transfusion – thereafter the patient did well and was discharged 10 days later.

Within an early follow-up period of six months, 5 patients were examined; in no case was a sign of restenosis detected.

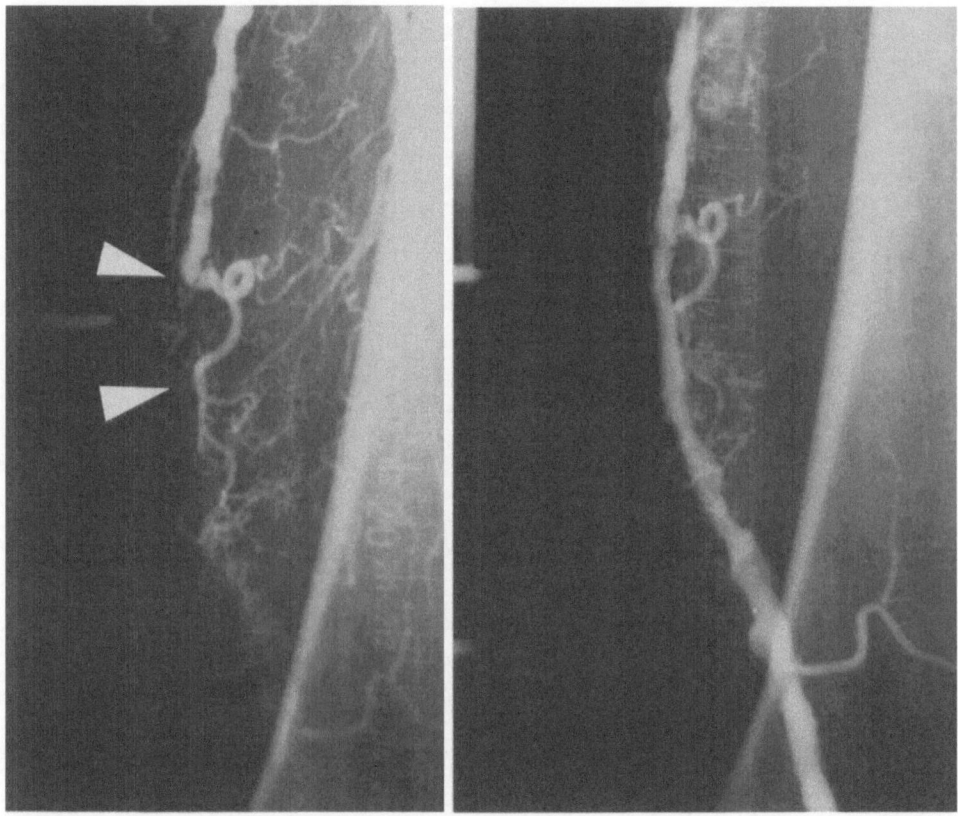

Fig. 3. Angiogram of a 72-year-old male with a superficial femoral artery occlusion before (left) and after (right) combined laser and balloon angioplasty

Discussion

Laser angioplasty has evolved into an accepted new therapeutic method for the treatment of peripheral arterial occlusive disease. A variety of different laser catheters for peripheral recanalization has been developed (2, 5, 12, 13, 16, 20). In clinical studies laser probes (hot-tip, sapphire-tip) were preferred to bare-fiberoptics, because early bare-fiber laser angioplasty was limited by frequent mechanical or thermal vessel wall perforation and only inadequate lumen improvement, followed by an increased rate of early reocclusion (1, 5, 14, 15). Nevertheless, bare fibers have certain advantages for tissue vaporization: the temperature at the fiber tip increases within less then 0.05 s to a maximum of at least 1500 °C, the cooling time amounts to approximately the same (10). Therefore, even short pulses of 0.2 seconds can be applied effectively and the thermal damage to surrounding normal tissue and blood cells can be minimized and a controlled application of laser energy is possible.

In comparison, the heat-up and cool-down times of thermal laser probes (hot-tip) are in a range of 3–5 s and the peak temperature is about 500 °C (2, 10). During heating and cooling the probe the risk of damaging normal parts of the vessel wall

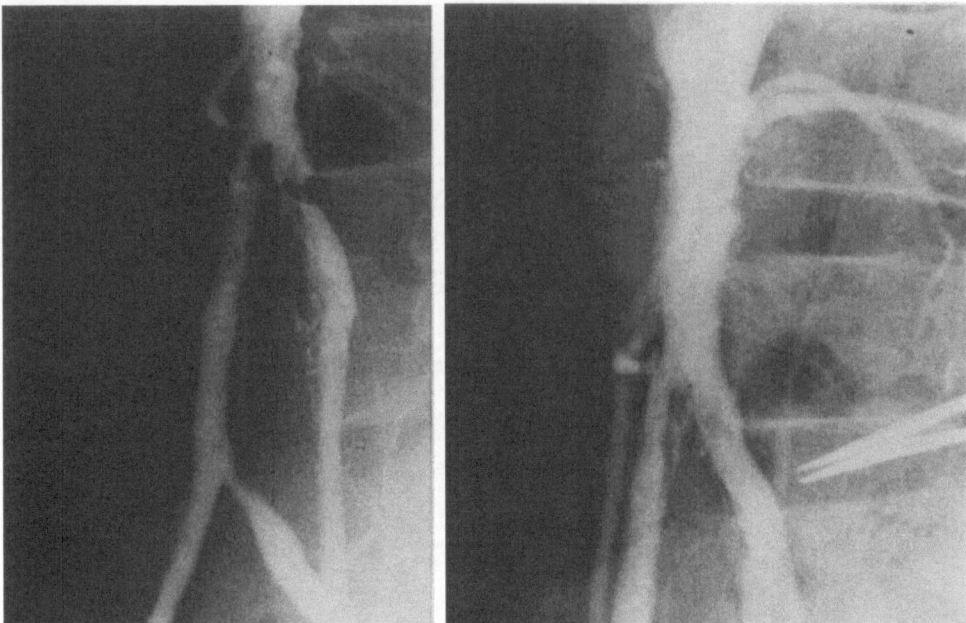

Fig. 4. Angiogram of a 43-year-old male with a high-grade eccentric stenosis of the common iliac artery before (left) and after (right) laser angioplasty *without* additional PTA

and the surrounding blood cells is markedly increased. A layer of coagulated blood or tissue may surround the probe and influence effective tissue vaporization (2). The risk of thermal damage to deeper layers of the arterial wall is increased (coagulation zones of up to 1 mm were observed [13]) and may probably result in shrinking of these treated segments with subsequent formation of restenosis. In conclusion, the recanalization properties of the hot-tip are influenced by numerous variables, and due to this fact the outcome of laser angioplasty using this system is uncertain.

Complications such as vessel wall perforation can be reduced by laser probe angioplasty compared to the formerly used bare-fiber methods, nevertheless, a perforation-rate of up to 14% is reported in the literature (13, 20). A recent publication cited a high incidence of significant peripheral embolization in 33% of the patients treated with the hot-tip system for a superficial femoral occlusion (11). Taking the advantages of bare fibers into account and knowing the possible complications of the method, a novel bare-fiber laser catheter was developed to allow safe and effective tissue vaporization (12, 16). The safeness of the new system was attained by use of a guidewire to prevent perforation, and application of only short laser pulses while the fibertip is cooled by flushing liquid, enabling controlled and localized vaporization of atherosclerotic tissue which reduces thermal damage to surrounding parts of the vessel. By rotating the laser catheter around the guidewire a large new lumen (compared to previous bare-fiber laser angioplasty without rotation) was achieved. The results of this clinical study proved the safety and efficacy of the described catheter system, there were no serious complications related to the laser treatment,

158

and the initial success rate for stenoses and occlusions in iliac and femoropopliteal arteries was 96%. In one case laser angioplasty failed in recanalization of a long and strongly calcified femoral obstruction. Previous studies demonstrated that Nd:YAG laser vaporization of calcified plaque is possible using melted fiber tips, but compared to fibrous plaque approximately 10-fold energy is required to achieve the same effect (12, 16). Therefore, today only patients with short calcified stenoses or occlusions were selected for laser treatment.

In our initial clinical study that included 19 patients with femoropopliteal lesions, laser angioplasty was completed by conventional balloon angioplasty as a part of the initial treatment protocol. It was suspected that balloon dilatation could reduce the remaining stenosis after laser angioplasty, smooth irregularities of the treated vessel wall, and thereby improve acute outcome and long-term success of the procedure. As can be seen by the values of mean percent stenosis, the major part of vessel recanalization was achieved by laser angioplasty (91% to 31%); subsequent balloon angioplasty further reduced the remaining stenosis (31% to 13%), but also caused dissections of the arterial wall in eight patients. In seven of eight cases dissections occured in patients with a 30%–50% residual stenosis after laser angioplasty; this may point out the necessity of effective lumen improvement by laser treatment even when laser angioplasty is performed as an adjunct to balloon dilatation.

In twelve of nineteen patients (63%) laser angioplasty alone improved the angiographic result to a residual stenosis of 30% or less, thus indicating a good functional result for vessel recanalization; further lumen improvement by additional balloon dilatation would not have been necessary in these patients.

In seven patients clinically insignificant peripheral embolization were detected on the control angiogram taken after balloon dilatation. Microembolisms have also been described after conventional balloon angioplasty. The patients had no clinical symptoms and in follow-up studies performed early after embolization spontaneous clot lysis could be demonstrated in most cases (22). It is not yet clear which mechanism caused microembolisms found in this study. There are two different in vitro studies dealing with surface thrombogenicity after laser angioplasty; Pollock et al. (17) reported an increased thrombogenicity after argon laser irradiation, Prevosti et al. (18) noted diminished thrombus formation after thermal laser angioplasty and direct Er:YAG laser application. If there is thrombus formation in clinical laser angioplasty, displacement of these thrombi by the balloon catheter may occur. Blood cell clotting induced by laser energy is another possible reason, but also ablation of larger atherosclerotic particles may be responsible. In the literature, embolization after laser angioplasty is reported to be low (13, 20) – only in one recent study was a 33% rate of significant peripheral embolization reported for hot-tip thermal laser angioplasty, and in 10 out of 12 cases surgical intervention was needed (11).

Laser angioplasty is likely to reduce the restenosis rate compared to conventional balloon dilatation by removing atherosclerotic tissue. In experimental studies performed in the atherosclerotic swine model a reduced incidence of restenosis was observed after laser angioplasty (19). Recently, Sanborn et al. reported on their results in 129 femoropopliteal laser recanalizations. In cases treated for stenoses and short occlusions (< 3 cm) the recurrence rate within one year was only 5% and 7%, respectively (20). Gailer and coworkers reported for cases of balloon dilatation for treatment of femoral artery stenoses (751 patients) and occlusions (518 patients) long-term success rates within two years of 76% and 72%, respectively (4). Within 12–24 months after PTA of femoropopliteal lesions, Schneider reported a cumulative patency rate of 69.3% (21).

In our initial clinical study we had to deal with all uncertainties of a new therapeutic strategy, nevertheless, the patency rate within a mean follow-up of 19.4 months was 76%, according to the number of treated patients, and 79% with respect to the number of treated lesions. These results are comparable with the patency rates of any well-established and multiply performed procedure such as PTA.

The reason for restenosis in our study is not clear. Probably the vessel wall irritation by combined laser and balloon technique is responsible. In three out of four recurrences dissections after PTA had occurred. To evaluate whether laser angioplasty alone is able to increase the long-term patency rate we have now started to treat patients by laser angioplasty without additional balloon dilatation. By an improvement of the catheter-technique even large iliac arteries could be recanalized with good angiographic and clinical results. In five patients no restenosis occurred within a short follow-up of six months (9).

In summary, laser angioplasty using the described technique is safe and effective for the treatment of peripheral arterial occlusive disease. Even in this early clinical study in a limited number of patients long-term results are comparable with those reported after conventional balloon angioplasty. Better knowledge of proper case selection, improvement of laser catheters, and increased technical skill of the operator will improve these results.

References

1. Abela GS, Norman S, Cohen D, Feldman RL, Geiser EA, Conti CR (1982) Effects of carbon dioxide, Nd-YAG and argon laser radiation on coronary atheromatous plaques. Am J Cardiol 50:1199–1205
2. Borst C, Verdaasdonk RM, Boulanger LHMA, Oomen A, Berengoltz SN, Mali WPTM, Westerhof PW, Robles de Medina EO (1988) Comparison of hot tip and sapphire tip recanalization. In: Biamino G, Müller GJ (eds): Advances in laser medicine I. First German symposium on laser angioplasty. Ecomed, Landsberg: 70–80
3. Dotter CT, Judkins MP (1964) Transluminal treatment of arteriosclerotic obstruction. Description of a new technique and a preliminary report of its application. Circulation 30:654–670
4. Gailer H, Grüntzig A, Zeitler E (1983) Late results after percutaneous transluminal angioplasty of iliac and femoropopliteal obstructive lesions – A cooperative study. In: Dotter CT, Grüntzig AR, Schoop W, Zeitler E (eds): Percutaneous transluminal angioplasty. Springer, Berlin: 215–218
5. Ginsburg R, Wexler L, Mitchell RS, Profitt D (1985) Percutaneous transluminal laser angioplasty for treatment of peripheral vascular disease. Radiology 156:619–624
6. Grüntzig A, Hopff H (1974) Perkutane Rekanalisation chronischer arterieller Verschlüsse mit einem neuen Dilatationskatheter. Modifikation der Dotter-Technik. Dtsch med Wschr 99:2502–2505
7. Heintzen MP, Neubaur T, Klepzig M, Richter EI, Zeitler E, Strauer BE (1988) Clinical experiences in Nd:YAG laser angioplasty in the periphery. In: Biamino G, Müller GJ (eds): Advances in laser medicine I. First German symposium on laser angioplasty. Ecomed, Landsberg: 103–113
8. Heintzen MP, Neubaur T, Klepzig M, Zeitler E, Strauer BE (1988) Nd:YAG laser angioplasty of peripheral arteries in humans: Acute results and follow-up. Eur Heart J 9, Suppl I:332

9. Heintzen MP, Neubaur T, Köhler M, Strauer BE (1988) Laser angioplasty of iliac artery stenoses. Heart and Vessels 4:53
10. Hessel S, Frank F, Ischinger T, Heintzen MP (1988) Possibilities for the use of Nd:YAG laser in vascular recanalization. In: Biamino G, Müller GJ (eds): Advances in laser medicine I. First German symposium on laser angioplasty. Ecomed, Landsberg: 89–95
11. Katzen BT, Kaplan JO, Schwarten DM, v. Breda A (1988) Complications of "hot-tip" laser assisted angioplasty. Circulation 78, Suppl II:417
12. Klepzig M, Neubaur T, Stellwaag M, Strauer BE (1986) Nd-YAG laser angioplasty: Vascular effects, catheter development and in vivo application. Circulation 74, Suppl II:203
13. Lammer J, Karnel F (1988) Percutaneous transluminal laser angioplasty with contact probes. Radiology 168:733–737
14. Lee G, Ikeda RM, Theis JH, Chan MC, Stobbe D, Ogata C, Kumugai A, Mason DT (1984) Acute and chronic complications of laser angioplasty: Vascular wall damage and formation of aneurysms in the atherosclerotic rabbit. Am J Cardiol 53:290–293
15. Lee G, Ikeda RM, Chan MC, Lee MH, Rink RL, Reis RL, Theis JH, Low R, Bommer WJ, Kung AH, Hanna ES, Mason DT (1985) Limitations, risks and complications of laser recanalization: A cautions approach warranted. Am J Cardiol 56:181–185
16. Neubaur T, Klepzig M, Strauer BE (1988) Perkutane transluminale Laserangioplastie bei arterieller Verschlußkrankheit – Entwicklung eines neuen Laserkathetersystems. Z Kardiol 77:245–250
17. Pollock ME, Eugene J, Hammer-Wilson M, Berns MW (1987) The thrombogenic potential of argon ion laser endarterectomy. J Surg Res 42:153–158
18. Prevosti LG, Lawrence JF, Leon MB, Kramer WS, Lu DY, Smith PD, Bonner RF (1987) Reduced surface thrombghenicity after thermal ablation of plaque. Circulation 76, Suppl IV:408
19. Sanborn TA, Faxon DP, Haudenschild CC, Gottman SB, Ryan TJ (1986) Laser thermal angioplasty: Reduced restenosis compared to balloon angioplasty. Circulation 74, Suppl II:6
20. Sanborn TA, Cumberland DC, Greenfield AJ, Welsh CL, Guben JK (1988) Percutaneous laser thermal angioplasty: Initial results and 1-year follow-up in 129 femoropopliteal lesions. Radiology 168:121–125
21. Schneider E, Grüntzig A, Bollinger A (1983) Long-term patency rates after percutaneous transluminal angioplasty for iliac and femoropopliteal obstructions. In: Dotter CT, Grüntzig AR, Schoop W, Zeitler E (eds): Percutaneous transluminal angioplasty. Springer, Berlin: 175–180
22. Seyfert W, Ernsting M, Grosse-Vorholt R, Zeitler E (1983) Complications during and after percutaneous transluminal angioplasty. In: Dotter CT, Grüntzig AR, Schoop W, Zeitler E (eds): Percutaneous transluminal angioplasty. Springer, Berlin: 161–169
23. Strauer BE, Neubaur T, Klepzig M, Heintzen MP, Zeitler E, Richter EI (1988) Perkutane periphere Laserangioplastie: Erste klinische Ergebnisse. Z Kardiol 77:29–35

Radiofrequency coronary angioplasty in patients with coronary artery disease – a new method for treatment of coronary artery stenoses

V. Hombach, M. Höher, M. Kochs, S. Wieshammer, W. Haerer, Th. Eggeling, A. Schmidt, H. W. Höpp, H. H. Hilger

Department of Cardiology-Angiology-Pneumonology, University of Ulm, FRG
Medical Clinic III, University of Cologne, FRG

Introduction

Balloon dilatation (PTCA) at present seems to be the standard procedure for non-surgical coronary angioplasty in patients with clinically significant stenoses (3, 5). Despite relatively high initial success rates of up to 90% and more (1), there are many patients with stenotic lesions (e.g., eccentric, calicified or longsized) that seem to be unsuitable for balloon dilatation. Moreover, recurrency rates after initial successful PTCA are in the range of 20%–30%. This may in part be due to a traumatization of the vessel intima by the balloon inflation, which may cause the release of aggregatory and vasoconstrictor substances, as well as of proliferatory factors that result in growing of the atheroma at the site of foregoing PTCA. Lastly, with balloon angioplasty atheromatous material will not be removed or condensed as could be accomplished by atherectomy or thermal angioplasty. Therefore alternative methods of coronary angioplasty are being developed, among which radiofrequency angioplasty (4) and laser angioplasty (8) seem to be the most effective and attractive methods. Based on experimental results with radiofrequency thermal recanalization of thrombotically occluded arteries in domestic pigs (4), we have designed a new catheter system for radiofrequency coronary angioplasty in patients with hemodynamically relevant coronary artery stenoses.

Patients

Thirteen patients, one female and 12 male, aged 30–60 years (mean: 54 ± 8 years) were treated with radiofrequency coronary angioplasty (RFCA). Twelve patients had stable angina pectoris of grade II–III according to CCS and one patient suffered from unstable angina. Nine patients had single-vessel disease, two patients double-vessel, and two patients triple-vessel disease. Four patients had suffered a myocardial infarction, (one non-transmural and three transmural infarctions), all located in myocardial regions that were dependent on the vessel approached for RFCA. In five patients regional hypokinesia was present on left ventricular angiography. Locations of stenoses were as follows: left anterior descending artery: n = 9, left circumflex artery: n = 2, and right coronary artery: n = 2. In eight patients RFCA was performed as the primary treatment, in three patients as a secondary treatment for restenosis of a successfully dilated stenosis, and in two patients as a tertiary treatment following re-restenosis. In six patients RFCA was applied exclusively, in another five patients followed by PTCA, and in two patients PTCA was performed first followed by RFCA.

Methods

The RFCA catheter consists of a flexible helical core, similar to those used as pacemaker electrodes, equipped with an electrode ring at the tip. The wire and the tip electrode are coated by polyurethane tubing so that the radiofrequency alternating current is delivered perpendicularly to the front line (cross-sectional area) of the ring electrode along the long axis of the vessel lumen. This prevents energy delivery and heating of the vessel wall in a radial direction and minimizes the risk for local thermal damage and perforation. This goal is supported by the use of a conventional guide wire, which can be advanced through the lumen of the RFCA-catheter, and placed distally to the targeted lesion, and thus will stabilize the catheter with it's tip in the central part of the vessel lumen ("over-the-wire technique"). Radiofrequency alternating current is delivered via the monopolar tip electrode in front of the atheromatous lesion, and is run through the tissue to the indifferent plate electrode located on the back of the patient. The electrodes are connected to the HAT 100 (Dr. Osypka GmbH, Grenzach-Wyhlen, FRG), which generates and delivers a radiofrequency current of about 600 kHz. The maximal energy delivered by the HAT 100 is 50 watt. In case of light arc production, the radiofrequency generator is automatically cut off by special electronic circuitry.

Following control coronary angiography, the steerable guide wire is placed in the vessel to be treated, advanced over the stenotic area and placed distally to the targeted lesion. Thereafter the RF catheter is advanced over the wire, until the tip of the catheter faces the lesion to be treated. Then the radiofrequency current is delivered for a short period of time (seconds), the catheter is advanced over the stenotic area, the radiofrequency current delivery is switched off and the RFCA catheter is withdrawn to a position proximal to the targeted lesion. Thereafter, control angiography is performed and the angioplasty procedure is repeated if necessary. In case of resistance to the advancing catheter, the delivery of radiofrequency current is immediately stopped in order to avoid vessel perforation. After repeat angiography with good anatomical result the catheter plus guide wire are withdrawn and final coronary angiography is performed. Pre- and post-medication of the patients is identical to that used for PTCA (aspirin 500 mg, nifedipin 20 mg, and isosorbide-dinitrate 60 mg per day).

Results

In 10 out of 13 patients (77%) a reduction of area of stenosis of equal or more than 20% was achieved. The mean area stenosis was $95 \pm 2\%$ before and $55 \pm 12\%$ after RFCA. In four patients initial RFCA results were about a 20% reduction of the stenotic area, but from an angiographic view it was incomplete, and subsequent PTCA further reduced the stenotic area significantly in two instances. In one patient

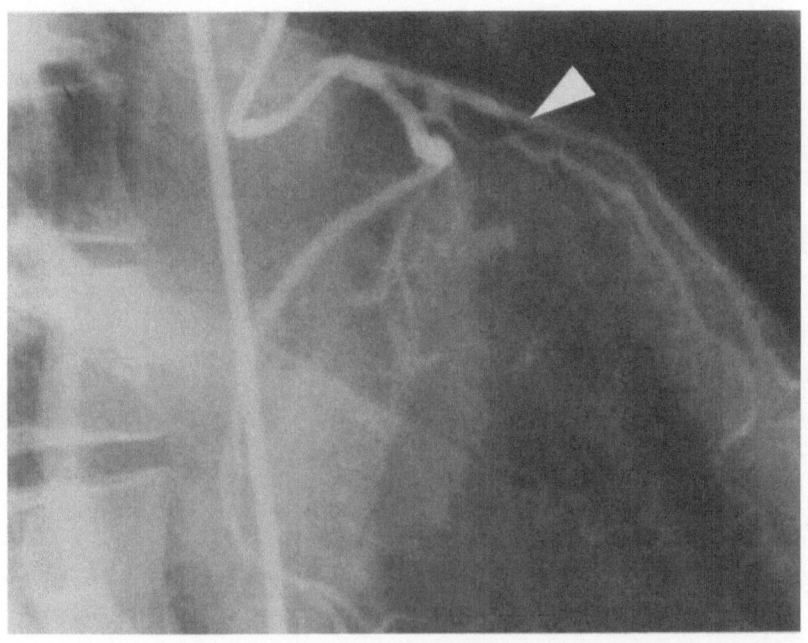

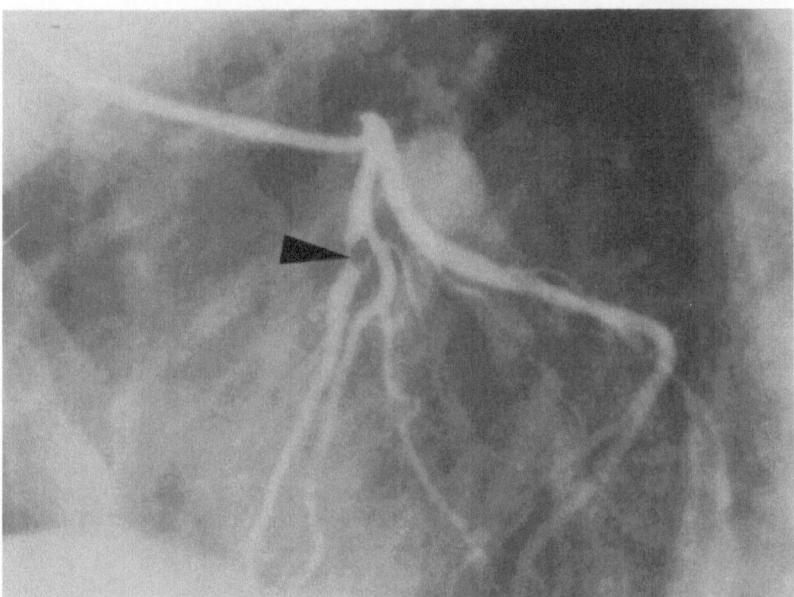

Fig. 1a. A 53-year-old patient with angina pectoris 3-CSS and high-grade stenosis of the LAD (97% area reduction, see arrow), prior to RFCA. Upper panel: 30°/20° RAO-projection; Lower panel: 45°/20° LAO-projection

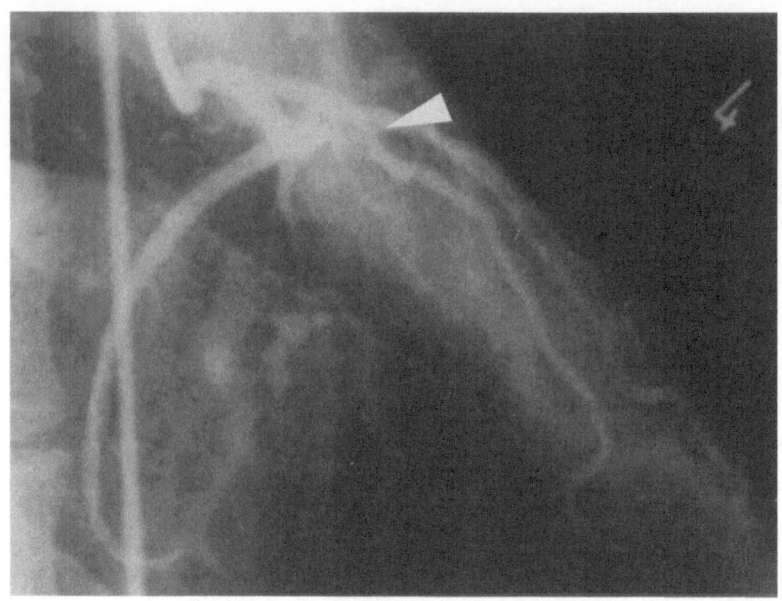

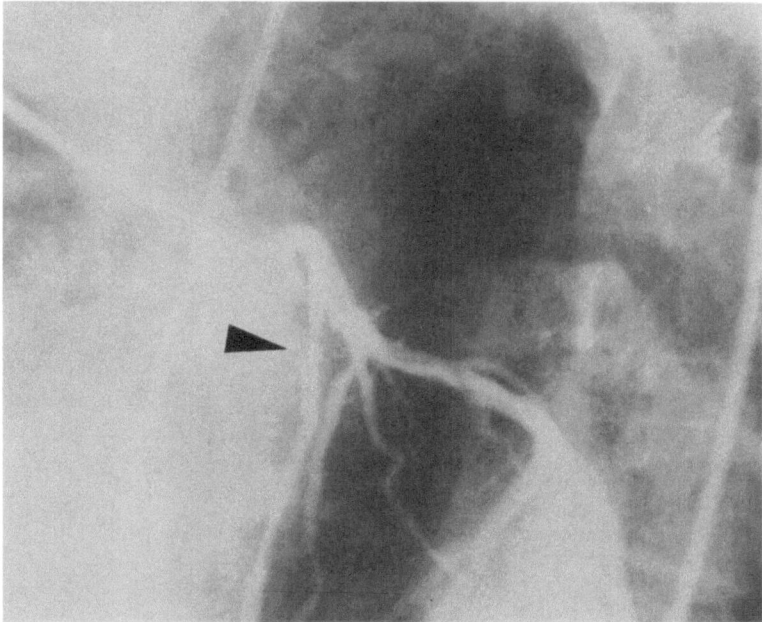

Fig. 1b. Same patient as in Fig. 1a following radiofrequency coronary angioplasty (alternating current application 4× up to 1.5 s). Reduction of the stenosis to 55% (area stenosis). Three months following RFCA the residual stenosis was 62% (not shown in this figure)

a subtotal reocclusion of the artery, whose stenosis area was initially reduced by a single FRCA procedure by more than 20%, occurred later on. The site of occlusion could be passed by a balloon catheter, and balloon inflation was performed twice. The reopened vessel showed the same area stenosis as was present following initial RFCA treatment, i.e., PTCA was not more efficient than RFCA for reduction of the targeted coronary artery stenosis in this patient. In two patients chronic vessel occlusions were reopened by balloon catheters, and the underlying stenoses were successfully treated by subsequent RFCA (an example is shown in Fig. 1).

In one patient only a short period of chest pain occurred during, and some minutes following, RFCA, and only mild ST segment elevations were seen at the end of RFCA treatment of a high-grade eccentric LAD stenosis. In none of the patients did chronic occlusion with subsequent myocardial infarction occur during or after RF-CA procedures.

A total of 3–12 episodes of radiofrequency current delivery were applied and the mean duration of RF current delivery was 2.1 ± 1.8 s. The total duration in an individual was 7.7 ± 6.7 s as a mean. One patient developed short episodes of ventricular arrhythmia only during the application of radiofrequency current, but these arrhythmias stopped immediately after termination of radiofrequency current delivery.

During a follow-up of three months, eight patients were restudied angiographically and in one of them restenosis occurred, in another reocclusion was present (total recurrency rate $2/8 = 25\%$). In six out of nine patients followed so far a significant improvement of the clinical status, particularly of angina pectoris grade, was observed.

Discussion

The initial experiences with RFCA reported here have demonstrated that hemodynamically significant coronary artery stenoses can be reduced by this technique. Regarding the side effects it is remarkable that in none of the patients was perforation of the vessel observed, and the procedure was absolutely painless in all but one of the patients. The former may be particularly due to the fact that the episodes of radiofrequency current delivery were relatively short and, moreover, that an "over-the-wire" technique was used with directing the long axis of the RFCA catheter within the central part of the artery. The painlessness of the procedure may be explained by the fact that the RFCA catheter did not occlude the vessel lumen prior to the treatment, when placed in front of the targeted lesion and the total occlusion time of the vessel during advancing the catheter over the stenosis was only a few seconds. Lastly, from our animal experiments and from theoretical reasons trauma of coronary artery vessel intima and vessel wall should be much less with RFCA than with balloon dilatation.

The primary success rates (equal or more than 20% reduction of area stenosis) are in a similar range as reported for balloon angioplasty (1, 2, 3, 5). However, the mean reduction of stenotic areas is smaller than that achieved by balloon angioplasty (RFCA: 50%–55% remaining stenosis, balloon angioplasty 25%–30%). The main reasons for this finding are technical peculiarities of the RFCA procedure itself used so far in our institution. In this series of patients RFCA catheters with fixed diameters (1.5 mm) of the tip electrode ring were used. There is no doubt that the effect of RFCA with these catheters will be much better in coronary arteries with smaller diameters (1.5–2.0 mm) than in those with larger diameters (2.0–4.0 mm). Therefore we have developed a new set of RFCA catheters with variable diameters of the "burning" tip that can be changed over a flexible guide wire ("over-the-wire" technique), which remains in place within the coronary artery with it's tip distal to the targeted lesion. We expect that with this new type of exchangable RFCA catheter stenotic lesions can be stepwise reduced by sequential application of larger diameters of the RFCA catheters.

The recurrency rates of RFCA so far seem to be in the same range as that reported for balloon angioplasty (RFCA: 25%, balloon angioplasty: 20%–30% of initially successfully treated coronary arteries). This may be partly explained by the use of the RFCA catheters with a fixed diameter that did not provide an optimal primary reduction of the stenotic lesion. An additional explanation may be that a number of patients treated with RFCA were those who already had experienced a re-stenosis or second re-stenosesis following an initial successful balloon angioplasty procedure. With the new RFCA catheters short- and longterm effects of balloon angioplasty and RFCA have to be compared in a randomized prospective trial in patients with primary treatment with either type of angioplasty. This study is now in the planning stage at our institution.

References

1. Cowley MJ, Block PC (1986) A review of the NHLBI-PTCA registry data. In: Yang GD (Ed.): Angioplasty. MacGraw Hill, New York 368
2. Detre KM, Myler RK, Kelsey SF, Raden van M, To T, Mitchell H (1984) Baseline characteristics of patients of the National Heart, Lung, and Blood Institute Percutaneous Transluminal Coronary Angioplasty Registry. Am J Cardiol 53:70
3. Grüntzig AR, Senning A, Siegenthaler W (1979) Non-operative dilation of coronary artery stenosis. New Engl J Med 301:61
4. Hombach V, Höher M, Arnold G, Osypka P, Kochs M, Eggeling Th, Höpp HW, Hirche HJ, Hilger HH (1987) Die Hochfrequenzangioplastie – Eine neue Methode zur Rekanalisation verschlossener arterieller Gefäße. CorVas 1:67
5. Ischinger T, Meier B Outcome of coronary angioplasty. In: Ischinger T (Ed.): Practice of Coronary Angioplasty (Springer, Berlin-Heidelberg-New York-Tokyo 1986), 194
6. Leimgruber P, Grüntzig AR Percutaneous transluminal coronary angioplasty. In: Hilger HH, Hombach V, Rashkind WJ (Eds): Invasive Cardiovascular Therapy (Martinus Nijhoff: Dordrecht-Boston-Lancaster 1987), 184
7. Meyer J, Schmitz HJ, Kiessling R, Erbel R, Krebs W, Schulz W, Bardos P, Minale C, Messmer BJ, Effert S (1983) Percutaneous transluminal coronary angioplasty in patients with stable and unstable angina pectoris. Analysis of early and late results. Am Heart J 106:973
8. Geschwind H, Boussignac G, Teisseive B, Vielledent C, Garton A, Becqemin JB, Mayiolini P (1984) Percutaneous transluminal laser angioplasty in man. Lancet 1:844

Angioscopy in the evaluation of interventional cardiovascular procedures

W. S. Grundfest, F. Litwak, J. Segalowitz, A. Hickey, J. Forrester

Department of Surgery, Divisions of General and Cardiothoracic Surgery and Department of Medicine, Division of Cardiology, Cedars-Sinai Medical Center, Los Angeles, California, USA

Introduction

Newly developed, high-resolution fiberoptic angioscopes allow direct percutaneous examination of the endothelial surface of the coronary artery during acute interventional therapy. Our initial experience with these devices was achieved during peripheral and coronary bypass surgery (1). Our present research is aimed at translating our intraoperative experience to percutaneous procedures. Coronary artery stenosis is known to cause angina pectoris but the etiology of acute changes in symptoms is not well defined. Coronary spasm, progressive stenosis, ruptured endothelium, and coronary thrombosis have all been implicated as causes of unstable angina. These same mechanisms may also play a role in the acute interventional setting. Systematic angiographic studies have shown that coronary thrombosis is present in as few as 2% or as many as 52% of patients with unstable angina. However, in a recent study, 96% of patients dying within 6 h of an acute ischemic event were found to have coronary thrombi or ulcerated plaque at autopsy (2). The cause of acute failure in the interventional setting remains poorly defined. The goal of our research is to define the sequence of events which occurs during acute angioplasty failure and the causes of acute ischemic syndromes.

Technology of angioscopy

Angioscopic technology is rapidly evolving. Less than four years ago the smallest available angioscope was 1.5 mm (3). To date we have performed percutaneous coronary angioscopy in 11 patients with prototype devices (AIS, Costa Mesa, California) that are 0.45 mm. in diameter with 3 000 pixels. This angioscope is housed in its own 5 French guide catheter and gives high resolution images (greater than 25 line pairs/mm at 5 mm). Similar devices are under development by Vascucare, Inc. (New York), ACS (Mountainview, California) and USCI (Massachusetts). Several other endoscopic manufacturers are considering development of percutaneous coronary angioscopes. The American Edwards Division of Baxter (Santa Ana, California) is developing digital angioscopy to improve image quality and decrease the number of pixels necessary for imaging. Olympus Corporation (Rye, New York) has developed an angioscopy pump for effective irrigation in both the percutaneous and the intraoperative setting.

To date no entirely integrated percutaneous angioscopic system exists, although all the parts and pieces are available from various manufacturers. Prototype devices to fit inside guidewires with a diameter as small as 200 mm are under development. Rapid progression of electro-optic technology will lead to more practical angioscopic systems. Until such practical systems are developed, angioscopy will remain a research tool.

Stable atheroma

In patients with chronic stable angina, the intimal surface is typically smooth, yellowish-white and glistening without evidence of disruption (4). The earliest nonobstructive lesions are oblong and oriented along the axis of flow; obstructive lesions can be concentric or eccentric. The small nonocclusive oblong protrusions are fatty streaks, which are composed predominantly of lipidladen macrophages. As the lesion enlarges smooth muscle cells migrate from the media into the subendothelium, and the lipid-laden macrophages are covered by a fibrous cap.

In patients with stable exercise-induced angina, balloon angioplasty causes stretching and disruption of the fibrous cap. Our angioscopic observations have revealed that the intimal surface may remain intact during angioplasty (5). Indeed, the intimal surface appears to stretch with the balloon in some cases. In other instances balloon angioplasty results in linear tears in the endothelium. The outcome of this tear depends upon the length and depth of the rent. Our observations of these tears, intimal flaps, and dissections lead us to believe that the pattern observed in unstable ischemic syndromes closely parallels the events observed during acute interventional therapies.

Endothelial ulceration

The distinguishing feature between acute and stable coronary disease at angioscopy is the endothelial ulcer (6). Thus far, all but one of our patients with accelerated angina examined angioscopically revealed disruption of the endothelium in the offending artery (7). In the case of acute ischemic syndromes, the cause of endothelial ulceration is not well established. However, in acute interventional therapies, abrasion of the intimal surface (either by mechanical trauma, wire abrasion, balloon overdistention, or rigid fibrotic vessels subjected to angioplasty) results in platelet deposition and aggregation. Interestingly, the mechanism by which ulceration leads to unstable angina may be through release of vasoconstrictive compounds from platelet aggregates and macrophages.

Angioscopic experience in failed PTCA

Endothelial disruption occurs in both successful and unsuccessful angioplasties. However, in successful angioplasties, the extent of this disruption appears to be limited to linear tears which do not invade the media. Our angioscopic experience during PTCA suggests that endothelial disruption that progresses beyond linear tears to circumferential lesions, dissections into the media, or denudation of the surface invariably results in thrombus formation. Both the endothelial disruption and the subsequent thrombus formation are poorly defined by angiography. Indeed, several patients who were initially thought to have had successful balloon angioplasty which subsequently closed acutely within 48 h were found on angioscopy to have thrombi (8).

Our previous experience in intraoperative angioscopy demonstrated that angioscopy provides information not available by angiography (9). This finding is reinforced by our observations during acute PTCA failures. In six patients who had acute PTCA failure, intimal flaps and thrombi were seen in all, but were detected angiographically only in two (10). Of the three failed PTCA patients with dissection, only one was seen angiographically. These angioscopic images lead us to believe that the process of endothelial disruption, platelet aggregation, and thrombus formation is a major cause of acute PTCA failure.

Thrombosis

Our intraoperative angioscopic experience has demonstrated that 87% of our patients with unstable rest angina have had subocclusive thrombus (6). These findings have been supported by the percutaneous observations of Hoher et al. (11) and Inoue et al. (12). In many cases irrigation removes the overlying thrombus to reveal an ulcerated intimal surface. In studies by Cowley et al. (13) and Park et al. (14), the presence of unstable angina and lesion thrombus was associated with an increased morbidity and mortality. The presence of thrombus suggests an underlying ulcerated thrombogenic surface. Balloon angioplasty appears to expose this surface to the blood stream and along with the thrombus already present, increases the potential for thrombotic reocclusion.

In animal experiments, our angioscopic observations have led us to believe that angioplasty of acute thrombotic occlusions leads to aggressive thrombosis despite adequate heparinization. We have observed a condition we term "malignant thrombosis" in patients with unstable angina or acute infarction. In these patients angioplasty of thrombotic lesions initiates activation of the clotting cascade which leads to abrupt vessel reclosure.

Studies by Ogilby et al. (15) and Pow et al. (16) suggest that pretreatment with heparin prevents abrupt closure and reduces propagation of intraluminal thrombus in acute PTCA. These studies are further supported by the results of Douglas et al. (17). Our angioscopic observations confirm that acute thrombus is present in almost all patients with acute myocardial infarction or unstable angina. In patients with previous myocardial infarction angioscopy performed between seven and 21 days post-infarction revealed spontaneous lysis, thrombus incorporation into the arterial wall, or recanalization of the artery.

Angioscopy for guidance of interventional therapies

In 1984, we used angioscopy in seven cases of argon laser angioplasty. Our angioscopic observations led us to realize that this laser source was inappropriate for vascular recanalization. In seven patients with occlusive arterial disease of the superficial femoral arteries, we demonstrated angioscopically that the argon laser was ineffective in vivo as it could not ablate calcified plaque. Despite vigorous irrigation, angioscopy clearly demonstrated the significant thermal damage produced by this continuous wave energy source (18).

Subsequent studies in our laboratory showed that angioscopy was effective for assessing the nature of the intimal surface, but without active steering it was ineffective in coaxially aligning the laser fiber. However, angioscopy after either laser angioplasty, or atherectomy clearly delineated the presence of flaps or thrombi which were not detected by angiography. Angioscopy revealed that excimer laser angioplasty both in the animal lab and in humans, produces smooth precisely cut channels with minimal, if any, flap formation. In contrast, rotational atherectomy tended to cause intimal disruption.

Conclusion

In summary, high-resolution ultrathin angioscopes permit direct visual examination of the intimal surface during interventional procedures. This information precisely delineates the presence of thrombi, intimal flaps, and eccentric stenoses and may help guide therapy. However, given the state of the art, routine angioscopic evaluation of angioplasty procedures is not yet a reality. Rapid progression of technology may improve the ease of use of these devices and permit direct evaluation in the post-interventional setting.

References

1. Grundfest WS, Litvack F, Sherman T et al. (1985) Delineation of peripheral and coronary detail by intraoperative angioscopy. Ann Surg 202:394
2. Falk E (1985) Unstable angina with fatal outcome: dynamic coronary thrombosis leading to infarction and/or sudden death. Autopsy evidence of recent mural thrombosis with peripheral embolization culminating in total vascular occlusion. Circulation 71:699
3. Litvack F, Grundfest WS, Lee ME et al. (1985) Angioscopic visualization of blood vessels interior in animals and humans. Clin Cardiol 8:65
4. Chaux A, Lee M, Blanche C et al. (1986) Intraoperative coronary angioscopy: technique and results in the initial 58 patients. J Thorac Cardiovasc Surg 92(6):972
5. Hickey A, Litvack F, Grundfest et al. (1986) In vivo angioscopy following balloon angioplasty. Circulation 74, Suppl II
6. Sherman C, Litvack F, Grundfest WS et al. (1986) Demonstration of thrombus and complex atheroma by in vivo angioscopy in patients with unstable angina pectoris. New Engl J Med 315:913
7. Hickey A, Kottler T, Berman D et al. (1988) Thallium–201 scintigraphy predicts instability of angioscopically visualized coronary arteries. 37th Annual Scientific Session. Am Coll Card
8. Grundfest WS, Litvack F, Hickey A et al. (1987) Coronary angioscopy: the spectrum of disease in the first 134 patients. 36th Annual Session. Am Coll Cardiol
9. Forrester WS, Litvack F, Grundfest WS et al. (1987) A perspective of coronary disease seen through the arteries of living man. Circulation 75(3):505
10. Grundfest WS, Litvack F, Hickey A et al. (1987) Coronary angioscopy correlation of intimal morphology with clinical syndromes. 2nd International Symposium on Coronary Arteriography (Rotterdam)
11. Höher M, Hombach V, Hopp HW et al. (1988) Percutaneous coronary angioscopy during cardiac catheterization. 37th Annual Scientific Session. Am Coll Cardiol
12. Inoue K, Kuwaki K, Ueda K et al. (1988) Angioscopic macropathology of coronary atherosclerosis in unstable angina and acute myocardial infarction. 37th Annual Session. Am Coll Cardiol
13. Cowley MJ, Kelsey SF, Holubkov R et al. (1988) Factors influencing outcome with coronary angioplasty: 1985–1986 NHLBI PTCA Registry. 37th Annual Session. Am Coll Cardiol

14. Park DD, Laramee LA, Teirstein P et al. (1988) Major complications during PTCA: an analysis of 5413 cases. 37th Annual Session. Am Coll Cardiol
15. Ogilby JD, Kopelman HA, Klein LW et al. (1988) Adequate heparinization during PTCA: assessment using activated clotting time. 37th Annual Session. Am Coll Cardiol
16. Pow TK, Varricchione TR, Jacobs AK et al. (1988) Does pretreatment with heparin prevent abrupt closure follwoing PTCA? 37th Annual Session. Am Coll Cardiol
17. Douglas JS, Lutz JF, Clements SD et al. (1988) Therapy of large intracoronary thrombi in candidates for percutaneous transluminal coronary angioplasty. 37th Annual Session. Am Coll Cardiol
18. Grundfest WS, Litvack F, Hickey et al. (1987) The current status of angioscopy and laser angioplasty. J Vasc Surg 5(4):667

Progress in intravascular real-time cross-sectional ultrasonic imaging at the Thoraxcenter

P. W. Serruys, E. Gussenhoven, N. Bom, J. R. T. C. Roelandt

Thoraxcenter, Erasmus University Rotterdam and University Hospital Rotterdam-Dijkzigt; Interuniversity Cardiology Institute of The Netherlands

Since the introduction by Grüntzig et al. (1) of nonoperative treatment of coronary artery stenosis (PTCA) significant progress has been made in methods for the treatment of arterial atherosclerotic disease. Currently many recanalization methods are being developed to reopen obstructed arteries during catheterization. New methods currently being studied include a rotating abrasive tip as suggested by Ritchie et al. (2), an atherectomy catheter tip method by Simpson et al. (3) and, for instance, a hot tip method as described by Sanborn et al. (4). In addition, direct laser application is also being considered for treating arterial obstruction (5, 6).

Complete removal of the obstruction might reduce the occurence of restenosis. Such techniques should, in addition, allow treatment of total occlusion not accessible by the current balloon dilatation techniques. But there is an increased need for a method to study the arterial wall beneath the endothelial surface in order to monitor plaque ablation in real-time thus providing the necessary operator feedback on the efficacy of this intervention. The steerability of the ablation process is as important as the removal of obstructing tissue and the healing response itself.

One of the main problems is arterial curvature and the asymmetry of the obstruction in relation to the arterial wall. In many of the newly proposed recanalization methods, this asymmetry introduces the risk of arterial wall perforation. For optimal use, knowledge of the localization and geometry of arterial obstruction is necessary. Catheter tip ultrasonic guidance seemed a good choice. On the other hand newer insights into the pathogenesis and pathophysiology of atherosclerosis and the potential of influencing the disease process with drugs further stimulated the development of methods to study the arterial wall. Ultrasonic intravascular imaging offers this unique potential and explains the increasing interest in this technique. This paper describes the technical aspects and first results of in-vitro experiments with high frequency intra-arterial echo imaging.

Early developments and early transducer for use inside the human body

As early as 1960, Cieszynski (7, 8) obtained echoes from within the heart with a single catheter mounted transducer introduced via the jugular vein in dogs. In 1964, Kimoto el al (9) reported their results with an intravenous transducer. After their first initial report, Omoto et al. (10) published their experience with an intravenous probe. The carrier of the probe consisted of a stainless steel tube with a 1.2 mm outside diameter and a wall thickness of 0.2 mm. Tomograms were obtained by rotation and withdrawal of the probe. Later, this method was extended by ECG triggering which allowed cross-sectional images to be obtained at a specific phase of the cardiac cycle. This method was similar to compound scanning (11).

The principle of a transducer mounted at the tip of a catheter from which the beam scans structures which are aligned perpendicularly to it offers the simplest approach to cross-sectional sonography. If the transducer rotates in synchronism with a display time-base, radial scanning produces images perpendicular to the catheter. This rotational technique was already used by Wild and Reid (12) in 1957 for intra-rectal scanning.

Early catheter tip work in Rotterdam

As early as 1969 we started a program to develop two-dimensional real-time invasive ultrasonic imaging using state-of-the-art technology. A 32-element circular array

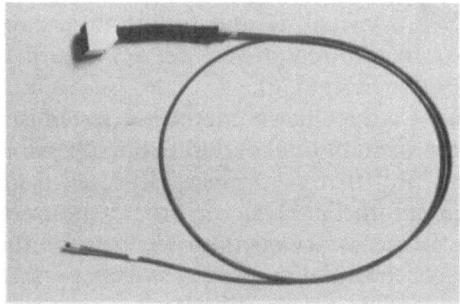

A

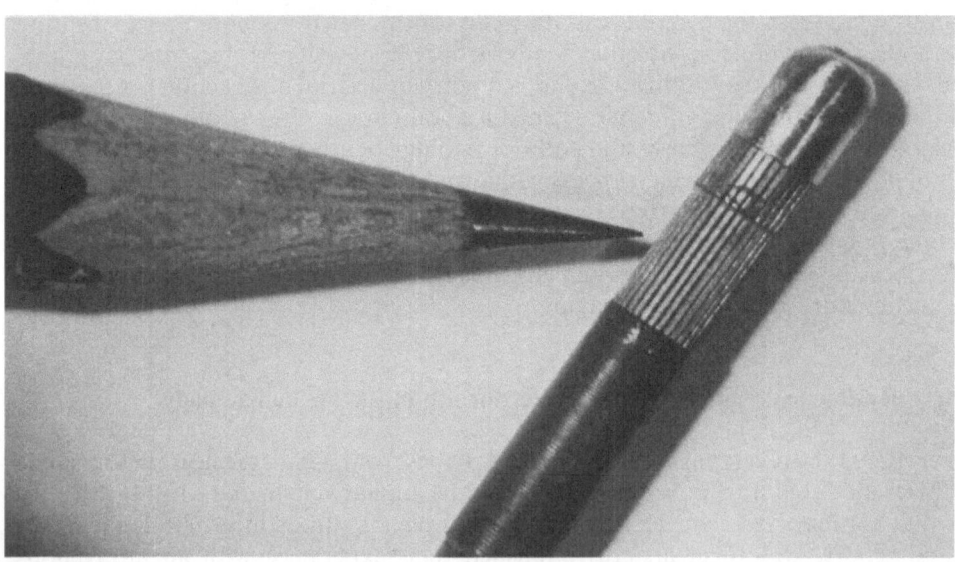

B

Fig. 1. Circular phased-array catheter for intracardiac ultrasonic real-time cross-sectional imaging. The catheter is 3 mm (9F) in diameter and is shown in the upper panel (A). An enlarged view of the 32-element catheter-tip is presented in the lower panel (B)

176

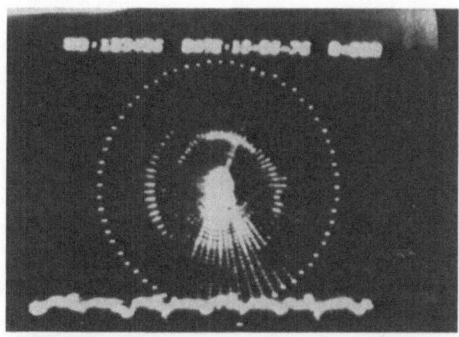

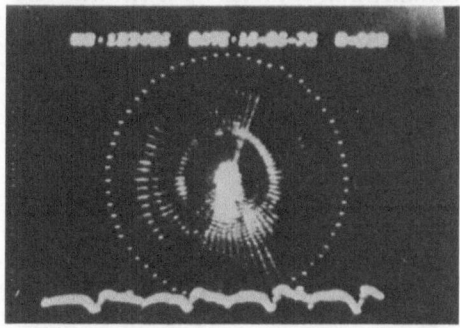

Fig. 2. Cross-sectional images of the left ventricle obtained during an experiment in a pig. The upper panel was recorded at the end-diastole and the lower panel in systole. The catheter artifact is in the middle and the outer cicle represents the viewing depth which is 4 cm. Note the ambiguous representation of the left ventricular cavity but there is clearly a systolic-diastolic change in surface area (ECG: electrocardiogram)

with an outer diameter of 3.2 mm mounted at the tip of a 9 French catheter, as illustrated in Fig. 1, was constructed (13, 14). As pointed out in the original paper (13), the array design had to be a compromise between the optimal design and the limitations imposed by technological constraints. The final design was chosen to operate at 5.6 MHz with a narrow main beam at the cost of a pronounced grating lobe at ± 56°. As a consequence the resulting display of an intracardiac scan was made up of three components: an image of echoes gernerated within the main beam and two superimposed images of reduced intensity from grating lobe echoes, but rotated over ± 56°. The net result is an ambiguous image as is illustrated in Fig. 2, obtained from within the left ventricular cavity of an experimental animal. A further reason not to adopt the multi-element course for intra-arterial imaging was the expected transmission pulse transient effect masking the nearby structures. The main limitations inherent in phased-array technology is that it is both complicated and expensive. Miniaturizing is difficult and poses serious technological problems both for the construction of the circular array of extremely small elements and the wiring through the limited lumen of the catheter. Lack of resolution in the near field and the size of the transducer continue to make circular phased-array systems unsuitable for intravascular imaging of smaller diameter vessels. In addition, for integration with spark erosion for the purpose of recanalization, the electronically steered phased array approach was not considered to be a first choice. Work has subsequently been focused on mechanical sector scan methods and we therefore opted for a 20 MHz single element construction in combination with an acoustic mirror. The diameter of the transducer element was selected to be 1 mm, using conventional technology. In a first set-up this element was provided with air backing and mounted onto a metal bar for study of sensitivity, working frequency, dead zone, echo pulse length and beam characteristics. Experience gained with these preliminary trials led us to the decision to design a mechanically rotating catheter-tip device that would provide cross-sectional two dimensional images. A single-beam A-mode display resulting from only one or a few forward looking acoustic elements at the tip was regarded too difficult to interpret.

Recent catheter tip work in Rotterdam

In Fig. 3, a schematic drawing of the echo/recanalization catheter tip is shown. The outer diameter is 2 mm. The mirror is mounted at the end of a flexible wire and can

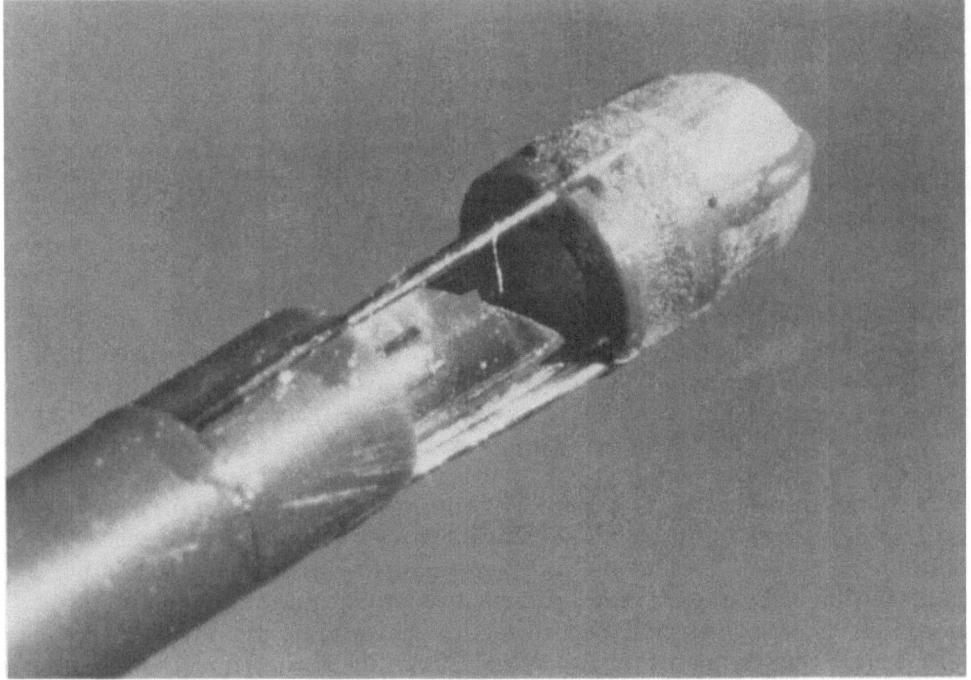

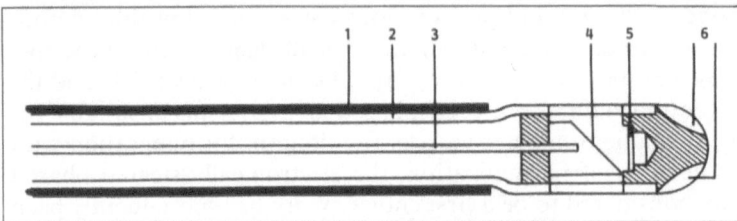

Fig. 3. Schematic drawing and photograph of a prototype spark erosion/ultrasonic imaging combination. Outer diameter is 2 mm. 1. catheter wall 2. electrode wire 3. rotating wire 4. acoustic mirror 5. acoustic element 6. electrodes

178

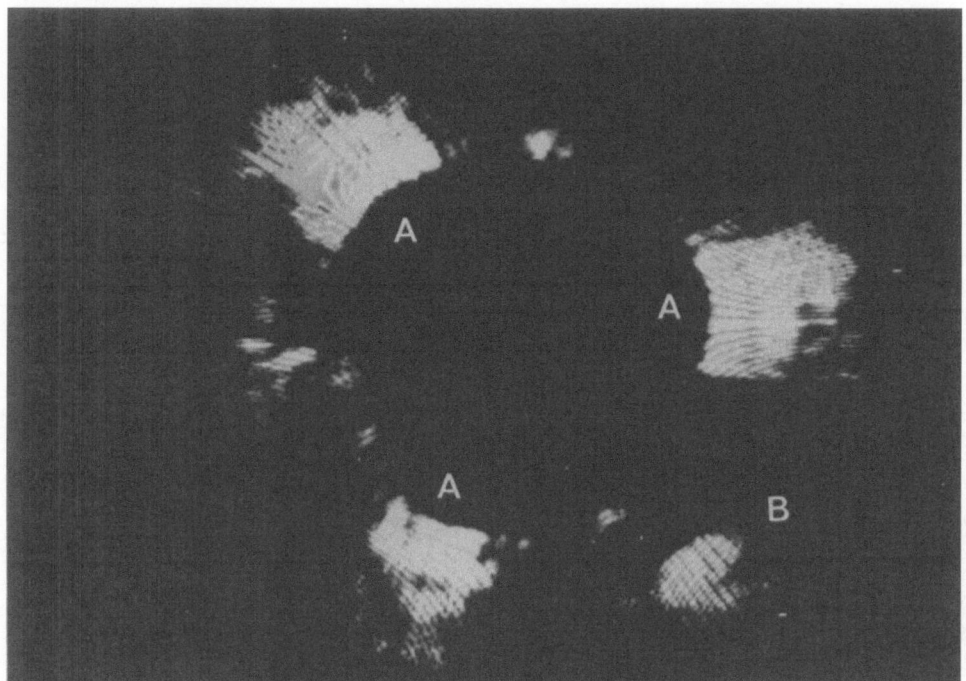

Fig. 4. First image obtained in vitro using the catheter shown in Fig. 3. On this image only the very strong echoes from the cage construction (A) and a plaque (B) are displayed

be rotated. The piezoelectric element is positioned over an airbacking for optimal sensitivity. The tip exists of three mutually isolated electrodes. The three electrodes' wires form an open cage for the echo signals and support the catheter tip. The three electrodes cause the cage echoes in some of the described results. The transducer wires are glued onto two of the isolated spark erosion electrodes. A first result from an in-vitro image as obtained with the catheter is shown in Fig. 4. In this image, the three cage echoes (A) and the echo of the calcified plaque (B) are clearly visible. These images show the possibilities of intra-arterial structure localization. Further studies taught us the limitations caused by the cage echoes and the design was modified. A rotating tip was designed and is illustrated in Fig. 5. Here the acoustic element is mounted at the fixed end of the catheter and the rotating tip is activated through a flexible shaft. In the tip a mirror for the ultrasound waves and an electrode for the spark erosion technique are incorporated. The first design features no contact of rotating mechanical parts with the internal arterial wall. The second design has the advantage that the image plane and the spark erosion plane are almost identical. An ultrasound intra-arterial image obtained from a specimen of the carotid artery is shown in Fig. 6. Water was used as a coupling liquid. The diameter of the lumen of this specimen approximates 5 mm. Inner and outer sides of the arterial wall are clearly visible. The two areas of plaque are clearly visible on the anatomic cross-section as well as on the echo image. This image was obtained with the in-vitro set-up as shown in Fig. 3.

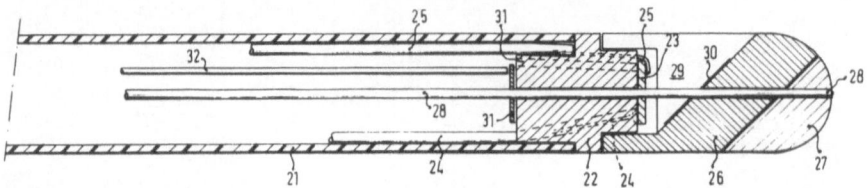

Fig. 5. A rotating tip design is illustrated in this figure. Here the acoustic element (23) is mounted at the fixed end of the catheter (21) and the rotating tip (26) is activated through a flexible shaft (28). In the tip a mirror (30) for the ultrasound waves and an electrode (27) for the spark erosion technique are incorporated

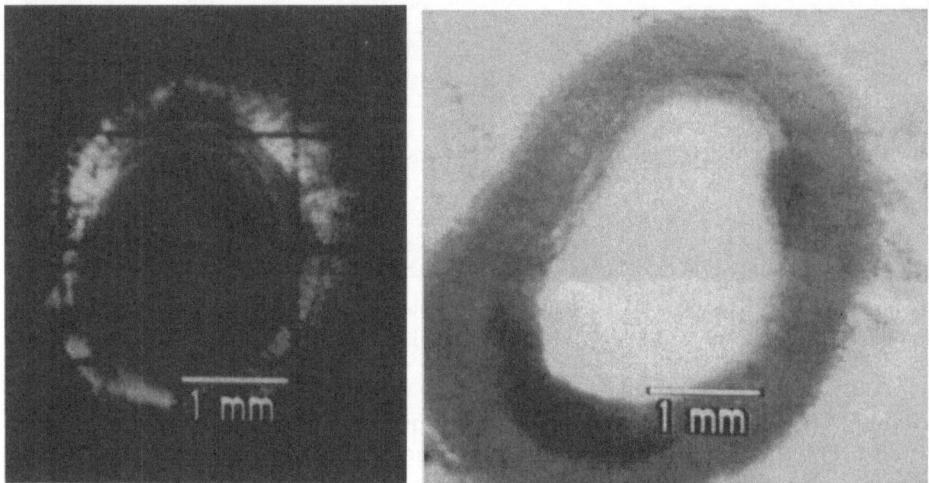

Fig. 6. First imaging results illustrated in an arterial specimen (A) and the corresponding intraarterial echo image (B) as obtained with the transducer assembly shown in Fig. 5.

The catheter diameter size required was based on work on the internal diameter of the coronary artery in normal adults. MacAlpin et al. (15) indicate that the lumen diameter of the right coronary artery ranges from 3.2 ± 0.6 mm (proximal) to 2.7 ± 0.7 mm (distal). The main left coronary artery lumen diameter was measured to be 4.0 ± 0.7 mm. For the left anterior descending artery a range was measured from 3.4 ± 0.5 mm (proximal) to 1.9 ± 0.3 mm (distal) and for the circumflex of 3.0 ± 0.7 (proximal). From this material it was concluded that in a first approach a 2 mm outer diameter catheter would be sufficiently small.

Recently, we constructed such a 2 mm (7F) catheter-tip-based single-element transducer system which operates at 40 MHz (16). An acoustic reflector rotating at 3 000 rpm sweeps the sound beam in a 360 ° arc. The transducer assembly is mounted at the tip of a 2 mm (7F) catheter and allows high resolution real-time imaging. A series of studies performed in vitro on human carotid arteries have accurately demonstrated both arterial lumen geometry and wall tissue abnormality including

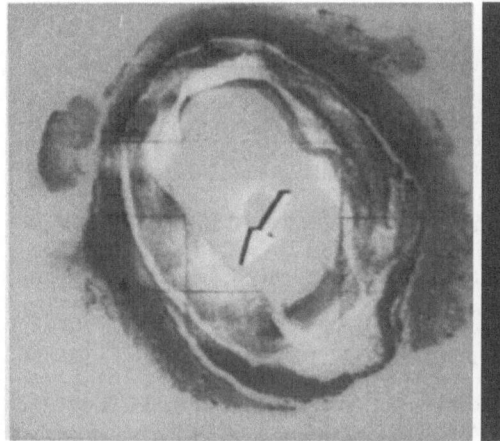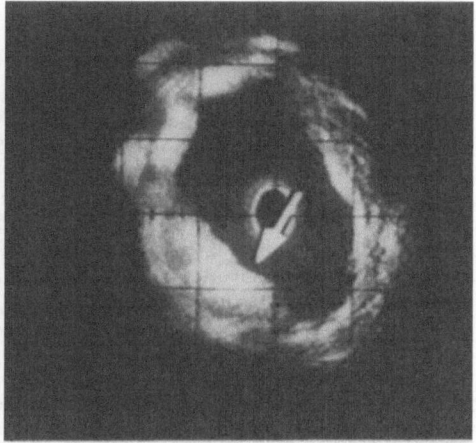

Fig. 7. An intravascular image of a human carotid artery with atherosclerosis obtained in in vitro experiment (A). The pathologic specimen is shown in the lower panel. Note the good histopathologic correlation. Two areas with atheroma are clearly visualized (arrows)

atheroma. The images show extremely good correlation with the histopathologic findings (Fig. 7). Subsequent intravascular studies of carotid arteries in experimental animals have demonstrated excellent clinico-pathologic correlation of both wall structure and dynamics.

The principle of a rotating single element transducer is simple and its construction can be made small enough to allow imaging of small diameter coronary arteries. This imaging system could in theory be combined with a desobliteration device. Equipped with a guide wire it could be manipulated into the required intravascular positions in a manner similar to a PTCA catheter. However, significant technical problems must still be solved such as an optimization of the driving mechanism while keeping the transducer fully flexible and steerable.

Conclusion

The need for better visualization of arterial obstructive lesions is a consequence of the rapid development of interventional radiology and cardiology, and in particular, the newer methods for angioplasty (laser, atherectomy, abrasion, spark erosion, etc.) of stenosed arteries. An imaging method which could show lumen morphology, extent of atheroma and other pathology within the vessel wall would have advantages for the diagnosis and treatment of arterial disease. Ultrasonic imaging offers this unique advantage since it allows the operator to see under the endothelial surface and to visualize the arterial wall components. In addition, the method has the potential for tissue characterization and this may provide further details of arterial wall pathology, especially the differentiation between various types of atheroma (calcified vs non-calcified), thrombus and the native vessel wall. Recent in vitro studies with a prototype intraluminal ultrasonic catheter support this possibility. The combination of intravascular ultrasonic imaging and sensing would be of major help before, during and after intravascular intervention as a guidance tool.

References

1. Grüntzig A, Senning A, Siegenthaler WE (1979) Non-operative dilatation of coronary artery stenosis: percutaneous transluminal angioplasty. N Eng J Med 301:61–8
2. Ritchie JL, Hansen DD, Vracko R, Auth D (1986) In vivo rotational thrombectomy. Evaluation by angioscopy. Circulation 74 Suppl II:457
3. Simpson JB, Hohnson DE, Braden LJ et al. (1986) Transluminal coronary atherectomy: results in 21 human cadaver vascular segments. Circulation 74 Suppl II:202
4. Sanborn TA, Faxon DP, Haudenschild CC, Ryan TJ (1985) Experimental angioplasty; Circumferential distribution of laser thermal energy with a laser probe. J Am Coll Cardiol 5:934
5. Choy DSJ, Stretzer S, Rotterdam HZ, Bruno MS (1982) Laser coronary angioplasty: experience with 9 cadaver hearts. Am J Cardiol 50:1209
6. Cross FW, Bowker TJ, Bown SG (1986) Contact saphire tip angioplasty with a pulsed Nd-Yag laser. In: proceedings Workshop, Laser Angioplasty with modified fiber tips. 3rd ELA Congress, Academic Medical Center, Amsterdam
7. Cieszynski T (1960) Intracardiac method for the investigation of structure of the heart with the aid of ultrasonics. Arch Immun Ter Dosw 8:551
8. Cieszynski T (1961) Intracardiac method of ultrasound heartstructure investigation. Polsk Przeglad Chirurg 33:1071
9. Kimoto S, Omoto R, Tsunemoto M et al. (1964) Ultrasonic tomography of the liver and detection of heart arterial septal defect with the aid of ultrasonic intravenous probes. Ultrasonics 2:82
10. Omoto R, Atsumi K, Suma K et al. (1963) Ultrasonic intravenous sonde 2nd report. Med Ultrason (Jpn) 1:11
11. Omoto R (1967) Ultrasonic tomography of the heart: an intracardiac scan method. Ultrasonics 5:80
12. Wild JJ, Reid JM (1950) Progress in techniques of soft tissue examination by 15 MC pulsed ultrasound. In: Kelly E (ed), Ultrasound in Medicine and Biology. Washington, American Institute of Biological Sciences, p 30
13. Bom N, Lanceé CT, Van Egmond FC (1972) An ultrasonic intracardiac scanner. Ultrasonics 10:72
14. Bom N. (1973) Apparatus for ultrasonically examining a hollow organ. Patent specification 1, 402,192
15. Mc Alpin RN, Abbasi AS, Grallman JA, Eber L (1973) Human coronary artery size during life. Radiology 108:567
16. Bom N, Lanceé CT, Slager CJ, De Jong N (1987) Ein Weg zur intraluminaren Echoarteriographie. Ultraschall 8:233

Current status of intracoronary stents

J. S. Douglas, Jr.

Andreas Grüntzig Cardiovascular Center, Departments of Medicine and Radiology, Emory University School of Medicine, Atlanta, Georgia, USA

Introduction

Although a decade of experience has resulted in improved initial success of percutaneous transluminal coronary angioplasty (PTCA) even in the presence of more difficult anatomic problems (1, 2), the technique fails to yield lasting results in a significant percentage of patients. Early failures occur due to abrupt coronary artery closure in approximately 5% – 7% of all patients (3, 4), and it is in these patients that most of the procedure related morbidity is encountered (3, 5). Restenosis appears in approximately a quarter of all patients within six months and in over one half of the patients undergoing vein graft PTCA (7, 8). Although a number of clinical, angiographic and procedural factors have been identified which appear to be associated with an increased risk of acute occlusion (3, 4, 9, 10, 11) and restenosis (6, 7, 8), the occurrence of these events in individual patients remains unpredictable. If one assumes that the results obtained in 14 experienced American centers participating in the 1985-86 NHLBI registry are similar to those in current practice, performance of 250 000 procedures annually world-wide would be expected to result in 19 000 acute closures (a 7.7% incidence) and 2 750 in-hospital deaths (a 1.1% incidence). Restenosis would be expected in at least 75 000 patients (assuming a 30% incidence). The enormous cost and morbidity related to these major limitations of PTCA have fostered innovative new invasive approaches aimed at maintenance of coronary luminal integrity. Placement of intracoronary stenting devices, a concept introduced by Dotter two decades ago (12), has been performed in several animal models and a number of different stent designs are currently undergoing clinical trials. Although still in an embryonic stage with respect to design features, determination of clinical utility and indications, and optimal adjunctive therapy, these new techniques have stimulated intense interest and may provide a method for treatment of patients who are now failures of PTCA or they may even become a routine component of angioplasty in some specific patient subgroups. The place of intravascular stenting in our therapeutic armamentarium will be determined by critical analysis of ongoing laboratory and clinical evaluations and technological improvements.

Stent design

Although a number of device prototypes are currently undergoing preliminary testing in Europe and the United States, most of the reported animal and human coronary experience has been with stents composed of stainless steel. In general,

Table 1. Characteristics of an ideal stent

- Simple accurate deployment
- Non-migrating
- Predetermined length and diameter
- Radial force to maintain lumen
- Non-thrombogenic
- Rapidly endothelialized
- Flexible
- Inert or absorbed
- Radiopaque
- Withstand motion stress
- Preserve side branches

these devices have either plastic qualities which permit them to be expanded by balloon inflation or elastic self-expanding characteristics. None of the current designs satisfy the requirements for an ideal stent (Table 1). Three stainless steel stents, the Medinvent stent (13), the balloon expandable etched tube of Palmaz (14, 15, 16) and the balloon mounted interdigitating coil stent of Gianturco have undergone preliminary animal and human testing. The Medinvent mesh stent is mounted on a 1.5 mm delivery catheter and released by withdrawal of a restraining membrane. This stent is reported to be awkward to deploy, somewhat inflexible, and poorly radio opaque. The Palmaz stent is inflexible and therefore unsuitable for tortuous coronary arteries. The Gianturco designed coil stent, although flexible and easily deployed, has the least ability to withstand elastic recoil forces tending to collapse the lumen and also is poorly radiopaque. All stents are inherently thrombogenic and only relatively inert. Each of these stents, however, is potentially capable of yielding a cylindrical lumen of predetermined diameter with more favorable flow characteristics than can be achieved by balloon angioplasty alone.

Animal models

In each stent design, implantation in animal models preceeded human application (13–17). No animal model, however, satisfactorily simulates human atherosclerosis. Using scanning electron microscopy, stents implanted in canine coronary arteries have been shown to be firmly imbedded in intimal trenches and covered by fibrin and a non-confluent endothelium at one week and by confluent but non-flow directed endothelial or pseudoendothelial cells at two to three weeks (18) (Fig. 1). After several months a mature confluent and flow directed endothelium is present. Stents are embedded in a neointima that on average is less than 300 μm (17) (Fig. 2).

Non-occlusive thrombus formation appears to be common shortly after stent placement and is reduced by antiplatelet and other antithrombotic therapy (9, 19). Gross and histologic documentation of early thrombus formation that is angiographically silent suggests that subclinical thrombus formation in human stenting may be common and the substrate for thrombotic stent occlusion. There is little thrombotic tendency once the stent is covered by endothelium. However, extrapolation of these results to diseased human coronary arteries is not possible. The generally good results in the canine model may be in part attributed to the normal arterial

184

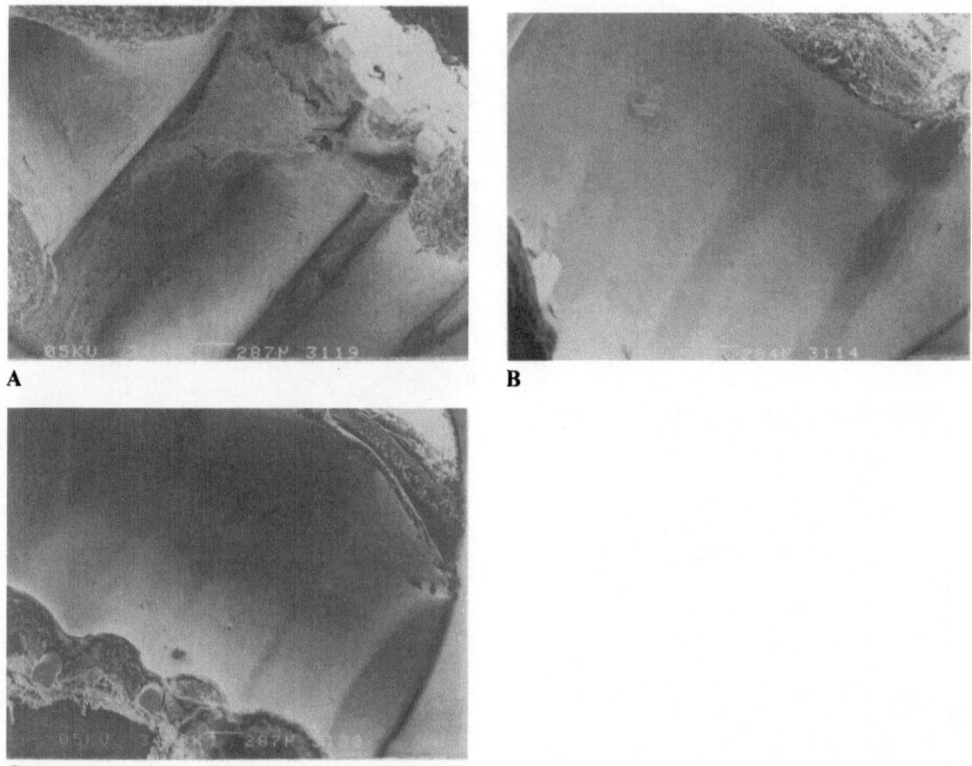

Fig. 1. Scanning electron micrographs of cut sections of stented canine coronary arteries showing luminal surfaces. (A) At three days after stent placement (35 ×), stent wires are seen "entrenched" with some overlying thrombus. (B) At four weeks after stent placement (35 ×), reendothelialization has occurred, minimal thrombus is present. (C) At 18 months after stent placement (35 ×), endothelial cells are confluent and flow-directed. Minimal intimal hyperplasia is present with no thrombus (Courtesy Keith A. Robinson)

surface underlying the stent and to the active canine fibrinolytic system. In addition, the time required for reendothelialization of stents in diseased human arteries may be significantly longer than in canine models.

Introduction of atherosclerosis in swine and rabbits has permitted testing of stent placement following PTCA in these models. Although a tendency for restenosis was documented in the rabbit, the larger initial lumen achieved by stent placement was maintained at late follow-up (20). In some animal models neointima covering the stent appeared to act as a barrier to atherogenesis, limiting atheroma progression to a position exterior to the stent. The relevance of this observation to human atherosclerosis is not known.

Anti-thrombotic therapy

Adjunctive therapy with antiplatelet agents, heparin, warfarin, dextran, thrombolytic agents, and other antithrombotic measures have not been systematically tested in

185

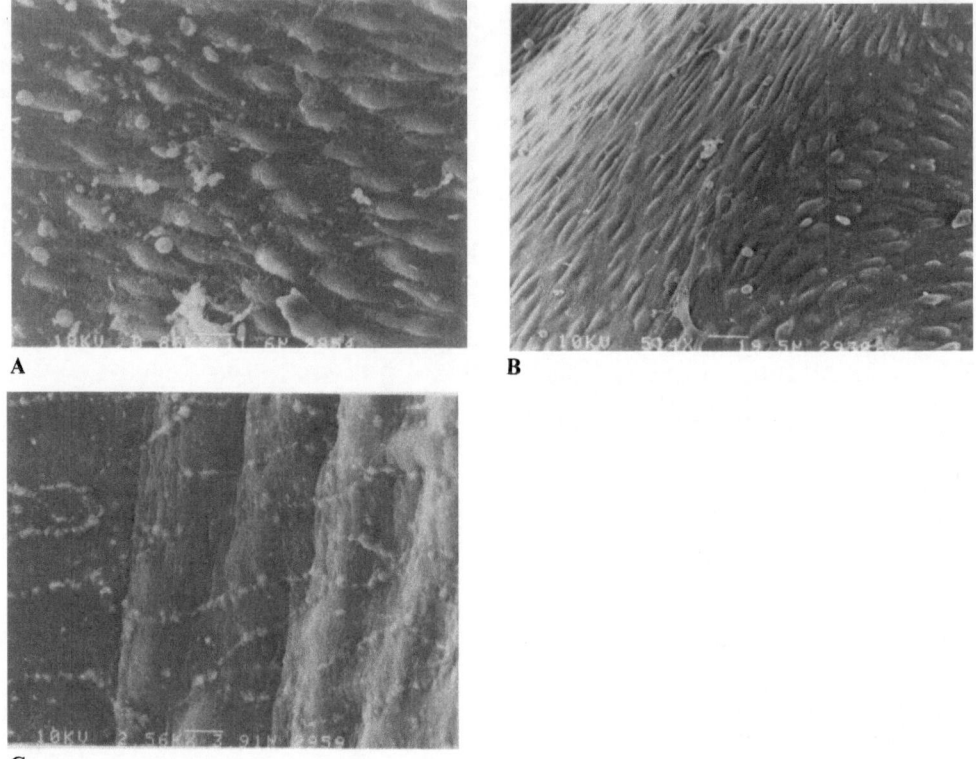

Fig. 2. Scanning electron micrographs of the luminal surfaces of stented canine coronary arteries. (A) At one week after stenting (860 ×), regenerating non-confluent endothelium is present with extended pseudopodia. Some adherent platelets and red blood cells are present. (B) At two weeks after placement (514 ×), endothelial cells are oriented circumferentially overlying the stent wires on the left of the micrograph and longitudinally outside the trench on the right. (C) At twelve months following stent placement (2,560 ×), endothelial cells directly over stent wires are now oriented in the direction of blood flow (note prominent cell junctions). (Courtesy Keith A. Robinson)

human subjects. Ideally, such therapy should be effective until reendothelialization occurs. Attempts are being made currently to reduce the thrombogenicity of stents by coating with a heparin substrate.

Human testing

Most of the clinical experience obtained with intracoronary stent placement has been with the Medinvent mesh stent (13). Initial results with this stent were marred by a significant instance of thrombotic occlusion within a few hours or days of placement (21). In 23 patients five acute thrombotic occlusions occurred immediately and five others in three-to-five days. Patients who are apparently at higher risk of acute thrombotic occlusion of the stented artery include those with slow coronary flow, i.e., following myocardial infarction and in cases of obvious intracoronary thrombus

186

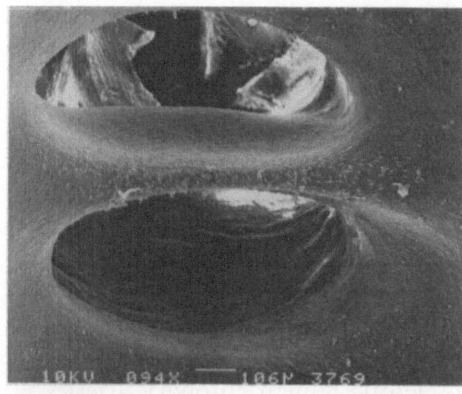

Fig. 3. Scanning electron micrograph of stented canine coronary artery at 15 months after stent placement (94 ×). This micrograph shows a stent wire spanning a side branch ostium completely covered with endothelium. (Courtesy Keith A. Robinson)

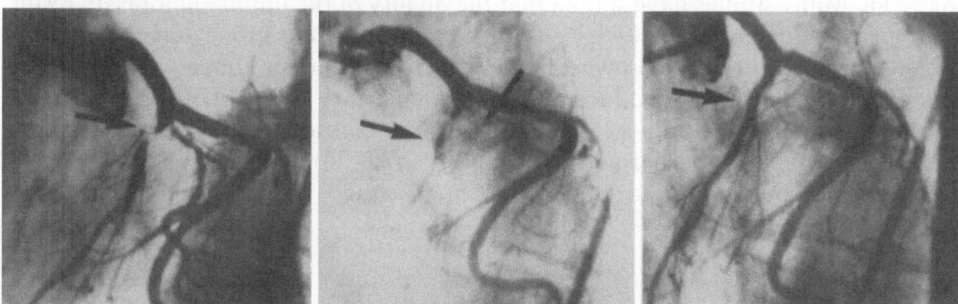

Fig. 4. Dilatation of the proximal left anterior descending coronary artery in an elderly lady was complicated by dissection of the proximal left anterior descending and diagonal coronary arteries. Acute occlusion was associated with chest pain and anterior ST segment elevation (center). Redilatation was not successful and a 3 mm stainless steel coil stent was placed in the proximal left anterior descending artery (right) restoring flow with relief of ischemia in the distribution of this artery. The patient underwent prompt coronary artery bypass grafting to the left anterior descending and diagonal coronary arteries as mandated by an FDA protocol. The electrocardiogram and ejection fraction following bypass surgery were normal. Placement of intracoronary stents as a "bailout" device in failed angioplasty appears to be safe and effective treatment minimizing ischemic injury associated with acute occlusion

formation. The best clinical results have been obtained in patients with acute closure following angioplasty and in vein graft stenosis. Sigwart has reported a low incidence of thrombotic stent occlusion in these patients and late restenosis has been infrequent (22). Very limited experience suggests that repeat angioplasty does not solve restenosis occurring within the stented segment. Percutaneous atherectomy has been performed successfully for this problem and long-term results are unknown. Histologic examination of the material removed revealed dense fibrosis (Gregory C Robertson – personal communication). Restenosis has been noted to occur at the ends of the somewhat inflexible stent. Whether this problem can be alleviated by design changes in the stent remains to be determined.

In our center six patients have received intracoronary flexible coil stents as therapy for acute occlusion occurring after balloon angioplasty. In all six of these patients the stent was quite effective in relieving chest pain and normalizing ST segment changes. In accordance with an FDA protocol these patients were subjected to emergency coronary bypass grafting. In all six patients the stent served as an effective bailout device which produced excellent coronary flow and relieved ischemia, and in all cases Q-wave myocardial infarction was avoided.

Some coronary experience has been obtained in the U. S. using the Palmaz stent. This stent is being inserted, under an FDA protocol, in patients with well collateralized native coronary arteries. Over 20 patients have been stented with no acute occlusions and no coronary artery restenosis (Richard A. Schatz, MD – personal communication). The results in this group of patients are quite preliminary. The use of stents in patients with a good collateral flow obviously provides a safer testing condition. However, the presence of the collaterals may permit silent coronary artery occlusion and the results of stenting will not be known until angiographic restudy has been accomplished.

The long-term result of stenting in atherosclerotic human coronary arteries is unknown. Many studies have shown that the quality of the initial angioplasty result is the primary determinant of long-term patency. By smoothing out the ragged, disrupted intimal surface and by exerting radial force, a larger lumen with improved flow conditions has been produced by human coronary artery stenting and documented by quantitative angioplasty, measurement of translesional pressure gradients and measurement of coronary flow reserve (23, 24). The degree to which the larger initial lumen, reduced turbulence, and stented arterial wall will prevent restenosis is unknown.

Conclusion

Because of acute closure and restenosis, PTCA is ineffective in many patients even when the coronary anatomy is ideal. Although the results of arterial stenting in animal models and in human iliac arteries is uniformly favorable, stent placement in human atherosclerotic coronary arteries has been complicated by acute thrombosis and associated morbidity in a significant percentage of cases. If this problem can be solved by improved stent design, adjunctive antithrombotic measures, or by other means, clinical trials will be needed to determine the efficacy of these stents in preventing restenosis. Favorable initial experience with the use of stents as temporary bailout devices in angioplasty complicated by acute occlusion suggests a continued roll for stents for this type of angioplasty failure.

References

1. Anderson H, Roubin G, Leimgruber P et al. (1985) Primary angiographic success rates of percutaneous transluminal coronary angioplasty. Am J Cardiol 56:712
2. Holmes DR, Vlietstra RE, Kelsey S and Detre K (1987) Comparison of current and earlier complications of angioplasty: NHLBI PTCA Resistry: J Am Coll Cardiol 9:19A
3. Bredlau CE, Roubin G, Leimgruber P et al. (1985) In-hospital morbidity and mortality in patients undergoing elective coronary angioplasty. Circulation 72:1044
4. Cowley MJ, Kelsey SF, Holubkov MS et al. (1988) Factors influencing outcome with coronary angioplasty: 1985–1986 NHLBI PTCA Registry. J Am Coll Cardiol 11:148A
5. Ellis SG, Roubin GS, King SB et al. (1988) In-hospital cardiac mortality after acute closure after coronary angioplasty: Analysis of risk factors from 8207 procedures. J Am Coll Cardiol 11:211–6

6. Leimgruber PP, Roubin GS, Hollman J et al. (1986) Restenosis after successful coronary angioplasty in patients with single vessel disease. Circulation 73:710–717
7. Douglas JS Jr, Grüntzig AR, King SB III et al. (1983) Percutaneous transluminal coronary angioplasty in patients with prior coronary bypass surgery. J Am Coll Cardiol 2:745–754
8. Douglas J, King S, Roubin G et al. (1986) Percutaneous angioplasty of venous aortocoronary graft stenoses: Late angiographic and clinical outcome. Circulation 74, Suppl II:281
9. Cowley M, Dorros G, Kelsey S et al. (1984) Acute coronary events associated with percutaneous transluminal coronary angioplasty. Am J Cardiol 53:12C
10. Sugrue DD, Holmes DR, Smith HC et al. (1986) Coronary artery throbus as a risk factor for acute vessel occlusion during percutaneous transluminal coronary angioplasty: improving results. Br Heart J 56:62
11. Ellis SG, Roubin GS, King SB et al. (1988) Angiographic and clinical predictors of acute closure after native vessel coronary angioplasty. Circulation 77:372
12. Dotter CT (1969) Transluminally-placed coilspring endarterial tube grafts. Long-term patency in canine popliteal artery. Inves Radiol 4:329
13. Sigwart U, Puel J, Mirkovitch V et al. (1987) Intravascular stents to prevent occlusion and restenosis after transluminal angioplasty. N Eng J Med 12:701
14. Schatz R, Palmaz J, Garcia F et al. (1986) Balloon expandable intracoronary stents in dogs. Circulation 74, Suppl II:458
15. Palmaz JC, Sibbitt RR, Tio FO et al. (1986) Expandable intraluminal graf:a feasibility study. Surgery 99:199
16. Palmaz JC, Windeler SA, Garcia F et al. (1986) Atherosclerotic rabbit aortas: expandable intraluminal grafting. Radiology 160:723
17. Roubin GS, Robinson KA, King SB et al. (1987) Early and late results of intracoronary arterial stenting after coronary angioplasty in dogs. Circulation 76:891
18. Robinson KA, Roubin GS, Apkarian RP et al. (1987) Short-term effects of intracoronary stenting in the canine: A descriptive scanning electron microscopic analysis. Circulation 76 Suppl IV:26
19. Palmaz JC, Garcia OJ, Kopp DT et al. (1987) Balloon expandable intra-arterial stents: Effect of anticoagulation on thronbus formation. Circulation 76, Suppl IV:186
20. Robinson KA, Siegel RJ, Brown JE et al. (1987) Effects of intra-arterial stenting on the progression of atherosclerosis in the rabbit. Circulation 76 Suppl IV:186
21. Puel J, Rousseau H, Joffre F et al. (1987) Intravascular stents to prevent restenosis after transluminal coronary angioplasty. Circulation 76 Suppl IV:27
22. Sigwart U, Golf S, Urs K et al. (1988) Analysis of complications associated with coronary stenting. J Am Coll Cardiol 11:66A
23. Surreys PW, Juilliere Y, Bertrand ME et al. (1987) Additional improvement in stenosis geometry by stenting human coronary arteries after angioplasty. Circulation 76 Suppl IV:232
24. Sigwart U, Kaufmann U, Goy JJ et al. (1987) Suppression of residual transstenotic pressure gradients after PTCA by implantation of self-expanding stents. Circulation 76, Suppl IV:186

4. Interventional techniques for arrhythmia control

Cardiac tachyarrhythmias: alternatives to medical treatment

G. Steinbeck

Department of Medicine I, Klinikum Großhadern, University of Munich, Munich, FRG

A simple clinical rule states: alternative treatment is indicated when drugs fail. This rule implies that antiarrhythmic drugs are and will remain the corner-stone of therapy for cardiac tachyarrhythmias. On the other hand, the definition of drug failure has expanded in the recent years because of various reasons to include not only refractoriness of disabling paroxysmal, incessant or even life-threatening tachyarrhythmias, but also non-compliance or limiting side effects. With the advent of new, possibly curative modes of treatment, it may be reasonable to take the one-time period of higher risk, which may in fact represent a lower cumulative risk in the long-term, compared to medical treatment (1).

In case of drug failure, the following non-pharmacologic alternatives may be offered to the patient: catheter ablation, implantation of antitachycardia devices and open heart surgery.

Catheter ablation

One option is to ablate a pathway of conduction or the area of the arrhythmogenic substrate directly by endocardial application of DC energy from standard defibrillators via electrode catheters. In 1982, Gallagher and Scheinman (2, 3) clinically introduced the method of transvenous catheter ablation of the His bundle by conventional DC energy in cases of drug resistant supraventricular tachyarrhythmias. Our own experience is reported elsewhere (4, 5). A world-wide registry for cases undergoing percutaneous attempt of His-bundle ablation in refractory supraventricular tachyarrhythmias has been set up; results and immediate as well as late complications of this procedure are illustrated in Table 1.

Based on our own experience, as well as on reports in the literature, this alternative is justified in cases of drug-resistant supraventricular tachyarrhythmias with rapid ventricular response, in which the impulses are conducted to the ventricles along the AV node-His bundle pathway (for example atrial fibrillation or atrial flutter with rapid ventricular response, AV node reentry). Only a minority of patients with accessory atrioventricular connections are suitable for this alternative (5).

Major complications and drawbacks of this method include the induction of myocardial necrosis (to a small extent), thrombus formation at the site of ablation, injury of the tricuspid valve and, last but not least, pacemaker implantation in all patients in whom a permanent third degree AV block can be achieved.

The treatment principle has also been further developed, as far as the energy source, as well as the arrhythmias being treated are concerned. As alternative energy

Table 1. Results and complications (immediate and late) of His bundle ablation for refractory supraventricular tachy-arrhythmias

Percutaneous His Bundle n = 127		Ablation Registry
Follow up		9.9 months ±8.2
AV block 3°:		71%
Arrhythmia control without drugs:		6%
Arrhythmia control with drugs:		13%
No improvement:		10%
Complication, immediate:	VT	n = 1
	Tamponade	n = 1
	Hypotension	n = 1
late:	VT	n = 3
	Sepsis	n = 3
	Hemothorax	n = 1
	Sudden death	n = 3

Scheinman et al., 1984

sources, radiofrequency and laser energy are being studied in order to circumvent some of the drawbacks of DC energy. Also, the method of delivering DC energy has been applied to patients with sustained ventricular tachycardia and accessory atrioventricular connections in order to directly ablate the arrhythmogenic substrate (7). Permanent success of this method demands precise localization of the origin of the arrhythmia by electrophysiological mapping techniques. Results in the latter patients are preliminary and far from perfect so that this indication is an experimental one at the present time.

Implantable antitachycardia devices

Whereas implantable pacemakers with antitachycardia stimulating capabilities have been shown to be fairly effective in selected patients with supraventricular tachy-arrhythmias, these devices without defibrillation back-up are generally felt to not be safe enough in patients with sustained tachyarrhythmias at the ventricular level (8). Therefore, the development of an implantable cardioverting or defibrillating device has been a major step for the alternative treatment of patients with drug refractory sustained ventricular tachycardia or ventricular fibrillation (9).

The study of Kelly et al. (10) constitutes the largest series, with 94 patients in whom AICD implantation was attempted, with the longest follow-up to date. Acute complications included three cases of perioperative death and in five cases the defibrillation threshold found intraoperatively was felt to be inappropriately high (greater than 25 J) so that implantation of the device had to be postponed or given up. Following hospital discharge, only five deaths occurred, including one sudden cardiac death during a mean follow up of 17 ± 10 months. Actuarial life table analysis, not including the perioperative mortality, however, gave a six month survival of 98.7%, and a 12 month survival of 95.4%, which quite favorably compares to the outcome of patients with these arrhythmias treated medically.

192

However, several improvements of the devices available at present are badly needed. These improvements include:

1) detection of the arrhythmia not only by analysis of rate, but also by rhythm, and analysis of the hemodynamic consequence of the arrhythmia;
2) easier mode of implantation;
3) intervention, first as antitachycardia stimulation, followed by low energy DC cardioversion and, finally, high energy DC defibrillation in case the prior steps do not terminate the arrhythmia; in addition, future devices should have the capability for antibradycardia stimulation;
4) full programmability of the device and a memory for the storage of the ECG strip showing the arrhythmia which led to the intervention of the device.

With the advent of these improvements together with lower costs, it is not difficult to foresee that such devices will play an increasing role in the treatment of patients with life threatening ventricular tachyarrhythmias.

Open heart surgery

Another major option for patients with drug-refractory life threatening ventricular arrhythmias is open heart surgery. The interested reader is referred to an excellent recent review (1). Surgery may be offered for the definitive treatment of the following

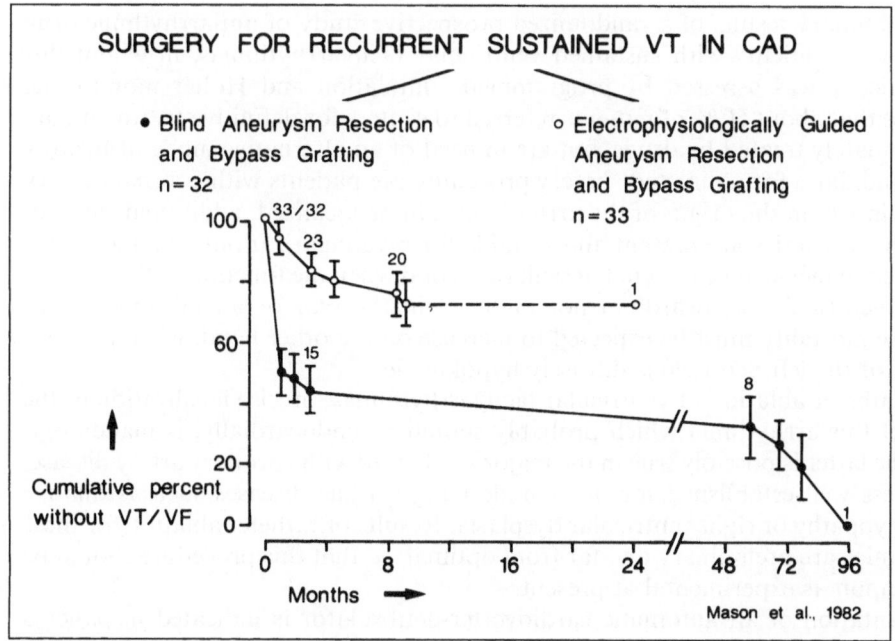

Fig. 1. Results of blind aneurysm resection (n = 32) as compared to electrophysiologically guided aneurysm resection (n = 33) for recurrent sustained VT in CAD; more than 50% of those with blind resection had a potentially life-threatening recurrence of the arrhythmia within four months of surgery

tachyarrhythmias: WPW-syndrome, AV nodal reentry, ventricular tachycardia, and ventricular fibrillation.

The procedures applied in open heart surgery may be either indirect (coronary bypass grafting, blind aneurysmectomy, transplantation) or direct ones such as encircling ventriculotomy (11), endocardial resection (12, 13), or cryosurgery. Direct approaches necessitate the prior localization of the origin of the ventricular tachyarrhythmia by electrophysiologic mapping techniques applied pre- or intraoperatively. In order to answer the question whether the direct approaches based on electrophysiologic mapping techniques are indeed superior to the indirect procedures, Mason and coworkers compared the results of surgery for recurrent, sustained ventricular tachycardia on the basis of coronary artery disease in 32 patients undergoing blind aneurysm resection and bypass grafting, with the results of 33 patients in whom electrophysiologically guided aneurysm resection was perfomed (14). Approximately four months after blind aneurysm resection, more than 50% of these patients had a potentially life-threatening recurrence of the arrhythmia (see Fig. 1). Although this study is not a controlled prospective one, most authors believe that mapping-guided surgical procedures are superior to the blind ones. Operative mortality and outcome of the various surgical techniques applied appear to compare favorably to the outcome of patients treated medically (15).

Guidelines for non-pharmacologic differential therapy in patients with sustained ventricular tachyarrhythmias

The preliminary results of a randomized prospective study of antiarrhythmic drug treatment in patients with sustained ventricular tachyarrhythmias, in whom this drug efficacy was assessed by programmed stimulation and Holter monitoring, indicates that about 50% of patients referred to centers for definitive treatment, are not adequately treated by drugs, but are in need of an alternative mode of therapy (16). Candidates for a directed surgery procedure are patients with coronary artery disease, in whom the origin of the arrhythmia can be localized, additional stenoses of coronary arteries are present and suitable for revascularization, and aneurysms are present which can be resected. Results are good when the function of the remaining left ventricular myocardium not involved in the scar or aneurysm is good; operative mortality must be expected to increase on the other hand, when the contraction of the left ventricle is diffusely hypokinetic.

For catheter ablation of ventricular tachyarrhythmias, precise localization of the origin of this arrhythmia which probably should be endocardially, is mandatory. While the latter is possibly true in the majority of cases with coronary artery disease, this is less well established for other underlying cardiac diseases such as dilative cardiomyopathy or right ventricular dysplasia. Results of catheter ablation for these arrhythmias are preliminary and far from optimal, so that this procedure should be looked upon as experimental at present.

Implantation of an automatic cardioverter-defibrillator is indicated in patients with drug refractory life-threatening ventricular tachyarrhythmias when the underlying cardiac disease is fairly constant (that is the patients who are not and will not be in the near future in class IV heart failure according to the NYHA classification). This treatment modality may be offered to patients in whom no localization of the arrhythmia origin is possible and, because of the lower operative mortality compared to open heart surgery, it may be offered also to older patients.

Finally, if drug refractory ventricular tachyarrhythmias occur on the basis of progressive cardiac disease with severe heart failure, especially in young patients, heart transplantation should be considered (17).

With the exception of heart transplantation, the application of all other types of treatment is based on the assumption that the occurrence of life-threatening ventricular tachyarrhythmias does not necessarily indicate irreversible heart failure, but may lead to premature death so that prevention or treatment of these "electrical accidents of the heart" is a difficult, but worthwhile task for these severely ill patients.

References

1. Gallagher JJ, Selle JG, Svenson RH, Fedor JM, Zimmern SH, Sealy WC, Robicsek FR (1988) Surgical treatment of arrhythmias. Am J Cardiol 61:27A
2. Gallagher JJ, Svenson RH, Kasell JH, German LD, Bardy GH, Broughton A, Critelli G (1982) Catheter technique for closed-chest ablation of the atrioventricular conduction system. A therapeutic alternative for the treatment of refractory supraventricular tachycardia. N Engl J Med 306:194
3. Scheinman MM, Morady F, Hess DS, Gonzalez R (1982) Catheter-induced ablation of the atrioventricular function to control refractory supraventricular arrhythmia. JAMA 248:851
4. Manz M, Steinbeck G, Gerkens U, Lüderitz B (1985) Supraventrikuläre Tachykardie: Ergebnisse der His-Bündel-Ablation. Dtsch med Wschr 110:576
5. Steinbeck G, Bach P, Haberl R, Markewitz A (1986) Ventricular preexcitation following catheter ablation of the His bundle in concealed WPW syndrome. Eur Heart J 7:444
6. Scheinman MM, Evans-Bell T, and the Executive Committee of the Percutaneous Cardiac Mapping and Ablation Registry (1984) Catheter ablation of the atrioventricular junction: a report of the percutaneous mapping and ablation registry. Circulation 70:1024
7. Fontaine G, Scheinman MM (1987) Ablation in cardiac arrhythmias. Mount Kisco. Futura Publishing
8. Fisher JD, Kim SG, Mercando AD (1988) Electrical devices for the treatment of arrhythmias. Am J Cardiol 61:45A
9. Mirowski M, Reid PR, Mower MM, Watkins L, Gott VL, Schauble JF, Langer A, Heilman MS, Kolenik SA, Fischell RE, Weisfeldt ML (1980) Termination of malignant ventricular arrhythmias with an implanted automatic defibrillator in human beings. N Engl J Med 303:322
10. Kelly PA, Cannom DS, Garan H, Mirabal GS, Harthorne JW, Hurvitz RJ, Vlahakes GJ, Jacobs ML, Ilvento JP, Buckley MJ, Ruskin JN (1988) The automatic implantable cardioverterdefibrillator: efficacy, complications and survival in patients with malignant ventricular arrhythmias. J Am Coll Cardiol 11:1278
11. Guiraudon G, Fontaine G, Frank R, Escand G, Etievent P, Cabrol C (1978) Encircling endocardial ventriculotomy. A new surgical treatment for life-threatening ventricular tachycardias resistant to medical treatment following myocardial infarction. Ann Thorac Surg 26:438
12. Harken AH, Horowitz LN, Josephson ME, Harken DE (1980) Comparison of standard aneurysmectomy and aneurysmectomy with directed endocardial resection for the treatment of recurrent sustained ventricular tachycardia. J Thorac Cardiovasc Surg 80:527
13. Josephson ME, Harken AH, Horowitz LN (1979) Endocardial excision: a new surgical technique for the treatment of recurrent ventricular tachycardia. Circulation 60:1430
14. Mason JW, Stinson EB, Winkle RA, Griffin JC, Oyer PE, Ross DL, Derby G (1982) Surgery for ventricular tachycardia: efficacy of left ventricular aneurysm resection compared with operation guided by electrical activation mapping. Circulation 65:1148
15. Borggrefe M, Podczek A; Ostermeyer J, Breithardt G, and the Surgical Ablation Registry (1987) Long-term results of electrophysiologically guided antitachycardia surgery in ventricular tachy-

arrhythmias: a collaborative report in 665 patients. In: Nonpharmacological Therapy of Tachyarrhythmias, G. Breithardt, M. Borggrefe, DP Zipes (eds) Futura Publishing Co, Inc. Mount Kisco, New York, p. 109

16. Steinbeck G, Andresen D, v. Leitner ER (1986) Sind Antiarrhythmika einem Betablocker überlegen in der Behandlung lebensbedrohlicher ventrikulärer Rhythmusstörungen? Vorläufige Ergebnisse einer kontrollierten Studie. Z Kardiol 75:47
17. Steinbeck G, Haberl R, Kemkes BM (1987) Herztransplantation bei therapieresistenten, rezidivierenden Kammertachykardien und Kammerflimmern. Z Kardiol 76:479

Catheter ablation: the state of the art

G. Fontaine

Service de Rhythmologie et de Stimulation Cardiaque du Pr. Y. Grosgogeat, Hopital Jean Rostand, Irvy, France

Introduction

Ablative techniques are causing major developments in the treatment of major cardiac arrhythmias. Large series have now demonstrated that, at least in supraventricular tachycardias, this approach is quite safe (2, 3). Its extension into other cardiac arrhythmias is a more recent and promising development. During the IVth International Symposium on the Ablative Techniques, organized by G. Fontaine and M. Scheinman and held in Monaco in June 1988, the state of the art of these techniques was presented by the most important international groups working in the field. The abstracts published in PACE 1988 and a few other nonpublished abstracts constitute the basis of the present report.

His-bundle fulguration

Ten cases of His-bundle ablation in which energies between 100 and 400 J were used and up to six shocks delivered in a single session have been assessed by echocardiography and Doppler by the group of Camm et al. (2). The authors conclude that His-bundle ablation has no effect on valvular or myocardial function.

This technique, which was first published in the early 1980s, has now been extended to a large number of cases. It is accepted as an interesting approach in the treatment of refractory SVT. The long-term results of the atrioventricular junction ablation can be assessed from the registry organized in France. Data have been collected by S. Levy from eight centers. The follow-up ranges from 10 to 76 months, with a mean of 31 months. Ninety-one patients underwent AV junctional ablation for atrial flutter or fibrillation (n = 54), reciprocating AV tachycardia (n = 25) and atrial tachycardia (n = 12). Eighty-six perccent of patients showed a long-term success and were asymptomatic either with or without (6%) antiarrhythmic therapy. Immediate complications included non-sustained ventricular tachycardia in 3 patients and ventricular fibrillation in one patient. One sudden death was reported on day eight after fulguration in a patient who experienced VT after the procedure. The late deaths observed were sepsis in one case, neoplasia in one, emboli in two and recurrence of pre-existing heart failure in two. This confirms that the technique should be reserved for patients with intractable supraventricular tachycardia (3).

A simplified technique has been proposed by Clementy et al. (4) in a series of 40 patients using a Josephson quadripolar catheter with electrodes 0.5 cm apart, from which it is possible to record the His amplitude between each pair of electrodes 1 – 2,

2–3, and 3–4, the shock being delivered by the couple recording the largest His bundle potential. The fulguration is performed after interconnecting the two corresponding electrodes. This new technique was compared with a control group which consisted of 30 patients in whom a regular USCI quadripolar catheter had been used and the His bundle localization performed with a unipolar system, the electrode working as a cathode. Although not significantly different, the results tend to favor the new technique, which is faster and easier to perform.

A highly effective technique has also been reported by Bredikis et al. in 140 procedures (5). The conventional technique was used for 60 patients with a success rate of complete AV-block in 60%. In a second group of 80 patients a specially designed electrode catheter with a surface of 40 mm was positioned under x-ray guidance of anatomical landmarks. This was achieved without His bundle recording and favorable results were observed in a significant number of cases.

Atrioventricular AV node reentrant tachycardia

The largest group has been reported on by Haissaguerre and Warin (6) on a series of 14 consecutive cases with a mean age of 56 ± 16 years, including 7 males suffering from AV junctional reciprocating tachycardia refractory to antiarrhythmic drugs. Four had coronary artery disease, two a cardiomyopathy and eight no structural heart disease. The first procedure was performed in March, 1985, before the surgical procedure reported by Ross and Johnson (7). In all patients retrograde atrial activation during AV node reciprocating tachycardia appeared earliest on the His-bundle lead. The second catheter used for fulguration was located around the perinodal atrium where one to eight cathodic transcatheter shocks of 160 to 240J were delivered to the selected site in one or two sessions. Complete AV block was observed in one patient, transient AV block in the other patients (1–28 min). EPS performed five days after the last procedure showed the abolition of retrograde conduction in 10 patients and modification was observed in 4 patients. In all of the cases except one, the AV conduction was preserved or was slightly modified. No echo or AV- nodal reciprocating tachycardia was inducible in 12 patients. AV- nodal reciprocating tachycardia did not occur in 13 patients during the follow-up period of 2–30 months. During the late follow-up AV-nodal reciprocating tachycardia was not inducible. These results demonstrate that catheter ablation of AV nodal reciprocating tachycardia is feasible with a high success rate without modification of anterograde conduction.

Good results have also been reported by Moro et al. in two patients in whom retrograde conduction was suppressed, while normal AV conduction was preserved with a follow-up period of 9.5 months. Both patients remain asymptomatic and without antiarrhythmic drug therapy (8).

Paroxysmal junctional reciprocating tachycardia (9)

This is the so-called almost permanent form of junctional reciprocating tachycardia, frequently observed in youngsters, with a typical ECG feature during the arrhythmia, a prolonged RP' interval, and negative P wave in leads 2, 3, and aVF. The substrate of this arrhythmia has been identified as a concealed AV accessory pathway with decremental properties, and slow retrograde conduction. The ablation of the AV node showed a long PR interval with the occurrence of a delta wave. Fulguration in the os of the coronary sinus could disturb the conduction in this long serpiginous retrogradely conducting accessory pathway without impairing normal AV conduction. In most recent developments, the anterograde bypass conduction has been disclosed in some cases by means of drug-induced AV block.

Atrial flutter fulguration

Chauvin and Brechenmacher have reported the use of endocavitary fulguration in the right atrium to ablate common recurrent atrial flutter resistant to drug therapy. Mapping the lower part of the right atrium demonstrated the area of slow conduction where a double potential was observed. A shock of 100 to 120 Joules was delivered. In two patients the flutter recurred after a few days and persisted despite two more fulgurations. Two patients are free of relapses without antiarrhythmic drug, with a follow-up ranging from 7 to 9 months. Two other patients needed one or two more procedures, but they have been free of arrhythmia and have not been taking anti-arrhythmic drug treatment. The follow-up ranges from 7 to 9 months and no mechanical complications were observed (10). This result confirms a previous report on the same subject.

Accessory pathway fulguration

Warin and Haissaguerre (11) reported on a series of 50 patients; indications were 36 patients with occurrence of malignant arrhythmia refractory to antiarrhythmic drugs, 12 patients who wanted to stop chronic medical therapy, and two patients who had no spontaneous tachycardia but did have atrial fibrillation with high ventricular response with a minimal RR interval in the range of 200 ms. Location of the accessory pathway was antero-septal in eight patients, right-lateral in seven patients, right posteroseptal in 20 patients, left posteroseptal in six, and left posterior or lateral in nine patients. These pathways were mapped by a catheter introduced through a patent foramen ovale in five patients, and after transeptal catheterization in four. Anterograde AP conduction was concealed in seven cases. Catheter position was guided by earliest retrograde atrial activation during reciprocating tachycardia, and recording of the discrete accessory pathway potential in 18 patients. Endocardial shocks were delivered directly to the AV annulus and not in the coronary sinus or its os. One to 12 cathodal shocks ranging from 80 to 160 Joules were delivered in one session in 32 patients, two sessions in 14, three sessions in three and four sessions in one patient. Following catheter ablation accessory pathway conduction was abolished in all patients. During the follow-up ranging from 1 to 36 months, all patients but one are free of cardiac arrhythmias. A pre-excitation has been observed in four patients with right posteroseptal accessory pathway. Three patients had no tachycardia, one required antiarrhythmic drugs, retrograde conduction was no longer present in 15 patients from 4 to 21 months after catheter ablation.

Therefore, intraatrial fulguration of accessory pathway seems to be extremely safe and effective in all locations. The authors conclude that this technique is the treatment of choice for patients with refractory arrhythmias and accessory pathways.

Ventricular tachycardia fulguration

The largest experience concerning 47 consecutive cases was reported by Frank et al. (12) during a period of 4 years, from 1983 to 1987. Etiologies of chronic VT were an old myocardial infarction in 17 cases, 13 cases of arrhythmogenic right ventricular dysplasia, cardiomyopathy in eight patients, idiopathic VT in eight patients and one case of right ventricular outflow tract surgical scar. Sixteen patients had an ejection fraction below 30 %. 236 shocks during 74 sessions were delivered in the left ventricle in 23 patients and in the right ventricle in 24 patients. When a first fulguration session was not effective, a new attempt of antiarrhythmic treatment was used and proved to be effective in several cases. It was finally necessary to group to four sessions in some patients, especially in those who had multiple VT morphologies. Four patients had transient relapses after hospital discharge, and these relapses disappeared spontaneously, leading to a success rate in the range of 90% after 3 months. Four deaths not related to the shocks were observed during the learning phase. Three patients died within 3 months of the progression of their underlying cardiac disease without VT relapses. Seven more patients died between 4 and 33 months after the procedure, with a mean value of 10 ± 4 months. Three late sudden deaths were observed during the follow-up.

Interesting results have also been observed by Klein (13) on a series of 41 patients. In 75 %, DC shocks were effective when performed in the area of slow conduction (nine out of 10 patients). In eight patients with incessant VT, five had a successful ablation. It is concluded that the catheter ablation is more successful when the energy is delivered in the area of slow conduction instead of the earliest endocardial activation as suggested by previous reports (14, 15).

The experience of Morady et al. (16) consists of a series of 39 selected patients. In 35 of those, only one configuration of VT was present. Coronary artery disease was the underlying pathology in 25 patients, cardiomyopathy in three, right ventricular dysplasia in two, tetralogy of Fallot in two, and no structural heart disease in seven patients. The mean left ejection fraction was 34 %; the mean VT cycle lengths was 418 ms. The VT exit site was identified by endocardial mapping and pacemapping and was in the left free wall in six patients, in the septum in 10 patients, and in the right ventricle in 13. One to four shocks of 100 to 300 Joules were delivered to the VT exit site in 37 patients or to the zone of slow conduction of the reentry circuit in two patients. There was no recurrence of symptomatic VT in 67% over a mean follow-up period of 20 ± 10 months. It is concluded that catheter ablation in selected patients with recurrent VT could achieve a long-term control of VT and is relatively safe.

Haissaguerre and Warin (17) also reported a consistent series of 28 patients with a mean follow-up of 27 months. The success rate of the procedure was in the range of 85 %. Patients are not taking antiarrhythmic therapy or are controlled after using the same regimen which was ineffective before fulguration. A better success rate was obtained when a premature potential in the range of 43 ± 29 ms was observed as compared with patients with earliest endocardial activation mean value of -5 ± 5 ms (p < 0.05).

Huang (18) reported interesting results on a series of 15 consecutive patients with history of myocardial infarction and recurrent VT refractory to many antiarrhythmic agents, with a mean follow-up of 18 months; 53% of patients are alive and off antiarrhythmic drugs. In 20% of the patients, VT has been controlled by previously ineffective antiarrhythmic drugs. Four patients (27%) died, one of sepsis, two of myocardial infarction recurrence without VT, one died suddenly 24 months after ablation.

A study by Kirkorian et al. (19) reported the comparison between two subgroups: group I with seven patients had amiodarone therapy, and group II of nine patients received from one to four cathodal shocks of 250 to 300 Joules at the site of VT origin without adverse effect. The follow-up was 15 months. One patient died suddenly, and two patients had recurrences in the fulgurated group, whereas no arrhythmic event occured in group I. Therefore, the fulguration was not considered as a first choice of therapy by these authors.

Other cases have been reported, for example by Sellers (20) in a series of six male patients. The success rate was 50% of fulguration alone, and with combination of antiarrhythmic drugs 33% more, and finally, ineffective in 17%. Late recurrences were related to probable technical difficulties.

Jordaens (21) reported one case in whom arrhythmogenic right ventricular dysplasia and refractory VT was ablated in the right ventricle with no untoward side effects. After the first shock the tachycardia cycle increased from 310 to 520 ms. After the second shock, VT was no longer inducible as well as during the follow-up period.

Akhtar reported as series of seven patients who had documented bundle branch reentrant ventricular tachycardia associated with syncope or sudden death, who underwent catheter ablation of their right bundle branch in a series of patients who previously failed treatment with antiarrhythmic medications. Two electric shocks of 170 to 310 Joules were delivered to the right bundle branch, which produced immediately a right bundle branch block pattern. No patient had inducible VT following ablation and follow-up of more than 45 months revealed no clinical recurrence of VT.

Similar excellent results were reported by Volkmann (22) in a 50-year-old patient after a single shock of 250 Joules which prevented reinduction of the tachycardia after ablation. Over a period of follow-up of 24 months the patients had no recurrence of ventricular tachycardia, and the right bundle branch block persisted.

Radio-frequency ablation

AV nodal ablation

Bowman et al. (23) reported different attempts of ablation of several parts of the AV conduction system: in three patients with atrial flutter or fibrillation, two patients with right bundle branch block and one patient with sustained bundle branch reentrant tachycardia and a segment of left bundle branch block for ventricular tachycardia in one patient. The power is in the range of 5 to 11 watts with an energy of 25 to 747 Joules per pulse.

In patients in whom AV junction ablation was attempted, complete AV block as achieved in all of them. In the patients with bundle branch reentrant tachycardia, the

His bundle and proximal right bundle branch were localized, and a right bundle branch block was produced with preservation of AV conduction. VT was not inducible 6 days later. One patient had frequent VT induced by exercise, which proved partially responsive to verapamil. Presystolic potentials suggesting left bundle branch potential were observed before the onset of the QRS complex, during VT as well as during sinus rhythm. No recurrence of VT was observed after a period of 6 weeks in that particular case. It is concluded that radiofrequency current is effetive for ablation of a selected segment of the AV conduction system.

In a series of seven patients with different forms of VT, Davis et al. (24) demonstrated that radiofrequency ablation could be effective in some patients with refractory arrhythmias, but when this procedure failed, the DC shocks could be more effective.

Borggrefe et al. (25) reported their experience in 17 consecutive patients in whom shocks were delivered to the atrium, AV node, and accessory pathway. In the atrium, the procedure was not effective; the long-term effect was satisfactory in one out of seven patients, and five out of 10 had AV node ablation. It was mentioned during the presentation that the same technique has been less successful in ventricular tachycardia.

Huang et al. (26) applied the technique of radiofrequency ablation in two patients. One patient had episodes of atrial flutter or fibrillation, the other had AV junction reciprocating tachycardia. This patient, who had concealed WPW syndrome, needed subsequent surgical ablation. It proved successful on a left lateral accessory pathway and suggested the evidence of multiple accessory pathways. It was concluded that catheter ablation was possible and safe but not the most effective form of therapy.

Kuck et al. (27) reported the modulation (and not ablation) of AV nodal conduction by radiofrequency current in order to decrease rapid AV conduction in nine cases with paroxysmal atrial fibrillation. Voltage and current were continuously monitored during the application of the current. The energy was delivered from 1–16 times during 20–40 s. During the follow-up period definite improvement was observed in seven cases.

Electro-thermal ablation

This technique was introduced by Narula (28). It consists of the heating of a resistor located at a catheter tip which functions as a kind of cautery, the thermal energy being produced by a 10-volt regular battery which delivers from 6 to 20 Joules. Five patients (age ranging from 57 to 65 years) with supraventricular tachycardia were managed by modification or interruption of a selected portion of the tachycardia pathway by the electro-thermal catheter technique. One patient had atrial flutter. After application of the technique, AH interval and effective refractory period of the AV node were prolonged. Three patients had AV junctional reciprocating tachycardia and one had His bundle tachycardia. In these patients the SVT cycle length ranged between 315 and 440 ms. In one patient, complete ventriculo-atrial block was induced with a slight lengthening of the AH interval and effective refractory period of the AV node. In two other patients, the Wenckebach point of the retrograde conduction was prolonged. In the latter two patients, PA, AH, and HV intervals remained unchanged. In the patient with atrioventricular junctional reciprocating tachycardia, the tachycardia was no longer inducible. In these four patients, the PA, HV, and QRS complex remained constant. In the patient with His bundle tachycardia, the conduction was interrupted in the distal His bundle, with unchanged AH and HA intervals. The patients were treated without general anesthesia; they felt no pain and they had no arrhythmias. There was no change in the enzymes, despite some changes during repeat electrophysiological studies. The patients remained asymptomatic during the 10–18 months of follow-up period. No drug therapy or pacemaker implantation was necessary after the procedure.

Conclusion

The ablative techniques using the catheter approach have demonstrated increased effectiveness in previously explored areas and their emergence in new cardiac arrhythmias. There is a tendency to exquisitely ablate the abnormal pathway instead of the His bundle in a significant number of SVT cases. Radiofrequency energy is extremely well tolerated, it does not require general anesthesia, and it has minor side effects. It is, however, less effective than properly used fulguration. Both techniques are still in their infancy. Their physical and biological basis are still poorly understood and major technical improvements are needed.

References

1. Scheinman MM, Evans-Bell GT (1987) Catheter electrocoagulation of the atrioventricular junction: a report of the percutaneous mapping and ablation registry. In: Ablation in cardiac arrhythmias. G. Fontaine, M.M. Scheinmann (eds), Futura Publishing C., Mount Kisco, New York, pp 161–169
2. Wafa S, Griffith M, Leech G, Camm AJ (1988) The effects of His-bundle ablation on myocardial and valvular function. Pace 11:918
3. Levy S, Bru P, Aliot E, Attuel P, Barnay C, Clementy J, Ebagosti A, Fauchier JP, Fontaine G, Leclercq JF (1988) Long-term Follow-up of transcatheter ablation of the atrioventricular junction. Pace 11:909
4. Clementy J, Coste P, Moreau C, Bricaud H (1988) His-bundle ablation. A simplified technique using Josephson catheter. Pace 11:909
5. Bredikis Y, Sakalauskas JJ, Benetis R (1988) Highly effective catheter technique for AV node His-bundle fulguration. Pace 11:917
6. Haissaguerre M, Warin JF (1988) Curative fulguration for atrioventricular node reentrant tachycardia: report of 14 patients. Pace 11:910
7. Ross DL, Johnson DC, Dennis AR, Cooper MJ, Richards DA, Uther JB (1985) Curative surgery for atrioventricular junctional (AV nodal) reentrant tachycardia. J Am Coll Cardiol 6:1383–1392
8. Moro C, Martinez J, Novo L, Nunez A, Pascual J (1988) Curative ablation for intranodal reentry without complete AV-block. Pace 11:919
9. Critelli G (1988) New trends in pathophysiology and treatment of the permanent junctional reciprocating tachycardia. Pace 11:907
10. Chauvin M, Brechenmacher C (1988) Treatment of recurrent atrial flutter by endocavitary fulguration (abstract). Pace 11:910
11. Warin JF, Haissaguerre M (1988) Catheter ablation of accessory pathway in all the locations: report of 50 patients. Pace 11:908
12. Frank R, Fontaine G, Tonet JL, Grosgogeat Y (1988) Long-term experience of fulguration for the treatment of ventricular tachycardia. Pace 11:912

13. Klein HO, Schroder E, Trappe HJ, Kuhn E (1988) Catheter ablation of ventricular tachycardia. How to define the area of ablation. Pace 11:911
14. Fontaine G (1986) Prevention of sudden arrhythmic death. Catheter ablation. In: Proceedings of the 1985 Sydney Opera House Symposium, Telectronics Vectors Pub., Sydney, pp. 18–21
15. Fontaine G, Frank R, Tonet JL, Grosgogeat Y (1988) Ablating the slow conduction zone during ventricular tachycardia: criteria for the critical circuit. Pace 11:911
16. Morady F, Scheinman MM, Griffin JC, Herre JM, Kou WH (1988) Results of catheter ablation of ventricular tachycardia using direct current shocks (abstract). Pace 11:912
17. Haissaguerre M, Warin JF, Le Metayer P, Guillem JP, Blanchot P (1988) Catheter ablation of ventricular tachycardia using high cumulative energy: results in 28 patients with a mean follow-up of 27 months. Pace 11:913
18. Huang SK, Bazgan ID, Ring ME, Lee MA (1988) Values of catheter ablation of refractory sustained ventricular tachycardia with direct-current energy. Pace 11:919
19. Kirkorian G, Atallah G, Lavaud P, Didier B, Zoheir F, Touboul P (1988) A randomized study comparing catheter ablation to medical therapy in patients with ventricular tachycardia. Preliminary results (abstract). Pace 11:911
20. Sellers TD, Dilorenzo D, Primerano P, Modesto T, Kirchoffer J, Conklin R, Kile J (1988) Catheter ablation of resistant ventricular tachycardia: immediate results and long-term follow-up (abstract). Pace 11:920
21. Jordaens L, van Wassenhove E, Roelandt R, Palmer A, Clement D (1988) Ablation with low-energy-shocks in arrhythmogenic ventricular dysplasia. Pace 11:913
22. Volkmann H, Kuhnert H, Dannberg G (1988) Successful therapy of ventricular tachycardia by catheter ablation of the right bundle branch (abstract). Pace 11:914
23. Bowman A, Fitzgerald DM, Friday KJ, Kuck KH, Naccarelli GV, Lazzara R, Jackman WM (1988) Catheter ablation of selected segments of the AV conduction system using radiofrequency current. Pace 11:908
24. Davis MJE, Murdock CJ, Cope GD, Kallas IJ, Lovett MD (1988) Radiofrequency catheter ablation for refractory arrhythmias. Pace 11:918
25. Borggrefe M, Podczeck A, Budde TH, Martinez-Rubio A, Breithardt G (1988) Catheter ablation of supraventricular tachycardia. Pace 11:910
26. Huang SK, Lee MA, Bazgan ID, Gorman G (1988) Initial experience with radiofrequency catheter ablation for intractable cardiac arrhythmias in man. Pace 11:919
27. Kuck KH, Kunze KP, Geiger M, Schluter M (1988) Modulation of AV nodal conduction in man by radiofrequency current. Pace 11:909
28. Narula OS, Salerno JA, Chimienti M, Finzi A, Pagnoni F (1988) Abolition of supraventricular tachycardia by an electro-thermal catheter: Follow-up observations (abstract). Pace 11:907

Preoperative and intraoperative mapping in patients with sustained ventricular tachycardia

R. Haberl, G. Steinbeck

Medical Hospital I, Klinikum Großhadern, University of Munich, Munich, FRG

Introduction

Patients with drug-resistant, life-threatening, and recurrent ventricular tachycardia have a poor prognosis. In recent years, invasive methods for ablation of the arrhythmogenic myocardial substrate have been developed and include: catheter ablation with DC-shock or radiofrequency energy, operative methods including endocardial resection, endocardial encircling, laser coagulation and cryothermal freezing. A prerequisite of these methods is the exact localization of the origin of ventricular tachycardia which sometimes is in the border zone of a myocardial infarction or aneurysm, but sometimes is located in apparently healthy myocardium (1, 4)

Patient selection

Electrophysiologic mapping should be performed in patients with ventricular sustained tachycardia, who are refractory to anti-arrhythmic drug therapy and in whom ablation of the arrhythmogenic substrate is possible. The best success rates are in patients after myocardial infarction, with or without ventricular aneurysm, who suffer from monomorphic sustained ventricular tachycardia which is hemodynamically tolerated during the time of mapping. The method should not be applied in patients in whom the arrhythmogenic substrate cannot be ablated (i.e., cardiomyopathy, severe right ventricular dysplasia) or in whom a mapping procedure is impossible (primary ventricular fibrillation, very fast ventricular tachycardia, very poor ventricular function, polymorphic ventricular tachycardia). In these cases, alternative methods like implantation of an automatic defibrillator or heart transplantation have to be considered.

Mapping techniques

Exact localization of the site of origin of ventricular tachycardia is only possible during ventricular tachycardia. The majority of tachycardias originate in the subendocardial layer, hence, epicardial mapping in general fails to identify the site of origin (2, 3).

1) Preoperative catheter mapping: all patients with ventricular tachycardia who are to be operated upon should undergo a preoperative mapping. This is because in some

205

patients ventricular tachycardia cannot be induced during operative conditions after ventriculotomy and cooling. A multipolar electrode catheter is placed via the femoral vein into the right ventricle; a second catheter is positioned in the left ventricle via the aorta. From multiple locations (exactly defined by multiplane x-ray) endocardial activation is recorded, along with the surface electrocardiogram during ventricular tachycardia. The site of earliest endocardial activation defines the origin of the tachycardia. The procedure requires about 30 min, and during this time the monomorphic sustained ventricular tachycardia must be tolerated by the patient. In patients with various documented clinical tachycardias, each must be induced and mapped (if possible).

2) Intraoperative mapping: currently, most centers perform mapping with a hand-held probe after ventriculotomy and induction of the ventricular tachycardia by programmed stimulation. The patient is on normothermal cardiopulmonary bypass. A map of ventricular activation is constructed from the data which are consecutively recorded from the endocardium in a circular manner (Fig. 1). Again, the earliest endocardial activation defines the site of origin of the tachycardia. Problems arise if the tachycardia cannot be induced (up to 30% of patients), or if the tachycardia is too fast and not hemodynamically tolerated, or the tachycardia is polymorphic. In order to overcome these limitations, computerized mapping systems are under development. A balloon with multiple electrodes (up to 192) is introduced into the left ventricle through the mitral valve (Fig. 2). The 192 unipolar channels are amplified,

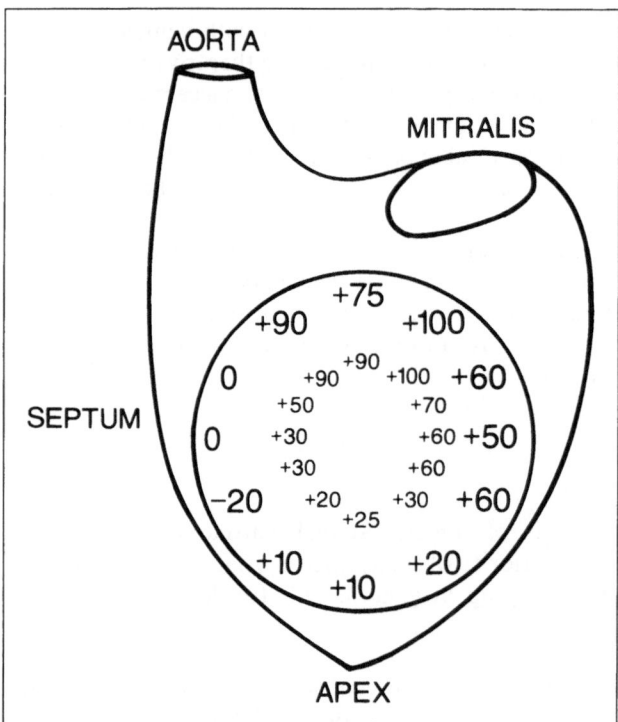

Fig. 1. Intraoperative mapping with a hand-held probe. Activation of multiple sites is recorded consecutively in a circular manner after ventriculotomy. At the lower septum, earliest endocardial activation (−20 ms compared to the beginning of the surface QRS) represents the site of origin of the ventricular tachycardia

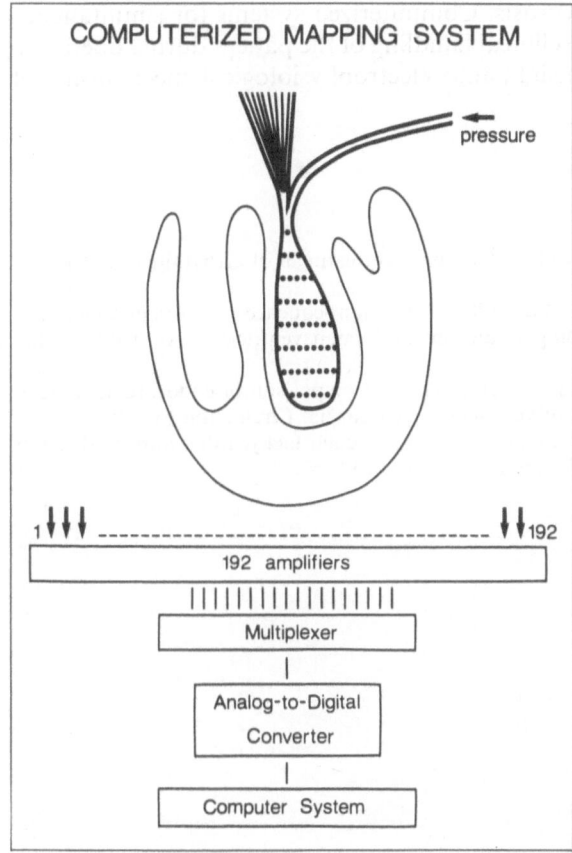

COMPUTERIZED MAPPING SYSTEM

← pressure

1 ↓↓↓ - ↓↓192

192 amplifiers

|||||||||||||||||||||

Multiplexer

Analog-to-Digital Converter

Computer System

Fig. 2. Computerized mapping system. The balloon with 192 electrodes is advanced into the left ventricle via the mitral valve. The multiplexing system and the analog-to-digital converter allow simultaneous recording of the 192 electrodes. Analysis is done automatically by the computer

multiplexed, and AD-converted (1000 Hz, 12 bit). The data are analyzed with a computer. This procedure has several advantages: induction of the ventricular tachycardia is facilitated in the absence of ventriculotomy and subsequent cooling; the spatial resolution is very high; simultaneous recordings of all channels enable the construction of a complete ventricular mapping during each beat of the ventricular tachycardia, thus, even short ventricular runs and polymorphic tachycardias can be mapped. The time of mapping is short, hence, bypass clamping time is shorter.

3) Pace mapping: during clinical spontaneous ventricular tachycardia, a 12-lead ECG is compared to a 12-lead ECG during paced rhythm with the pacing electrode at various ventricular sites. If the morphology of the clinical and paced ventricular tachycardia is identical, the pacing site represents the origin of the ventricular tachycardia.

Conclusion

Mapping procedures serve as a guideline for a directed ablation of arrhythmogenic substrate by transferring an electrically inhomogeneous myocardial tissue into an

207

electrically stable, homogeneous necrosis. Computerized systems for simultaneous multi-channel analysis will improve clinical handling of the patient during operation and will allow a more accurate insight into electrophysiological mechanisms of ventricular tachycardia.

References

1. Gallagher JJ, Selly JG, Swenson RH et al. (1988) Surgical treatment of arrhythmias. J Am Coll Cardiol 61:27
2. Harris L, Downar E, Mickleborough L et al. (1987) Activation sequence of ventricular tachycardia; endocardial and epicardial mapping studies in the human ventricle. J Am Coll Cardiol 10:1040
3. Josephson ME, Horowitz LN, Spielman SR et al. (1980) Comparison of endocardial catheter mapping with intraoperative mapping of ventricular tachycardia. Circulation 61:395
4. Krafchek J, Lawrie G et al. (1986) Surgical ablation of ventricular tachycardia: improved results with a map-directed regional approach. Circulation 73: 1239

Surgical therapy of ventricular tachycardia

E. Kreuzer

Department of Cardiothoracic Surgery, Klinikum Großhadern,
University of Munich, Munich, FRG

Although new surgical techniques are being developed in the modern laboratory and the understanding of the pathophysiology of rhythm disturbance is growing, the surgical therapy of rhythm disturbance is one alternative useful only for a handful of rhythm disorders. Although arrhythmias still remain in the field of cardiology, we have noticed an abrupt increase in the frequency of surgical interventions since 1978; nevertheless controversy still remains.

The discrepancy between the complexity of a rhythm disturbance and its simple surgical treatment, or viceversa, results from the fundamental difference between the anatomical substrate and the clinical expression of ventricular or supraventricular tachyarrhythmias. The anatomical substrate – the endocardial fibrosis which is associated with most ventricular arrhythmias – can be identified. Its surgical approach is relatively simple, although the ventricular arrhythmia often does not

Table 1. Non-specific surgical techniques for treatment of rhythm disturbance

---

Indirect surgical procedure

---

1. Sympatectomy ($+\beta$-blockers) (left ganglion stellatum)
2. Coronary-bypass-operation
3. Aneurysmectomy $\genfrac{<}{}{0pt}{}{\text{blind}}{\text{map-guided}}$
4. Replacement of mitral valve (prolapse of mitral valve)
5. Resection of tumors

Table 2. New direct surgical procedures for the treatment of refractory rhythm disturbance

---

Direct surgical procedure for refractory ischemic tachycardia

---

1. Endocardresection $\genfrac{<}{}{0pt}{}{\text{local}}{\text{extended}}$ >directed or sequential
2. Encircling endocardial ventriculotomy $\genfrac{<}{}{0pt}{}{\text{local}}{\text{extended}}$
3. Cryosurgery – ablation
4. Coagulation
5. Laser-ablation
6. Combination 1–5

---

permit an exact localization since the pathophysiological origin remains unclear. Surgery does, however, offer the therapeutic option of diminishing symptoms, or of at least intensifying the effect of drug therapy.

The surgery of ventricular tachyarrhythmias can be divided into the non-specific surgical techniques and map-guided procedures. The former include thoracic sympathectomy, coronary bypass grafting, the resection of scarred myocardium, and a combination of the above (Table 1) involving an overall mortality of 27%. The success rate was about 56% and 17% of the cases remained without a positive result. On the other hand, the new direct techniques (Table 2) include Guiraundon's first endocardial encircling ventriculotomy in 1978, Harken's focal endocardial resection, cryoablation which preserves collagen tissue and the integrity of the ventricle, coagulation, laser ablation, and chemical ablation. It is important to recognize the generating mechanism of many tachycardias. In the ischemic state, a limited local event may be etiologic and therefore, a more localized map-guided technique is preferable to a more extended one. In addition, a map-guided localized procedure may result in less impairment of myocardial function.

Despite advances in surgical technique, there are still some limitations. The subendocardial encircling ventriculotomy or the enodardial resection ventriculotomy (Fig. 1) cannot reach all sections of the endocardium. The base of the two papillary muscles, for example, as well as the annuli of the aortic and mitral valve are not suitable for these procedures. Cryosurgery (Fig. 2) in combination with other techniques is one solution since healing occurs in 85% of cases. Another problem is the

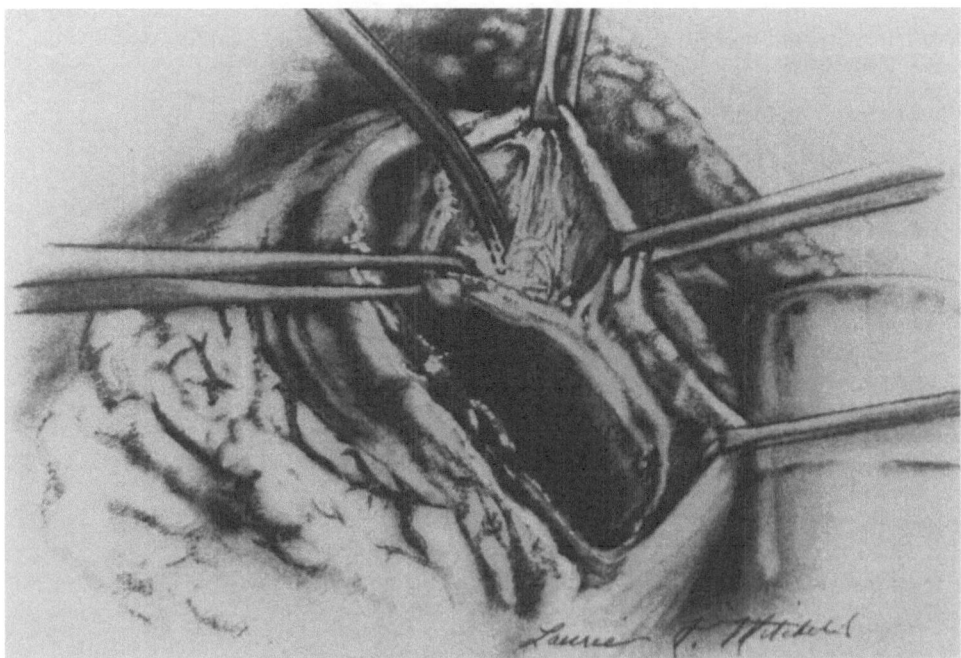

Fig. 1. Sharp endocardial resection after ventriculotomy in the center of an aneurysm; (after Cox, 1985).

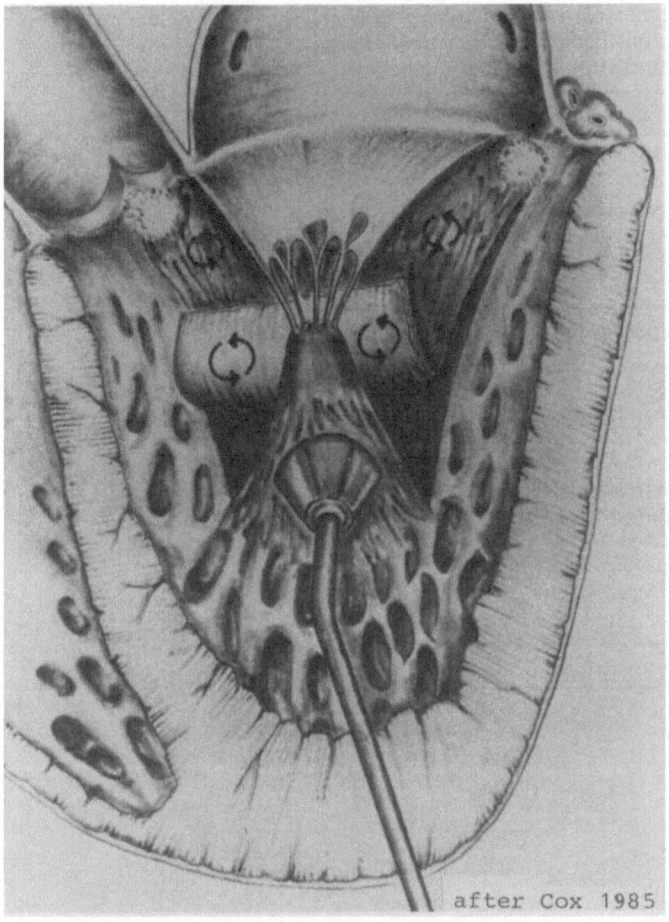

Fig. 2. Application of the intraoperative cryosurgical technique, which can be performed alone or in combination with other techniques; (after Cox, 1985).

development of ventricular septal rupture after an invasive approach. In general, however, the results are acceptable as compared with the indirect methods. According to Cox, the overall mortality is 12%, with a success range between 83% – 87%. The number of failures is negligible.

In our own collective, 10 patients with tachycardia required heart transplantation (performed by Kemkes), 10 patients received a defibrillator and 20 patients were treated with one of the above mentioned direct methods. A larger perspective on surgical therapy of ventricular arrhythmias can be found when looking at data from the International Voluntary Registery; the results on 665 patients undergoing electrophysiologically guided operations at eight centers were reported by Borggrefe (1) in 1987 (Table 3). In addition to these direct approaches, coronary bypass grafting was performed in 55% of patients and aneurysmectomy in 73% (Table 4). The overall operative surgical mortality, including intraoperative and hospital mortality

Table 3. Results on 665 patients undergoing electrophysiologically guided operations (from the international Surgical Ablation Registry as reported by Borggrefe et al. (1)

Antitachycardia surgical procedures applied in 665 patients	
● Localized ER	33.2%
● Partial EEV	16.8%
● Localized ER + cryosurgery	16.1%
● Complete EEV	9.3%
● Cryosurgery	7.4%
● Others	12.5%

EEV = encircling endocardial ventriculotomy; ER = endocardial resection.

Table 4. In addition to a direct electrophysiologically guided procedure, CABG was performed in 55% and aneurysmectomy in 73% of patients (Surgical Ablation Registry, Borggrefe et al. (1))

Additional surgical procedures	
● CABG (55%)	
no grafts (45%)	
1	24.2%
2	19.9%
3	8.5%
≥4	2.7%
● Aneurysmectomy	73%
● Valve replacement	
primary indication	1.6%
secondary indication	0.2%

CABG = coronary artery bypass grafts.

Table 5. The overall surgical mortality within 30 days of operation is shown according to the procedure performed (Surgical Ablation Registry, Borggrefe et al. (1))

Complete endocardial encircling ventriculotomy	13%
Extended endocardial encircling ventriculotomy	8%
Local endocardial resection procedure	10%
Extended endocardial resection procedure	27%
Endocardial encircling ventriculotomy in combination with endocardial resection procedure	23%
Local endocardial resection in combination with cryosurgery	16%
cryosurgery	8.5%

212

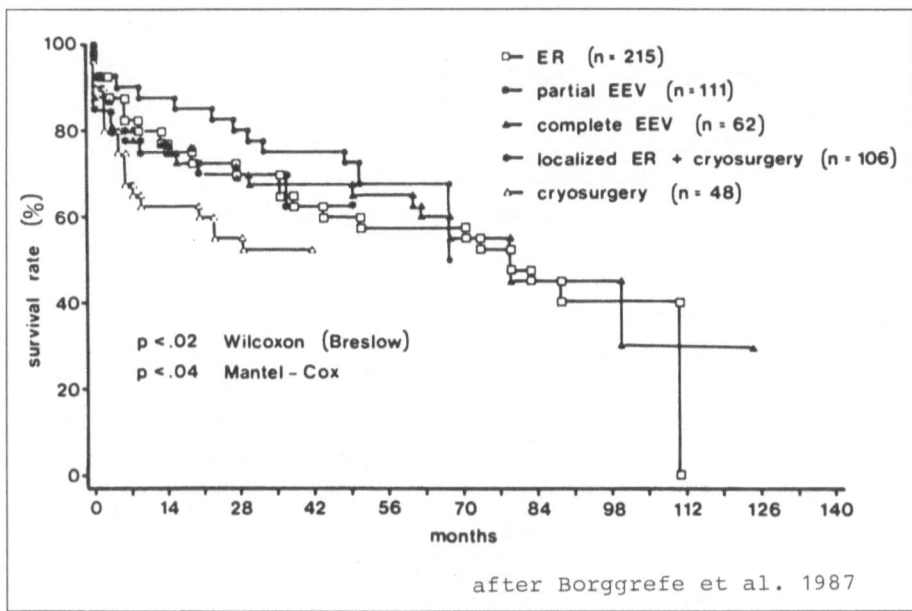

Fig. 3. Surgical Ablation Registry (modified from Borggrefe et al. (1987): Long-term survival after electrophysiologically guided operation; similar results were obtained after endocardial resection (ER), complete endocardial encircling ventriculotomy (EEV) and localized endocardial resection combined with cryosurgery (ER + cryosurgery). Partial subendocardial encircling ventriculotomy (partial EEV) offered a significantly better survival while cryosurgery alone had a significantly less favorable outcome

defined as death within 30 days after operation was analyzed for the different types of approaches (Table 5).

It seems that the more localized procedures are associated with a lower surgical mortality rate as opposed to surgical methods creating greater myocardial damage, such as extended endocardial resection or combined procedures. In the actuarial survival curves of cardiac mortality, 72% of patients were alive after two years and 57% have survived up to years, with a continuing risk of death over the following years (1).

One might assume that late mortality may be related to the type of operation performed, however, apparently overall long-term survival seems to be similar for endocardial resection, complete endocardial encircling ventriculotomy and localized endocardial resection combined with cryosurgery (Fig. 3). In contrast, patients treated by partial subendocardial encircling ventriculotomy offer a significantly better survival whereas patients who underwent cryosurgical treatment alone had a significantly less favorable outcome.

The underlying cardiac disease as well as the preoperative left ventricular ejection fraction influence the survival rates significantly (Fig. 4). The most common causes of death are heart failure, fatal reinfarction, and sudden death. The overall out-of-hospital recurrence rate of ventricular events was 16%. Postoperatively 64.7% of the patients did not require antiarrhythmic therapy. A significantly lower incidence of

213

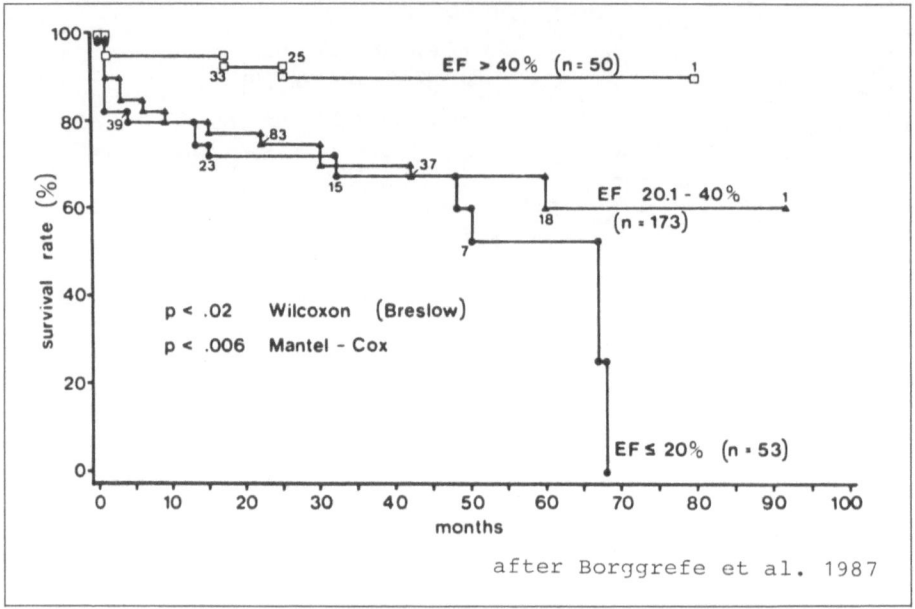

Fig. 4. Surgical Ablation Registry (modified from Borggrefe et al. (1987): Underlying cardiac disease and preoperative left ventricular ejection fraction significantly influenced the long-term survival rate

postoperative inducibility was found only after complete endocardial encircling ventriculotomy, whereas the other surgical procedures were equally effective.

Conclusion

Most ventricular tachycardias can be successfully treated surgically with an acceptable surgical mortality and a relatively high long-term survival rate in high-risk groups of patients suffering from life-threatening ventricular arrhythmias, when surgery is guided by an electophysiologic stimulation protocol. It is therefore our opinion that each patient with therapy-resistant ventricular tachycardia should undergo an electrophysiological investigation as a potential candidate for antitachycardia surgery. Perhaps additional insight into the causes of these tachycardias and resultant sudden cardiac death can thus be acquired.

Reference

1. Borggrefe M, Podczek A; Ostermeyer J, Breithardt G, and the Surgical Ablation Registry (1987) Long-term results of electrophysiologically guided antitachycardia surgery in ventricular tachyarrhythmias: a collaborative report in 665 patients. In: Nonpharmacological Therapy of Tachyarrhythmias, G. Breithardt, M. Borggrefe, DP Zipes (eds) Futura Publishing Co, Inc. Mount Kisco, New York, p. 109

Interventional cardiology today

S. King

Andreas Grüntzig Cardiovascular Center, Department of Medicine (Cardiology), Emory University, School of Medicine, Atlanta, Georgia, USA

It is fascinating to see the interest in aortic valvuloplasty which has grown from a curiosity to nearly 100 communications being submitted to the American Heart Association on the subject. One point of confusion has been the differing results between the Rouen group and the groups in the United States. However, as one considers patients who are truly inoperable from the group in Rouen, we see that the results are very similar to those from groups in the United States who have taken on valvuloplasty only when surgery is rejected. The results of valvuloplasty based on a number of individual communications and also the registries that have been instituted show similar trends. The in-hospital mortality to this point in the U.S. has ranged somewhere between 5% and 10%. What is the cause of that mortality? In our group, we do not have a vast experience with valvuloplasty because we have a very aggressive surgical group who will operate on almost all patients who could be candidates for valvuloplasty. If they reject the patient for surgery, we then do valvuloplasty.

Serious catastrophic complications at the time of the procedure have not been common but in one 88-year old, a trefoil balloon was tried, followed by a 23 mm balloon; the result was a disruption of aorta at the level of the valve. The valve was densely calcified without commisural fusion. The experience by Robiscek in the operating room dealt with this sort of valve without commissural fusion and with actual bone formation. In this patient, the 23 mm balloon resulted in disruption of the aorta and catastrophic bleeding into the pericardial space.

What happens, however, to the patients who survive aortic valvuloplasty? The one-year mortality in the experiences currently being presented, which admittedly includes some of the learning curve, is about 20%–25%. How many patients get better? Those patients who are functionally improved range from 25%– 50%. For those patients who are asymptomatic or improved following valvuloplasty, objective measures at recatheterization show restenosis has occurred in about half. Also, objective evidence is lacking for improvement in myocardial function. With valve surgery, there is regression in left ventricular mass, however this has not been documented in valvuloplasty.

There has been a recent comparative trial of valvuloplasty and aortic valve replacement from the University of Michigan. Survival was not different at one year. There was 71% survival in the surgical group and 57% in the valvuloplasty group but it was not significantly different (1). However, there was an increase in congestive heart failure at follow-up in the valvuloplasty group and there was a marked difference in the number of asymptomatic patients. Sixty-nine percent of the surgically treated patients were asymptomatic compared to 31% of the valvuloplasty patients.

215

This is a comparison of patients who are operable. These results might be even less satisfactory in patients who are not operable.

Finally, in aortic valvuloplasty the best predictor of a good result is the pre-dilatation valve area. If the valve area is large, then we can expect very good hemodynamic results and good survival. If the valve area is very tight, we do not expect very good results. All this is a little bit depressing but as has been emphasized, aortic valvuloplasty remains a very palliative procedure for patients who cannot have valve surgery.

The mitral valvuloplasty, on the other hand, works. The mitral valve has commissures that are fused and if they are split and the valve is opened, the results are predictable. There is a recent randomized trial comparing mitral valvuloplasty to closed mitral commissurotomy and the results are comparable between the two approaches (2).

With regards to the selection of patients for coronary angioplasty or coronary bypass surgery, I think it is worth examining the long-term results of the initial group treated by Gruentzig, the inventor of interventional cardiology. The Zurich patients, some followed for over 10 years, have done well. They continue to have an excellent survival as well as functional result. The survival overall at six years, was 96 % (3). At Emory, the patients treated in 1981 were followed completely at five years and again we saw excellent cardiac survival of 97 % and freedom from the major events, cardiac mortality, myocardial infarction, or death of 80 % (4). These were primarily single-vessel disease patients. I do not think a randomized trial of single-vessel disease is needed. I believe the results of angioplasty have been quite satisfactory in single-vessel disease throughout the world. There are a few arguments that can be raised, particularly about ostial lesions that have a high restenosis rate. The right ostium and the very origin of the LAD have a high restenosis rate, and there is a need for improved technology to deal with these areas.

The results of our experience, gathered together with Douglas and Grüntzig, illustrate that complications continue to occur as more complex case selection counterbalances improved technology. Multi-vessel cases have a mortality rate of around one half of 1 %, single-vessel about one-tenth of 1 %. If we look at our multivessel experience, we see that the results are somewhat different than found in single-vessel disease. The total success in multivessel disease has been 88 %. Partial success occurs in another 6 % (5). Although the mortality is higher than in single-vessel disease, the overall outlook for these patients has been surprisingly good. Patients with multivessel disease who underwent angioplasty prior to 1987, a time when we began a randomized trial, have been followed. These were selected multivessel patients and they have more similartiy to single-vessel patients than patients who are currently being operated with multivessel disease. Eighty-nine percent of them had double-vessel disease and only 11 % had triple-vessel disease. The survival was 97 % at four years, and freedom from death, myocardial infarction or bypass surgery was 72 % at that same time interval.

There are four things one must consider in selecting patients for angioplasty (6). First, whether angioplasty can be done; second, what will the success rate be; third, how safe is it for the patient; and finally, will it last? In addition, the value of angioplasty vs the alternatives, namely bypass surgery and medical therapy, must be considered. When we are evaluating angioplasty and bypass surgery, we are really comparing angioplasty to internal thoracic artery surgery. At our center, 90 % of the patients undergoing bypass surgery receive internal thoracic artery grafts and many of them receive bilateral internal thoracic artery grafts. There are acute differences between angioplasty and surgery and there are late differences. The acute differences have to do with the morbidity of the operation itself, however with angioplasty there is morbidity as well, which is related to many factors, not the least of which is the morphology of the obstructions, the number of obstructions, and the amount of myocardium affected. The late outcome is influenced by the restenosis problem. The two major problems of angioplasty remaining are acute closure and late restenosis.

So, given this choice between two therapies, we have a dilemma that needs some rational approach. If, for example, a patient has sequential lesions in the right artery, a high grade lesion in the anterior descending branch, and a total occlusion of a circumflex marginal branch, will that patient be best served by having angioplasty, perhaps dilating both these lesions in the right, also the LAD, perhaps not trying to pass the total occlusion of the marginal which may be chronic, or would the patient be better served by going directly to bypass surgery? The obvious difference of avoiding a sternotomy and reducing the time in the hospital may be overcome by the recurrent ischemia that may take place with restenosis. On the other hand, if bypass surgery is complicated by cerebrovascular complications, pulmonary complications, or infection, then obviously angioplasty would have been a better choice.

When such a dilemma exists, the only real solution is a randomized trial. At Emory, the National Institutes of Health have funded a trial of angioplasty compared to surgery in patients with multivessel disease: E.A.S.T. Patients who traditionally would have had bypass surgery are being randomized. The hard endpoints from this trial will be anatomic, namely angiography, and functional in the form of exercise tomographic thallium scans. Additional endpoints will be very important, particularly the cross-over rates and costs. In other words, will the starting strategy of angioplasty be sufficient or will a large percentage of the patients go to surgery anyway? This will be investigated in the E.A.S.T. trial, as well as in a multicenter trial in the United States, the B.A.R.I., and importantly the C.A.B.R.I. trial, which is sponsored by the European Cardiac Society. I do not think the answers are in, but we have a headstart trying to determine which of our patients should have angioplasty and which should have bypass surgery.

References

1. Holland K, Brown K, Kirsh M, et al. (1988) One Year clinical follow-up of balloon aortic valvuloplasty vs aortic valve replacement in elderly operative candidates. Circulation 78
2. Reyes VP, Raju BS, Raju ARG, Turi ZG (1988) Percutaneous balloon mitral valvuloplasty vs surgery: results of a randomized clinical trail. Circulation 78
3. Gruentzig AR, King SB III, Schlumpf M, Siegenthaler W (1987) Long-term follow-up after percutaneous transluminal coronary angioplasty. N Engl J Med 316:1127–32
4. Talley JD, Hurst JW, King SB III et al. (1988) Clinical outcome 5 years after attempted percutaneous transluminal coronary angioplasty in 427 patients. Circulation 77:820–829
5. Roubin G, Weintraub WS, Sutor C, et al. (1987) Event free survival after successful angioplasty in multi-vessel coronary artery disease. J Am Coll Cardiol 9:15A
6. Ryan TJ, Faxon DP, Gunnar RM, et al. (1988) ACC/AHA task force report. Guidelines for percutaneous transluminal coronary angioplasty. J Am Coll Cardiol 12:529–545

Cardiac Valve Allografts 1962–1987

Current Concepts on the Use of Aortic and Pulmonary Allografts for Heart Valve Substitutes

A. C. YANKAH, Berlin, FRG; R. HETZER, Berlin, Germany; C. MILLER, Stanford, USA; D. N. ROSS, London, UK; J. SOMERVILLE, London, UK; M. H. YACOUB, Harefield, UK (Eds.)

Foreword: J. KIRKLIN, Birmingham, USA

1988. XVI, 390 pp.
Cloth. DM 150,–; US $ 86.00

It is now 25 years since the first successful orthopic aortic allograft transplantation was performed, and allograft valves and conduits are now in clinical use. However, very few everyday clinical questions in this area have been answered with sufficient exactitude. At this stage of perfecting the allograft valve, precision, maximum longevity, and reduced patient morbidity are to be desired. These can only be achieved through continued investigation and interdisciplinary work; this book contributes to reaching these aims.

The editors and other leading researchers discuss their work on cardiac valve allografts and problems in their use. Detailed information is presented under the following broad headings:

– Procurement and preservation techniques and cryobiology
– Use of viable and non-viable allografts
– Surgical implant techniques
– Assessment of late survivals
– Immunologic aspects

"...The present book may be designated as an exeedingly accomplished congress volume of major informative value, and should be compulsory reading for everyone working in the field of cardiac surgery."

(The Thoracic and Cardiovascular Surgeon)

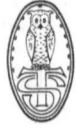

Steinkopff **Dr. Dietrich Steinkopff Verlag**
P.O.Box 11 14 42, D-6100 Darmstadt, FRG